AF767164

HIGH ALTITUDE CARDIOLOGY

LEONIDA COMPOSTELLA
Prevention of Cardiovascular Diseases at High Altitude,
University of Padua's Feltre Campus.

WILEY

This edition first published 2026

© 2026 by John Wiley & Sons Ltd

All rights reserved, including rights for text and data mining and training of artificial intelligence technologies or similar technologies. No part of this publication may be reproduced, stored in a retrieval system, or transmitted, in any form or by any means, electronic, mechanical, photocopying, recording or otherwise, except as permitted by law. Advice on how to obtain permission to reuse material from this title is available at http://www.wiley.com/go/permissions.

The right of Leonida Compostella to be identified as the author of this work has been asserted in accordance with law.

Registered Offices
John Wiley & Sons, Inc., 111 River Street, Hoboken, NJ 07030, USA
John Wiley & Sons Ltd. New Era House, 8 Oldlands Way, Bognor Regis, West Sussex, PO22 9NQ, UK

For details of our global editorial offices, customer services, and more information about Wiley products visit us at www.wiley.com.

The manufacturer's authorized representative according to the EU General Product Safety Regulation is Wiley-VCH GmbH, Boschstr. 12, 69469 Weinheim, Germany, e-mail: Product_Safety@wiley.com.

Wiley also publishes its books in a variety of electronic formats and by print-on-demand. Some content that appears in standard print versions of this book may not be available in other formats.

Trademarks: Wiley and the Wiley logo are trademarks or registered trademarks of John Wiley & Sons, Inc. and/or its affiliates in the United States and other countries and may not be used without written permission. All other trademarks are the property of their respective owners. John Wiley & Sons, Inc. is not associated with any product or vendor mentioned in this book.

Limit of Liability/Disclaimer of Warranty

The contents of this work are intended to further general scientific research, understanding, and discussion only and are not intended and should not be relied upon as recommending or promoting scientific method, diagnosis, or treatment by physicians for any particular patient. In view of ongoing research, equipment modifications, changes in governmental regulations, and the constant flow of information relating to the use of experimental reagents, equipment, and devices, the reader is urged to review and evaluate the information provided in the package insert or instructions for each chemical, piece of equipment, reagent, or device for, among other things, any changes in the instructions or indication of usage and for added warnings and precautions. While the publisher and the authors have used their best efforts in preparing this work, including a review of the content of the work, neither the publisher nor the authors make any representations or warranties with respect to the accuracy or completeness of the contents of this work and specifically disclaim all warranties, including without limitation any implied warranties of merchantability or fitness for a particular purpose. No warranty may be created or extended by sales representatives, written sales materials or promotional statements for this work. The fact that an organization, website, or product is referred to in this work as a citation and/or potential source of further information does not mean that the publisher and authors endorse the information or services the organization, website, or product may provide or recommendations it may make. This work is sold with the understanding that the publisher is not engaged in rendering professional services. The advice and strategies contained herein may not be suitable for your situation. You should consult with a specialist where appropriate. Further, readers should be aware that websites listed in this work may have changed or disappeared between when this work was written and when it is read. Neither the publisher nor authors shall be liable for any loss of profit or any other commercial damages, including but not limited to special, incidental, consequential, or other damages.

Library of Congress Cataloging-in-Publication Data has been applied for:

Hardback: 9781394420896
ePDF: 9781394420919
epub: 9781394420902
obook: 9781394420926

Cover Design: Wiley
Cover Image: © Buena Vista Images/Getty Images

Set in 10 x 12 STIXTwoText by Lumina Datamatics

Table of Contents

Foreword

High Altitude Cardiology is a long-awaited text and reference book that will appeal to anyone involved in alpine medical training, care or mountain rescue activities – focusing on the cardiovascular system. It is also ideal for individuals with a personal interest in the subject who wish to delve deeper.

This book was written by Dr. **Leonida Compostella**, an Italian cardiologist who specialises in preventing cardiac diseases at high altitudes. His extensive scientific, clinical and practical experience makes him the ideal author of this book. He provides a comprehensive review of the latest available information on the physiology and diseases of the heart related to mountaineering activities and exposure to high altitudes. This book is intended to educate students and help cardiologists, general practitioners and nurses provide the best possible care for mountaineers.

I firmly believe that it will importantly enhance the existing body of knowledge in alpine medicine and serve as an essential resource.

Martin Burtscher, MD, PhD
Professor (retired)
Department of Sport Science, University of Innsbruck, Innsbruck, Austria

Abbreviations

AED	Automated External Defibrillator
AMI	Acute Myocardial Infarction
AMS	Acute Mountain Sickness
AMSL	Above Mean Sea Level
BLS	Basic Life Support
BP	Blood Pressure
bpm	Beats per minute
CAD	Coronary Artery Disease
CCS	Canadian Cardiovascular Society
CHF	Congestive Heart Failure
CMS	Chronic Mountain Sickness
COPD	Chronic Obstructive Pulmonary Disease
CPR	Cardiopulmonary Resuscitation
CV	Cardiovascular
DES	Drug Eluting Stent
DM	Diabetes Mellitus
ECG	Electrocardiogram
EEG	Electroencephalogram
EPO	Erythropoietin
FiO_2	Fraction of O_2 in the inspired air
HACE	High-altitude Cerebral Oedema
HAPE	High-altitude Pulmonary Oedema
Hb	Haemoglobin
HR	Heart Rate
ICD	Implantable Cardioverter Defibrillator
IDF	International Diabetes Federation
INR	International Normalized Ratio
LV	Left Ventricle
LVEDD	Left Ventricle End-diastolic Diameter
LVEF	Left Ventricle Ejection Fraction
METs	Metabolic equivalents
mmHg	Millimetres of Mercury
Nt-proBNP	N-terminal pro B-type Natriuretic Peptide
NYHA	New York Heart Association
OR	Odd Ratio
$PaCO_2$	Partial pressure of Carbon Dioxide in the arterial blood
PAO_2	Partial pressure of O_2 in the alveoli
PAPm	Mean Pulmonary Artery Pressure
PB	Barometric Pressure
PEA	Pulseless Electrical Activity
PFO	Patent Foramen Ovale

PH_2O	Partial pressure of water vapour
PiO_2	Partial pressure of oxygen in the inspired air
PM	Pacemaker
R/E	class of Recommendations and level of Evidence
RAA	Renin–Angiotensin–Aldosterone
RV-RA	Right Ventricle – Right Atrium
RVSP	Right Ventricle Systolic Pressure
SaO_2	Arterial Oxygen saturation
SCD	Sudden Cardiac Death
SpO_2	Peripheral Oxygen saturation
STEMI	ST-elevation Myocardial Infarction
TIA	Transient Ischemic Attack
UIAA	Union Internationale des Associations d'Alpinisme (International Climbing and Mountaineering Federation)
VO_2Max	Maximal Oxygen Consumption; Maximal Oxygen Uptake
WADA	World Anti-doping Association

PART 1

Background

CHAPTER 1

Definitions of Mountain Altitude

Altimetric Classification

Different mountain altitudes have variable consequences on the physiology of the cardiovascular system, that vary with the absolute elevation and the atmospheric pressure, the rapidity of ascent and the individual capacity of adaptation.

One **common definition** reports that:[1]

- **Sea and hill levels** generally refer to altitudes lower than 500 m AMSL.
- **Low altitude** is the altitude between 500 and 1,800–2,000 m AMSL.,
- **Medium altitude** is between 2,000 and 3,000 m AMSL.,
- **High altitude**: 3,000–5,500 m AMSL.,
- **Very high or extreme altitude**: >5,500 m AMSL..

Another, most widely accepted, **classification** includes (Figure 1.1):[2]

- **Low altitude** from 0 to 1,500 m AMSL,
- **Moderate or intermediate altitude**: 1,500–2,500 m AMSL. Arterial oxygen saturation lowers to 90%; some physiological changes may be detectable and in susceptible individuals may already appear symptoms of mountain sickness, especially in case of rapid ascent.
- **High altitude**: 2,500–3,500 m AMSL; more common appearance of mountain sickness, especially in case of rapid ascent.
- **Very high altitude**: 3,500–5,800 m AMSL; arterial oxygen saturation reaches levels much lower than 90%, and hypoxaemia worsens during effort as well as during sleep.
- **Extreme altitude**: 5,800–8,000 m AMSL, where marked hypoxaemia is present already at rest; hypocapnia is present.
- **Deadly altitude, also called 'death zone'**: above 8,000 m AMSL. Arterial oxygen saturation reaches the very low levels of about 55%, so that most mountaineers require oxygen supplementation and/or previous prolonged acclimatization, and can stay at such an altitude only for very short period of time.

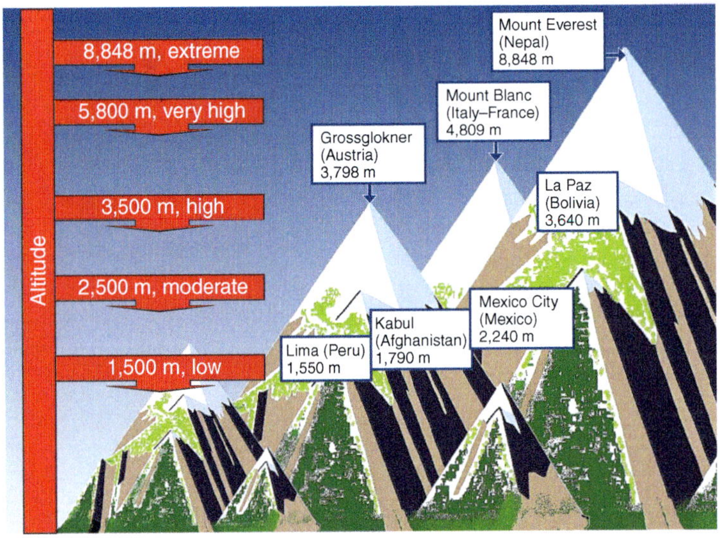

FIGURE 1.1 Mountain altitudes, indicated for exemplification purpose only (see text).

These subdivisions are only conventional and differ among various scholars; there is no European or international legal definition in this respect. They only serve to give an idea of the altitudes which we are referring to, altitudes whose physiological effects could be very different among individuals.

Physiological Classification

Different individuals behave differently at altitude, depending on their general health conditions, their age, the use of drugs and the possible presence of lung or heart diseases. Thus, a 'physiological' definition of high altitude has been proposed, which attempts to take into account the body's responses to the hypobaric hypoxia that is linked to mountain ascent. So, from a physiological point of view, **high altitude is defined as an altitude at which the O_2 saturation of haemoglobin (SaO_2) drops below 90%.**[3]

For people in normal health, at intermediate latitudes this altitude corresponds approximately to 2,500 m above sea level.

Above these altitudes (in relation to the drop of SaO_2, especially below 90%), a series of cardiovascular and pulmonary adjustments are triggered, which will be described in the following chapters. The main physiological effects include increased ventilation at rest, decreased exercise performance, and a more common occurrence of acute mountain sickness especially during rapid ascents.

References

1 Vanoni L, for CAI Club Alpino Italiano, Commissione Centrale Medica. L'alta quota e gli effetti sull'organismo [High altitude and its effects on the body], November 07, 2020. https://www.cai.it/organo_tecnico/commissione-centrale-medica/lalta-quota-e-gli-effetti-sullorganismo./

2 Imray C, Booth G, Wright A, Bradwell A. Acute altitude illnesses. BMJ 2011; 343:d4943. https://doi.org/10.1136/bmj.d4943. https://www.researchgate.net/publication/259452664_Acute_altitude_illness

3 Rimoldi SF, Sartori C, Seiler C, Delacrétaz E, Mattle HP, Scherrer U, Alemann Y. High-altitude exposure in patients with cardiovascular disease: risk assessment and practical recommendations. Prog Cardiovasc Dis 2010; 52(6):512–524. https://doi.org/10.1016/j.pcad.2010.03.005.

CHAPTER 2

General Data, Relevance of the Problem

All over the world, mountains occupy 24% of the earth's landscape; it is generally assumed that over 389–500 million people live at >1,500m and that over 81.6–140 million humans live permanently at elevations above 2,500m AMSL and 14.4 million at ≥3,500m.[1]

High-altitude Populations

While it is clear that the number of people living at altitude decreases faster than exponentially with increasing elevation,[2] the proportion of people who permanently reside at high altitudes is nevertheless not negligible. In the year 2000, it was estimated that:

- 56% of the world's high-altitude population lives in Asia. The countries of Afghanistan, Bhutan, China, India, Kyrgyzstan and Nepal have 2–45% of their populations living above 2,500m. In four high plateaus of China (Qinghai–Tibet, average altitude 4,380m; Inner Mongolia, average altitude 1,200m; Yun-Gui, average altitude 2,000m; and Yellow Land Plateau, average elevation 1,200m), it is reported that nearly 80 million people are living.[3] China also has the greatest absolute population in the world living at altitudes ≥3,500m (estimated at more than 3 million people).[1, 4]
- 26% of the world's high-altitude population lives in Central and South America. In South America, three capitals are located at high altitude: La Paz, Bolivia, 3,650m; Bogotá, Colombia, 2,640m; Quito, Ecuador, 2,850m. Some 35 million people are living above 2,500m; Bolivia also has the greatest population living at ≥2,500 and ≥3,500m and has the highest major city (El Alto, 4,150m; population c. 940,000); Peru has the highest city in the world (La Rinconada, 5,052m, population c. 50,000).
- 17% in Africa: Ethiopia has the largest absolute population (estimated at 85%) living at ≥1,500m and ≥2,500 m; Addis Ababa (c. 2.5 million population) is located at 2,355m; Debre Birhan (c. 140,000 population), located at 2,840m AMSL, is the highest town in

Africa. Lesotho has the greatest percentage of its population above 1,500m. Nairobi (Kenya) is located at 1,795m AMSL; approximately 4.4 million people are permanently living there. Johannesburg, the most populous city in South Africa, is located in the eastern plateau of Highveld, at an altitude of 1,753m.

- Less than 1% in North America and an even lower percentage in Europe.[5]

To have a closer look at North America, Mexico City (Mexico) is the most elevated and the most populated mountain city, located at an average altitude of 2,216m AMSL with a population of 8.84 million people as of 2013; Guadalajara (Mexico), with a population of almost 1.5 million inhabitants and about 5 million inhabitants in its metropolitan area, is located at an average altitude of around 1,500m AMSL.

In USA,[1, 6] the most elevated cities are Alma (the 'two miles high' city), Montezuma, Leadville, Blue River and Fairplay (Colorado), all located at altitudes greater than 3,000m; together these cities have a very limited population, with a total of around 5,000 residents. Another 146 cities are located at altitudes above 2,000m, the most populous being Santa Fe (New Mexico; 85,000 inhabitants), Flagstaff (Arizona, 75,000 inhabitants) and Laramie (Wyoming, 31,000 inhabitants). Denver (Colorado), located at 1,610m AMSL is the so-called 'Mile High City'; it has a population of approximately 700 thousand permanent residents. Two Utah cities, Salt Lake City (1,288m AMSL; more than 200 thousand inhabitants) and Provo (1,387m AMSL; more than 117 thousand inhabitants), are part of the highest cities in USA, as well as El Paso (Texas: 1,140m AMSL and almost 682 thousand inhabitants) and Albuquerque (New Mexico: 1,619m AMSL and approximately 560 thousand inhabitants). From available data, it may be calculated that approximately 313 thousand people live at altitudes greater than 2,100m.

In the wide European region (that includes the 27 countries of the European Union as well as other countries of 'geographical' Europe), estimates made in 2008 indicate that 118.4 million people (17.1% of the continent's population) live in mountainous areas of varying altitudes, but mostly at low altitudes.[7]

In Europe, the highest and most extensive mountains are the Alps, a mountain range spanning eight countries: Austria, France, Germany, Italy, Liechtenstein, Monaco, Slovenia and Switzerland. Based on the *Alpine Convention*, these countries have cooperated since 1991 in activities aimed at supporting a way for sustainable life in the Alps and a sustainable development and protection of the entire mountain range.[8] In the wide Alpine area, approximately 14 million inhabitants are living, with a number that has almost doubled in the last 150 years. This makes the Alps one of the most densely inhabited mountain areas in the world. Due to orographic constraints, most of this population is, however, living at low altitudes, in the more easily accessible mountain valleys, while higher altitudes are becoming progressively less populated.[9]

So, how many people do live permanently at high altitude on the Alps?

Europeans Living at Altitude: Italy

The Italian National Institute of Statistics (ISTAT) regularly provides a statistical description of the geographical characteristics of the national territory.[10] Based on ISTAT and other data,[11, 12] there are 104 municipalities located at an altitude ≥1,000m AMSL, but only 6 have their municipal headquarters located at an altitude equal to or greater than 1,500m above sea level. However, it should be considered that there are a total of 1,535 municipalities (i.e. 19% of the total of 7,901, data from January 2023)[13] that have some localities within their territory at altitudes equal to or well above 1,500m AMSL; and 463 with altitudes above 2,500m above sea level. As regards the permanently resident population, the top 50 municipalities by altitude (located between 1,385 and 2,035m AMSL) have a resident population of just under 39,000 inhabitants. The overall permanent resident population in these municipalities is therefore clearly very limited.

Europeans Living at Altitude: France

In France, the available data indicate that 29 departments have inside their area some mountains that reach altitudes higher than 1,500m AMSL and in 13 of them altitudes are higher than 2,500m AMSL. The highest located municipalities are Saint-Véran (Hautes-Alpes) at an altitude of 2,042m AMSL with slightly less than 400 inhabitants, and Tignes (Haute-Tarentaise) with localities scattered at altitudes between 1,550 and 2,150m AMSL and total resident population of approximately 2,000 persons.[14] Briançon (Hautes-Alpes), located at an altitude of 1,326m, is the highest city in France with more than 2,000 inhabitants (in 2018, its population was just over 11,000).

Europeans Living at Altitude: Switzerland

In Switzerland, which is a completely mountainous country, there are at least 9 municipalities located at altitudes higher than 1,500m AMSL, with areas that reach altitudes as high as 4,634m AMSL in Pointe Dufour (Dufourspitze) in the Massif of Mount Rosa, in Zermatt municipality. On the Jungfraujoch, marketed as Top of Switzerland, there is the highest railway station in Switzerland and Europe, located at 3,454m AMSL.

As in Italy, both in France and Switzerland the resident population in such highly elevated areas is very limited, counting to a total of a few tens of thousands.

A study made at the University of Eastern Piedmont in 2016 by Bartaletti[15] reports that all together the population permanently resident at altitudes higher than 1,500m AMSL in Italy, France, Switzerland, and Austria amounts to approximately 84,000 inhabitants, thus confirming the scarcity of the population permanently resident at those altitudes (Figure 2.1).

However, we must consider two other main factors:

- In Europe as well as in other parts of the world, many municipalities include places of high altitude within them, even if the main municipal seat is located at a modest altitude; their population usually frequents the higher areas both for work reasons (agriculture, tourist activities) and for pleasure (practice of mountain sports).;
- Mountain resorts see a significant influx of tourists at various times of the year, so much so that in many cases their population even increases tenfold or more during the winter or summer seasons.

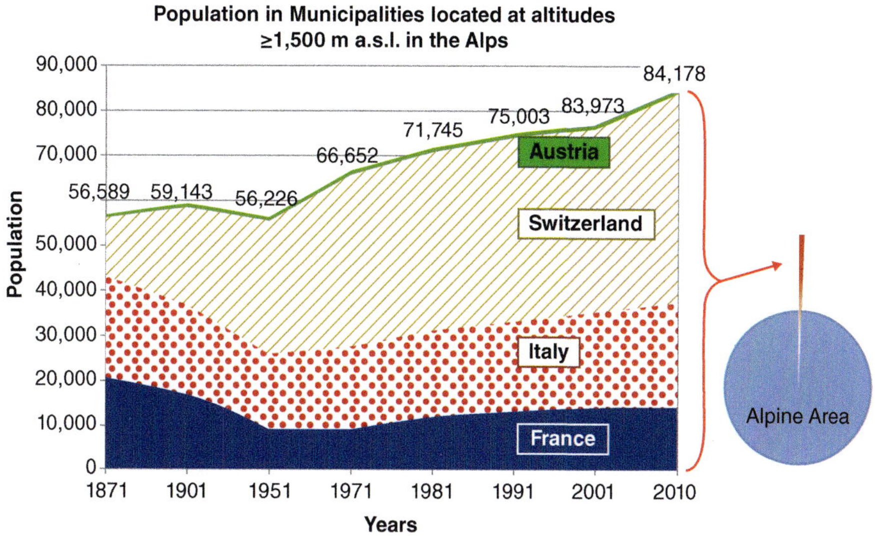

FIGURE 2.1 Resident population in the municipalities located at altitudes ≥1,500m a.s.l., in France, Italy, Switzerland and Austria; [15].

Tourists to Moderate or High Altitudes

Globally, it has been reported that mountain areas are second only to coasts and islands as popular tourism destinations, generating 15–20% of annual global tourism.[16] It has been estimated that more than 100 million lowlanders visit areas above 2,500m annually.[17] The relevance of mountain tourism is evident both for the economy of the areas involved and for the environmental, social and health implications that this movement entails.

All over the Alpine range, a total of around 120 million people (calculated as overnight stays) are estimated to visit the mountains each year; certain areas experience a relevant tourist pressure (Figure 2.2).[18] For instance, a recent publication[19] reports that the mountainous region of Bozen, in the Alps in northern Italy, is the European region with the greatest number of nights spent by tourists in 2021 (a total of 23.8 million nights, with more than 10 million nights spent by international tourists, in a province that counts slightly more than 500,000 permanent residents).

A similar tourist movement is also recorded in the United States, where every year more than 100 million people travel to high-altitude regions for work or pleasure.[20] In the United States, as in Europe, small mountain towns host large numbers of tourists every year; for example, the town of Vail (Colorado), which lies between 2,353 and 4,139m AMSL, is home to approximately 10,000 residents but welcomes approximately 1.5 million visitors annually.[21]

In China, the Huangshan Mountains (with altitudes up to 1,840m, some of which are easily accessible by cable car) are one of the top tourist destinations, attracting over 3 million tourists every year.[21] More challenging mountains can be found in Tibet, where anyway trips are regularly organized for winter sports, for sightseeing in Lhasa (3,650m AMSL) and visits to the highest peaks, including trekking across passes at 4,700–5,000m and setting up camps at

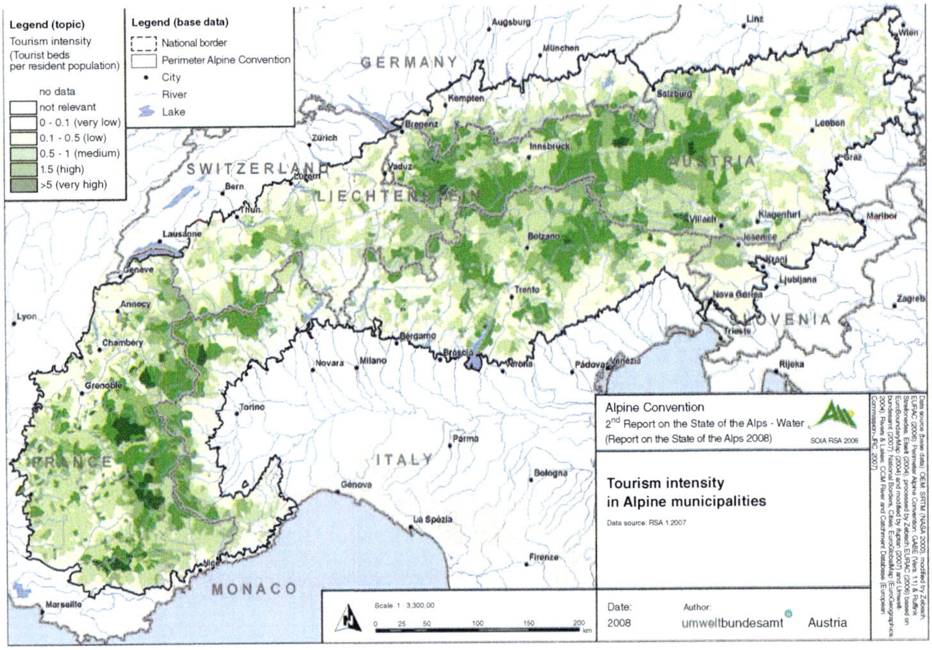

FIGURE 2.2 Tourism intensity (tourism beds per resident population) in Alpine municipalities. [18]/Permanent Secretariat of the Alpine Convention.

5,100m (Everest Base Camp). According to data from the Tibet Autonomous Region, in 2023 Tibet welcomed the astonishing number of 55 million domestic tourists (over 15 times the local population!) and nearly 20,000 foreign tourists.[22]

In Nepal, the Himalayas attract travellers from around the world, and overtourism has become a problem in some destinations; in addition to attracting approximately 45,000 mountaineers, Nepal attracts 30,000 trekkers every year, due to its 1,700 Km long High Route (at an average altitude of 3,000–5,000 m) and the Cultural (or Low) Route (1,500 Km through mid-mountains between 1,500 and 2,500 m).[23]

On Mount Kilimanjaro (Tanzania), tourists are offered 6–8 day excursions, starting from 1,640 or 2,100 m AMSL to reach the summit of the mountain at 5,895 m; more than 30,000 people tackle the climb every year. Similarly, on Mount Kenya (Kenya), various trekking routes lead to its highest trekking peak, Point Lenana at 4,985 m, a climb attempted by 15,000 hikers every year. In South Africa,[24] the Amphitheatre (located at altitudes between 1,830 and 3,050 m) in the northern Drakensberg region is visited by around 15,000 trekkers each year.

In South America, in the Andes, the annual number of visitors may be relatively low in some protected areas, but it is much larger in other areas: in the World Heritage Site of Machu Picchu in Peru (at altitudes ranging between 2,200 and 6,271 m; 900,000 tourists annually), in Nahuel Huapi National Park (Patagonia, Argentina; altitude 700–3,554 m) with 300,000 tourists every year, as well as 50,000 tourists in Colombia's Los Nevados (altitude 2,600–3,261 m) and 4,000 tourists in Bolivia's Sajama National Park (altitude 4,200–6,548 m).[25]

Age of Mountain Tourists

We should pay particular attention to the fact that a significant proportion of tourist presences is made up by adults and – in some areas – even by older people. The average age of mountain users varies depending on the area: it seems to be lower in those areas that allow more challenging excursions, while it is modestly higher in those areas that are generally chosen for summer 'rest' or family holidays. In the Italian Alps, a publication by the Autonomous Province of Bozen (South Tyrol)[26] reports that the most representative group of tourists is that made up of people aged between 45 and 64 (45.7%), while the over-65s represent 20.0%; the younger class (25–44 years) constitutes 22.2% of tourists. Therefore, two-thirds of tourists in South Tyrol are adults or elderly; furthermore, in the years between 2007/08 and 2012/13, the older age groups (45–64 and over 65) recorded an increase of 9.0 and 3.9%, respectively. In the United States, the situation is quite similar; the median age of mountain tourists (especially skiers) has increased over the years, and recently the number of mountain tourists aged 65 and over has tripled.[27] Younger ages are reported for tourists trekking in the Himalayan mountains, with an average age of 48 years, but with some tourists as old as 76.[28]

Comorbidities in High-mountain Tourists

It has been calculated that approximately 9–14% (and up to 28%) of people who frequent the Alps suffer from some form of cardiovascular disease (with increasing prevalence for older ages); this means that every year there are approximately 4–5 million hikers and skiers who frequent the Alps despite suffering from known cardiovascular diseases.[29, 30] Also, in the high mountains of the Himalayas, one-third of trekkers report pre-existing medical conditions and 41% of the entire group studied by Keyes et al. needed to take one or more medications.[28]

There is no doubt that some factors pose significant prevention challenges and urge for early recognition of cardiovascular diseases: the high number of presences in mountain areas, the average adult or elderly age of tourists, the history of pre-existing diseases, combined with the fact that a good portion of them engage in more or less intense physical activity (for which they are sometimes not adequately trained).

Cardiovascular Diseases in Mountain Residents

What has been presented so far concerns those who visit the mountains occasionally.

But what is the prevalence of cardiovascular diseases for permanent residents at more or less high altitudes?

Among the inhabitants of the Italian provinces of the Alpine arc, the standardised mortality rate[i] for cardiovascular diseases (which represent the leading cause of death in the adult population, constituting 27.0% of deaths in 2022, progressively decreasing, however, in the last 15 years)[31] and the standardised rate of diseases of the cardiovascular system appear to be significantly lower than in other areas of Italy.[32]

It must be taken into account that the population living in Alpine provinces is generally younger than the national average, has a lower smoking habit, a lower level of obesity and is more likely to practice some sporting activity. This could mean a lower prevalence of cardiovascular risk factors in these populations.

This also appears to be confirmed by a recent prospective study carried out in Spain[33] and by an observational study performed in Ecuador,[34] in which residents at higher altitudes would have a lower prevalence of metabolic syndrome. In Ecuador, living at high altitudes may have protective effects also on cerebrovascular events, but this effect only remains evident in residents at altitudes between 1,500 and 3,500m, while, above these elevations, the risk seems to rise again.[35] Another study made in 2017 in La Paz and El Alto (Bolivia; altitudes ranging from 3,100 to 4,100m of altitude) observed a longer duration of life of persons chronically resident at higher altitudes.[36]

The reported data are clearly not conclusive, but they make us recall what was stated by Heath D and Williams DR in their 1989 book: '... *the prevalence of cardiovascular diseases is lower in high altitude dwellers than in sea level inhabitants*'.[37]

References

1 Tremblay JC, Ainslie PN. Global and country-level estimates of human population at high altitude. Proc Natl Acad Sci USA 2021;118(18):e2102463118. https://doi.org/10.1073/pnas.2102463118. https://www.pnas.org/doi/epub/10.1073/pnas.2102463118.

2 Cohen JE, Small C. Hypsographic demography: the distribution of human population by altitude. Proc Natl Acad Sci USA 1998; 95(24):14009–14014. https://doi.org/10.1073/pnas.95.24.14009. https://www.pnas.org/doi/epdf/10.1073/pnas.95.24.14009.

3 León-Velarde F, Maggiorini M, Reeves JT, Aldashev A, Asmus I, Bernardi L, Ge RL, Hackett P, Kobayashi T, Moore LG, Penaloza D, Richalet JP, Roach R, Wu T, Vargas E, Zubieta-Castillo G, Zubieta-Calleja G. Consensus statement on chronic and subacute high altitude diseases. High Alt Med Biol. 2005; 6(2):147–157. https://doi.org/10.1089/ham.2005.6.147.

4 Paik C, Shawa TW. Altitude and adaptation: a study of geography and ethnic division. Appl Geogr 2013; 40:212–221. https://doi.org/10.1016/j.apgeog.2013.02.003.

[i]The **Standardized Mortality Rate** represents an artificially constructed indicator which does not correspond exactly to the real value, but which is suitable for comparing mortality values between different periods and territorial realities by age structure in resident populations. It represents the value that the crude mortality rate would have assumed if the population under study had a distribution of the variable for which it is standardized [in this case: cardiovascular diseases] equal to that of the reference population.

5 Jodry MA, Santoro CM. Walking closer to the sky: high-altitude landscapes and the peopling of the New World. Quaternary Intern 2017; 461: 102–107. https://www.sciencedirect.com/science/article/abs/pii/S1040618217313587.
6 U.S. Department of the Interior, U.S. Geological Survey, Educational Resources. Elevations of the 50 largest cities (by population, 1980 census). https://www.usgs.gov/educational-resources/elevations-50-largest-cities-population-1980-census. And: a map of the 346 U.S. cities with higher elevations than the 'mile high city'. https://blog.batchgeo.com/highest-elevation-us-cities.
7 European Environmental Agency. Report No 6/2010. Europe's ecological backbone: recognising the true value of our mountains. EEA, Copenhagen, 2010. https://www.eea.europa.eu/publications/europes-ecological-backbone.
8 The Alpine Convention: https://www.alpconv.org/en/home./.
9 Permanent Secretariat of the Alpine Convention. Demographic changes in the Alps. Report on the state of the Alps. Special Edition 5. Innsbruck, 2015. https://www.alpconv.org/fileadmin/user_upload/Publications/RSA/RSA5_EN.pdf.
10 Istituto Nazionale di Statistica (ISTAT), Istituto Nazionale della Montagna (IMONT). Atlante statistico della Montagna Italiana [Statistical Mountains Atlas]. Bologna: Bononia University Press; 2007. https://www.istat.it/it/archivio/138206; downloadable as zip version from: http://www.istat.it/storage/cartografia/atlante-statistico-montagna/volume-atlante-montagna.zip.
11 Istituto Nazionale di Statistica (ISTAT). Principali statistiche geografiche sui comuni. Altitudine dei Comuni tramite DEM [Main geographical characteristics of Italian Municipalities], Updated on February 25, 2026. https://www.istat.it/classificazione/principali-statistiche-geografiche-sui-comuni/.
12 Tuttitalia. Comuni italiani per altitudine: https://www.tuttitalia.it/comuni/altitudine/.
13 ISTAT. Codici Statistici delle Unità Amministrative Territoriali: Comuni, Città Metropolitane, Province e Regioni [Statistical codes of the territorial administrative units: municipalities, metropolitan cities, provinces and regions], Updated on January 17, 2023. https://www.istat.it/it/archivio/6789#:~:text=Nota.,la%20soppressione%20di%20cinque%20comuni.
14 INSEE, Institut national de la statistique et des études économiques. Populations de référence, 2022. https://www.insee.fr/fr/statistiques/8290072?sommaire=8290669.
15 Bartaletti F. La popolazione delle Alpi per fasce altimetriche. Distribuzione spaziale e variazioni [The alpine population broken down by altimetric belts. Spatial distribution and changes]. AST - Ambiente Società Territorio, Geografia nelle Scuole 2016; 1:3–11.
16 United Nations Environment Programme. Tourism and mountains, a practical guide to managing the environmental and social impacts of mountain tours. Paris, 2017. https://www.oneplanetnetwork.org/sites/default/files/tourism_and_mountains_a_practical_guide_to_managing_the_social_and_environmental_impacts_of_mountain_tours.pdf.
17 Burtscher M, Bachmann O, Hatzl T, Hotter B, Likar R, Philadelphy M, Nachbauer W. Cardiopulmonary and metabolic responses in healthy elderly humans during a 1-week hiking programme at high altitude. Eur J Appl Physiol 2001; 84(5):379–386. https://doi.org/10.1007/s004210100393.
18 Permanent Secretariat of the Alpine Convention. The Alps. People and pressures in the mountains, the facts at a glance. Vademecum. Innsbruck, 2010. https://www.alpconv.org/fileadmin/user_upload/Publications/Vademecum_EN.pdf.

19 Eurostat, Statistics explained. Tourism statistics at regional level. March 2023. https://ec.europa.eu/eurostat/statistics-explained/index.php?title=Tourism_statistics_at_regional_level#Number_of_nights_spent_in_tourist_accommodation.

20 Cornwell WK 3rd, Baggish AL, Bhatta YKD, Brosnan MJ, Dehnert C, Guseh JS, Hammer D, Levine BD, Parati G, Wolfel EE. American Heart Association Exercise, Cardiac Rehabilitation, and Secondary Prevention Committee of the Council on Clinical Cardiology; and Council on Arteriosclerosis, Thrombosis and Vascular Biology. Clinical implications for exercise at altitude among individuals with cardiovascular disease: a scientific statement from the American heart association. J Am Heart Assoc 2021;10(19):e023225. https://doi.org/10.1161/JAHA.121.023225. https://www.ncbi.nlm.nih.gov/pmc/articles/PMC8649141/pdf/JAH3-10-e023225.pdf.

21 Romeo R, Russo L, Parisi F, Notarianni M, Manuelli S, Carvao S. Mountain Tourism - Towards a More Sustainable Path. Rome: FAO – UNWTO; 2021. https://doi.org/10.4060/cb7884en. https://openknowledge.fao.org/server/api/core/bitstreams/f7257ef4-0b45-4c2b-b47f-80502c9e53f1/content.

22 Eagan K. Tibet's tourism revenue reached a record in 2023. Tourism Review News, May 27, 2024. https://www.tourism-review.com/tourism-revenue-of-tibet-hit-a-new-record-news14438.

23 Upadhayaya PK. Sustainable management of trekking trails for the adventure tourism in mountains: a study of Nepal's great Himalaya trails. J Tour Advent 2018; 1(1):1–31. https://www.nepjol.info/index.php/jota/article/view/22748/19325.

24 Linde J, Grab S. Regional contrasts in mountain tourism development in the Drakensberg, South Africa. Mt Res Dev 2008; 28(1):65–71. https://doi.org/10.1659/mrd.0937.

25 Barros A, Monz C, Pickering C. Is tourism damaging ecosystems in the Andes? Current knowledge and an agenda for future research. Ambio 2015; 44(2):82–98. https://doi.org/10.1007/s13280-014-0550-7. https://pmc.ncbi.nlm.nih.gov/articles/PMC4329127/pdf/13280_2014_Article_550.pdf.

26 Provincia Autonoma di Bolzano – Alto Adige. Indagine sul turismo in Alto Adige, Anno turistico 2012/13 [Survey on tourism in South Tyrol, Tourist Year 2012/13]. AstatInfo 10/2015 n. 56. 2015. https://astat.provinz.bz.it/de/aktuelles-publikationen-info.asp?news_action=300&news_image_id=827929.

27 Silk R. Ski resorts are urged to reach out to Gen Z. Travel Weekly, March 30, 2023. https://www.travelweekly.com/Travel-News/Hotel-News/Ski-resorts-urged-to-reach-out-to-Gen-Z.

28 Keyes LE, Mather L, Duke C, Regmi N, Phelan B, Pant S, Starling J, McElwee M, Cole D, McConnell T, Paudel P, Sallade TD, Sheets A, Twillman D, Young DS, Basnyat B. Older age, chronic medical conditions and polypharmacy in Himalayan trekkers in Nepal: an epidemiologic survey and case series. J Travel Med 2016; 23(6):taw052. https://doi.org/10.1093/jtm/taw052.

29 Faulhaber M, Flatz M, Gatterer H, Schobersberger W, Burtscher M. Prevalence of cardiovascular diseases among alpine skiers and hikers in the Austrian Alps. High Alt Med Biol 2007; 8(3): 245–252. https://doi.org/10.1089/ham.2007.1005.

30 Faulhaber M, Gatterer H, Burtscher M. Preexisting cardiovascular diseases among high-altitude mountaineers in the alps. J Travel Med 2011; 18(5):355–337. https://doi.org/10.1111/j.1708-8305.2011.00536.x.

31 ISTAT Istituto Nazionale di Statistica. Noi Italia 2025, Salute e Welfare > Sanità e Salute [ISTAT Italian Institute of Statistics, We Italy 2025, Health and Welfare]. Rome, 2025. https://noi-italia.istat.it/pagina.php?id=3&categoria=6&action=show&L=026.

32 ISTAT Istituto Nazionale di Statistica. Noi Italia, 100 statistiche per capire il Paese in cui viviamo, 2014. https://www.istat.it/it/files//2014/03/Noi-Italia-2014.pdf.

33 Lopez-Pascual A, Bes-Rastrollo M, Sayón-Orea C, Perez-Cornago A, Díaz-Gutiérrez J, Pons JJ, Martínez-González MA, González-Muniesa P, Martínez JA. Living at a geographically higher elevation is associated with lower risk of metabolic syndrome: prospective analysis of the SUN cohort. Front Physiol. 2017; 7:658. https://doi.org/10.3389/fphys.2016.00658. https://www.frontiersin.org/articles/10.3389/fphys.2016.00658/full.

34 Lopez-Pascual A, Arévalo J, Martínez JA, González-Muniesa P. Inverse association between metabolic syndrome and altitude: a cross-sectional study in an adult population of Ecuador. Front Endocrinol (Lausanne) 2018;9:658. https://doi.org/10.3389/fendo.2018.00658. https://pmc.ncbi.nlm.nih.gov/articles/PMC6240603/pdf/fendo-09-00658.pdf.

35 Ortiz-Prado E, Espinosa PS, Borrero A, Cordovez SP, Vasconez JE, Barreto-Grimales A, Coral-Almeida M, Henriquez-Trujillo AR, Simbaña-Rivera K, Gomez-Barreno L, Viscor G, Roderick P. Stroke-related mortality at different altitudes: a 17-year nationwide population-based analysis from Ecuador. Front Physiol 2021; 12:733928. https://doi.org/10.3389/fphys.2021.733928. https://pmc.ncbi.nlm.nih.gov/articles/PMC8525493/pdf/fphys-12-733928.pdf.

36 Zubieta-Calleja GR, Zubieta-DeUrioste NA. Extended longevity at high altitude: benefits of exposure to chronic hypoxia. BLDE Univ J Health Sci 2017; 2:80–90. https://www.zuniv.net/pub/Longevity.pdf.

37 Heath D, Williams DR. Heart and coronary circulation. In: Heath D, Williams DR (Eds.). High-Altitude Medicine and Pathology. 2nd ed. London: Butterworths; 1989. pp. 186–195.

PART 2

Physiology of the Cardiovascular System at High Altitude

CHAPTER 3

Cold Environment and the Heart

The influence of the mountain environment on the physiological conditions of the organism could be roughly divided into two groups: positive factors and negative factors.

The positive factors and their effects are essentially attributable to psychological and physical well-being, linked to the healthiness of the air and the amenity of the landscape.

On the other hand, however, there are important problems due to potentially adverse environmental characteristics, such as orography (and consequent physical fatigue when travelling) and isolation (difficulty in solving any arising problems; worsening of possible stress and depression).

As regards problems related to the cardiovascular system, two other factors are present, linked, respectively, to meteorology (cold, rain and snow...) and – most important – to reduced atmospheric pressure (and consequent reduction in the partial pressure of oxygen).

With the ascent to mountains, the ambient temperature decreases by an average of about 0.65–0.7 °C for every 100 m of ascent (*elevation-dependent temperature lapse rate*). However, the actual temperature change varies depending on factors such as humidity, geographic features (localised microclimates), and weather conditions (presence of sun, cloud cover, temperature inversions and pre-monsoon period in the Himalayas); the effects of **cold** are much more intense when combined with the presence of **wind**.[1]

Wind Chill Effect

The perceived temperature is decidedly lower than the real temperature in the presence of wind (*wind-chill effect*) (Figure 3.1). For example, an environmental temperature of 0 °C in the presence of wind at a speed of 5 km/h ('light breeze') is perceived as −2 °C; at the same absolute temperature of 0 °C, a wind of 15 km/h ('breeze') creates a sensation of cold corresponding to −4 °C. If the absolute temperatures are lower, as often encountered at moderate and high altitudes, a temperature of −10 °C is perceived – for the same wind speeds reported above – as if it was −13 °C and −17 °C, respectively. More detailed data are reported in a paper by Castellani JW et al., that we recommend to read.[2]

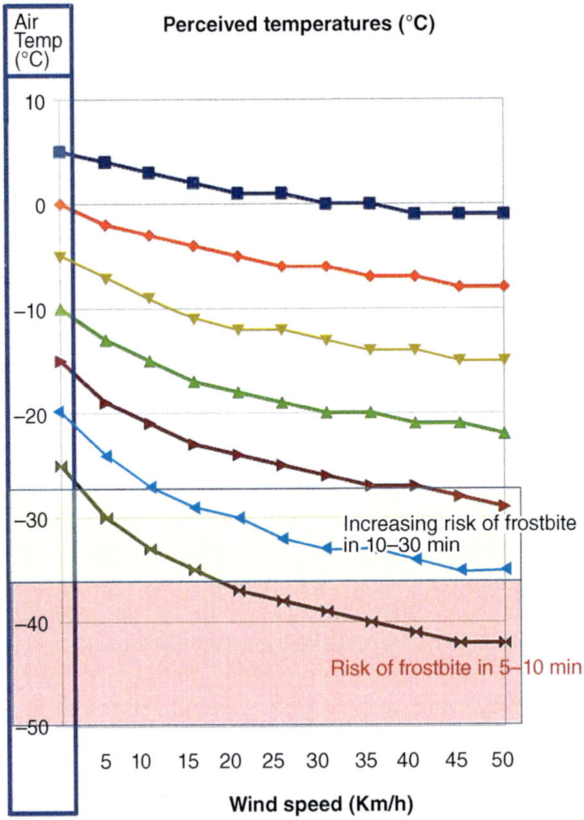

FIGURE 3.1 'Wind chill' temperature index – perceived temperature (in °C) and risk of frostbite on exposed facial skin (according to the Meteorological Society of Canada/Environment Canada). [3]/with permission of Sage Publications.

Athletes who participate in winter events, such as cross-country skiing, downhill skiing, winter triathlon, sled racing and winter climbing, must take into account the phenomenon of wind chill and its consequences on the body.

It has been reported that cold-related skin damages (chilblains, cold urticaria, frostbite) can have a significant incidence in winter sports, affecting up to 20% of cross-country skiers, 31% of sled racers and 36% of mountain climbers;[3] adverse effects can occur already at temperatures of −0.5 °C. Their incidence increases in the presence of wind or by contact with surfaces or liquids at low freezing temperatures (metals or liquids such as petrol and fuels, alcohol; wet clothing).

When the entire body is surrounded by snow (as in the case of avalanche victims), the cooling of the body can be approximately 9 °C per hour,[4] and in the case of immersion in water at +2 °C, hypothermia can be about 0.35 ± 0.14 °C for each minute of immersion.[5]

Hypothermia and the Heart

When heat dispersion exceeds the body's capacity to produce heat (via shivering-induced thermogenesis and other forms of thermogenesis), the effects of low temperature manifest throughout the body, with a core temperature that can reach as low as below 35 °C (**hypothermia**). During this phase, the body produces a high amount of catecholamines, which lead to generalised vasoconstriction and increase in peripheral vascular resistance and, consequently, to an increase in blood pressure and heart rate. This translates into a significant increase in O_2 consumption by the heart, a fact that – obviously – can be very pernicious in patients with heart disease.

The sequence of phenomena that appear with varying degrees of hypothermia is summarised in Table 3.1.

TABLE 3.1 **Summary of the main effects of different degrees of hypothermia.**

Core Temp.	Physiological and clinical effects
36 °C	Sensation of cold, shivering. Confusion / disorientation. Uncertain gait. Drowsiness. Skin extremely cold to the touch. Increased blood pressure. (Tachycardia).
34 °C	Incoordination, similar to drunkenness. Amnesia. Dysarthria, Indistinct speech. Poor judgment. Cardiac arrhythmias (most frequently atrial fibrillation). Progressive bradycardia. QT prolongation, and ST-T abnormalities.
32 °C	Cyanosis. Ataxia, apathy, stupor. Shivering becomes muscle stiffness. Blood pressure difficult to be measured. Atrial fibrillation, junctional bradycardia, and other arrhythmias.
30 °C	Progressive reduction of cardiac output. Dilated pupils. Hypoventilation (3-4 respiratory acts per minute). Lactic acidosis. Unconsciousness.
28 °C	Reduced blood flow to the kidneys. Cold induced diuresis. Ventricular fibrillation likely. Hypoventilation. Pulmonary oedema. Absence of tendon reflexes and voluntary motion.
26 °C	Severe hypotension. Ventricular fibrillation, or asystole, or PEA. No muscle stiffness (flaccid muscles). Reduced cerebral blood flow. Fixed miosis. Apparent clinical death.

(continued)

TABLE 3.1 (continued)

Core Temp.	Physiological and clinical effects
24°C	Hypoventilation. Ventricular fibrillation. Areflexia, no corneal reflexes.
22°C	Apnoea.
20°C	Cardiac arrest.

With **mild hypothermia** (i.e. with a core temperature between **35°C and 32°C**), the person presents with increasing shivering, social detachment and other behavioural changes.

From a cardiovascular point of view, what happens with a further drop in temperature to **32°C – 28°C (moderate hypothermia)** becomes extremely relevant. In addition to general signs (dilation of the pupils, loss of ability to shiver, confusion and loss of consciousness), cardiac signs appear:

- Conduction disorders.
- Progressive bradycardia (up to less than 50% of baseline heart rate at a body temperature of 28°C, due to a reduction of spontaneous depolarisation of the pacemaker cells);[6] in these cases, the administration of atropine is ineffective.
- QT prolongation, ST segment depression, T wave abnormalities, appearance of J wave on the electrocardiogram (also called Osborn wave or hypothermic hump; although this abnormal extra deflection at the end of the QRS complex is not specific for hypothermia,[i] its amplitude is linearly correlated with the degree of hypothermia).[7, 8]
- Cardiac arrhythmias, such as the appearance of atrial premature contractions, wandering pacemaker, atrial fibrillation, ventricular extrasystoles, ventricular tachycardia and nodal rhythm.[9]
- Risk of ventricular fibrillation or cardiac arrest;[10, 11] ventricular fibrillation may develop without any previous changes of rhythm.[7]
- Progressive reduction of cardiac output: at body temperatures below 30°C, cardiac output is significantly reduced, up to 45% at a temperature of 25°C. Depression of cardiac function may persist long after the patient has been rewarmed.

With core temperatures **below 28°C (severe hypothermia)**, it becomes very likely:

- the appearance of asystole or ventricular fibrillation or PEA ('pulseless electrical activity'), as well as
- pulmonary oedema,
- severe hypotension,
- acid-base balance disorders.

[i]A J wave is present also in hypocalcaemia, early repolarization and Brugada syndrome, as well as in subarachnoid haemorrhage and brain injury.

At a temperature of **18°C**, asystole is described;[2] the ECG trace is flat (as is the EEG) and the patient may appear clinically dead (however, these are not sufficient signs to declare death until the patient's body has not been warmed).

In addition to the reduction of body temperature, the phenomena described above are favoured by a combination with hypovolaemia (in hypothermia there is a shift of liquids from the intravascular to the extravascular space, in addition to the suppression of the release of antidiuretic hormone with consequent cold diuresis), with hypoxia, and with alteration of pH and serum electrolytes.

It is therefore generally strongly recommended that coaches and athletes should know the risk factors for hypothermia and how to identify symptoms linked to it at an early stage, use adequate clothing, check the temperature index linked to the 'wind chill' phenomenon and practice special surveillance when the perceived temperature is very low; for instance, for an environmental temperature of −15°C and wind at 40km/h ('cool wind') the perceived temperature is as low as −27°C. Careful monitoring is needed of people who suffer from asthma or cardiovascular diseases.[3]

Cold Environment and Cardiovascular Risk

Low temperatures, such as those found in high mountains and even at low-moderate altitudes during the winter season, can have relevant cardiovascular implications, although the effects of cold may be difficult to distinguish from the effects of high-altitude hypoxia. Among acute high-altitude travellers, it has been observed that cardiovascular workload increased as they ascended from low to high altitude, most noticeably during winter, with greater increases in systolic and diastolic blood pressure and heart rate in winter compared to summer.[12]

It is known that exposing the hands or face to cold, as in the 'cold pressor test', causes intense sympathetic stimulation and increased cardiac workload, both in healthy subjects and in those with coronary artery disease. A study by Gavhed et al. demonstrated an increase in systolic and diastolic blood pressure of an average of 15 and 13mmHg, respectively, (and up to 51 and 45mmHg!) when the forehead, cheek and nose of volunteers were exposed to a temperature of −10°C and a wind speed of 5m/s; the observed blood pressure responses may pose a serious health risk for hypertensive individuals and patients with angina.[13] It is therefore advisable to cover cheeks, forehead, nose and neck during exposure to temperatures ≤−10°C especially in the presence of wind speeds greater than 5m/s.

Furthermore, in coronary artery disease, exposure to cold (particularly exposing the chest to cold or inhaling cold air) reduces myocardial oxygen supply, which can lead to myocardial ischaemia.

Carrying out physical activity in a cold environment (think, for example, of an adult/elderly person shovelling snow in front of their house) leads to a greater increase in cardiac work than would occur if the effort were performed in less rigid temperature conditions. Together with reduced myocardial perfusion, this can lead to the onset of ischaemia and angina at lower workloads, and reduced exercise tolerance, both in people with coronary artery disease and those with heart failure, thus contributing to an increased morbidity and mortality among these patients during cold seasons.[14]

Even at sea level, low temperatures are associated with an increased cardiovascular risk due to a combination of multiple risk factors;[15] in 2013, a review by Fares reported that in addition to low temperatures and physical activity, other factors (which may also be triggered when frequenting high mountains) contribute to increased morbidity and mortality during the cold season: variations in plasma levels of fibrinogen, stress hormones and vasoactive substances.[16] Another study conducted in New York City between 2005 and 2013[17] demonstrated that perceived temperatures ('wind-chill temperatures') ≤ −12.2 °C (in the previous 4–6 days) were associated with an increase in emergency room visits for cardiovascular diseases. The study also confirmed the existence of an association between perceived temperature ≤ −12.2 °C and incidence of acute myocardial infarction in winter, as well as a progressive increase in emergency room visits for hypertensive crises, in direct relation to the reduction in perceived temperature.

A large-scale study presented at the European Society of Cardiology Congress in 2022, involving 2.28 million adults from five European countries, found that a 10 °C drop in temperature (from 5 °C to −5 °C) resulted in a 19% higher risk of death from cardiovascular disease and a 22% higher likelihood of death from ischaemic heart disease; an 11 °C drop in temperature (from 2 °C to −9 °C) resulted in a 4% higher risk of new-onset ischaemic heart disease. The correlation between cold temperatures and deaths was more pronounced among women and people over 65.[18]

We do not know if these findings also apply to winter athletes and to people travelling from sea level to mountain resorts during the winter season, but they suggest that some additional risks may be present. The risk may be higher in vulnerable subgroups, such as the elderly and people with pre-existing cardiovascular diseases or with metabolic syndrome, due to their reduced thermoregulatory capacity and impaired autonomic function.

A review paper by Gatterer et al. focuses on various aspects of the body's response to sport activities performed in cold environment; its reading is recommended.[19]

Most research studies on the effects of cold environments describe the physiological consequences of acute exposure. Adaptation to cold has been reported to take approximately 2 weeks, after which physiological responses to cold attenuate and cold exposure is subjectively considered less stressful.[20] Very limited data are available on chronic high-altitude residents, who in theory should be somehow accustomed to lower ambient temperatures. A study conducted in China[21] found no significant changes in mortality during cold spells in the vast Southwestern Chinese region, which includes Tibet, without unfortunately reporting specific data on high-mountain populations.

There is a clear lack of information on the effects of exposure to a cold environment among people living in low- and middle-income countries, as well as in socio-economically disadvantaged areas.

In conclusion, mountain travellers (especially vulnerable populations such as individuals with hypertension, coronary artery disease, or a history of stroke) should take particular care not to expose themselves to excessively low temperatures, to pay attention to protecting themselves adequately from the cold, and to avoid strenuous physical exertion as much as possible.

References

1 Lankford HV, Fox LR. The wind-chill index. Wilderness Environ Med 2021; 32(3):392–399. https://doi.org/10.1016/j.wem.2021.04.005.

2 Castellani JW, Young AJ, Ducharme MB, Giesbrecht GG, Glickman E, Sallis RE; American College of Sports Medicine. American college of sports medicine position stand: prevention of cold injuries

during exercise. Med Sci Sports Exerc 2006; 38(11):2012–2029. https://doi.org/10.1249/01.mss.0000241641.75101.64.

3 Fudge J. Preventing and managing hypothermia and frostbite injury. Sports Health 2016; 8(2):133–139. https://doi.org/10.1177/1941738116630542.

4 Pasquier M, Moix PA, Delay D, Hugli O. Cooling rate of 9.4 °C in an hour in an avalanche victim. Resuscitation 2015;93:e17–e18. https://doi.org/10.1016/j.resuscitation.2015.05.009.

5 Proulx CI, Ducharme MB, Kenny GP. Effect of water temperature on cooling efficiency during hyperthermia in humans. J Appl Physiol 2003; 94(4):1317–1323. https://doi.org/10.1152/japplphysiol.00541.2002.

6 Covino BG, D'Amato HE. Mechanism of ventricular fibrillation in hypothermia. Circ Res 1962; 10:148–155. https://doi.org/10.1161/01.res.10.2.148.

7 Coniam SW. Accidental hypothermia. Anaesthesia 1979; 34(3):250–256. https://doi.org/10.1111/j.1365-2044.1979.tb06303.x.

8 Ambesh P, Hollander G, Shani J. Osborn waves of hypothermia. Cleve Clin J Med 2017; 84(10):746–747. https://doi.org/10.3949/ccjm.84a.16134.

9 Bjørnstad H, Tande PM, Refsum H. Cardiac electrophysiology during hypothermia. Implications for medical treatment. Arctic Med Res 1991;50 (Suppl 6):71–75.

10 Caldini P. Ventricular fibrillation in induced hypothermia. Postgrad Med J 1959;35(408):538–542. https://doi.org/10.1136/pgmj.35.408.538.

11 Dietrichs ES, McGlynn K, Allan A, Connolly A, Bishop M, Burton F, Kettlewell S, Myles R, Tveita T, Smith GL. Moderate but not severe hypothermia causes pro-arrhythmic changes in cardiac electrophysiology. Cardiovasc Res 2020; 116(13):2081–2090. https://doi.org/10.1093/cvr/cvz309. Erratum in: Cardiovasc Res 2020;116(7):1322. https://doi.org/10.1093/cvr/cvaa048.

12 Tsao TM, Hwang JS, Tsai MJ, Lin ST, Wu C, Su TC. Seasonal effects of high-altitude forest travel on cardiovascular function: an overlooked cardiovascular risk of forest activity. Int J Environ Res Public Health 2021; 18(18):9472. https://doi.org/10.3390/ijerph18189472.

13 Gavhed D, Mäkinen T, Holmér I, Rintamäki H. Face temperature and cardiorespiratory responses to wind in thermoneutral and cool subjects exposed to −10 degrees C. Eur J Appl Physiol 2000; 83(4–5):449–456. https://doi.org/10.1007/s004210000262.

14 Ikäheimo TM. Cardiovascular diseases, cold exposure and exercise. Temperature (Austin) 2018; 5(2):123–146. https://doi.org/10.1080/23328940.2017.1414014.

15 Ni W, Areal AT, Lechner K, Breitner S, Zhang S, Woeckel M, Slesinski SC, Nikolaou N, Dallavalle M, Schikowski T, Schneider A. Low and high air temperature and cardiovascular risk. Atherosclerosis 2025; 406:119238. https://doi.org/10.1016/j.atherosclerosis.2025.119238.

16 Fares A. Winter cardiovascular diseases phenomenon. N Am J Med Sci 2013; 5(4):266–279. https://doi.org/10.4103/1947-2714.110430.

17 Lin S, Lawrence WR, Lin Z, DiRienzo S, Lipton K, Dong GH, Leung R, Lauper U, Nasca P, Stuart N. Are the current thresholds, indicators, and time window for cold warning effective enough to protect cardiovascular health? Sci Total Environ 2018; 639:860–867. https://doi.org/10.1016/j.scitotenv.2018.05.140.

18 American College of Cardiology, ACC News Story. EXHAUSTION project finds extreme temperatures associated with CV death, Stroke. August 26, 2022. https://www.acc.org/Latest-in-Cardiology/Articles/2022/08/25/19/13/fri-837am-EXHAUSTION-esc-2022.

19 Gatterer H, Dünnwald T, Turner R, Csapo R, Schobersberger W, Burtscher M, Faulhaber M, Kennedy MD. Practicing sport in cold environments: practical recommendations to improve sport performance and reduce negative health outcomes. Int J Environ Res Public Health 2021; 18(18):9700. https://doi.org/10.3390/ijerph18189700.
20 Rintamäki H. Human responses to cold. Alaska Med 2007; 49(2 Suppl):29–31.
21 Wang L, Liu T, Hu M, Zeng W, Zhang Y, Rutherford S, Lin H, Xiao J, Yin P, Liu J, Chu C, Tong S, Ma W, Zhou M. The impact of cold spells on mortality and effect modification by cold spell characteristics. Sci Rep 2016; 6:38380. https://doi.org/10.1038/srep38380.

CHAPTER 4

Altitude, Atmospheric Pressure and Physiopathological Phenomena on the Cardiovascular System

Altitude and Barometric Pressure

The most relevant pathophysiological phenomenon related to climbing to high altitude is the progressive **decrease in atmospheric pressure** with the associated **decrease in the partial pressure of oxygen**.

As we gradually leave sea level to rise to increasingly higher altitudes (Figure 4.1), the barometric pressure (P_B) decreases due to the progressive reduction of the column of air above us. If at sea level in temperate zones the atmospheric pressure is around 760 mmHg (around 1,013 hPa),[i] at the top of Everest it is around 253 mmHg (337 hPa),[1] a truly significant reduction to around one-third! (Note: these values may change by 8 mmHg between summer and winter, as well as in relation to the variability of atmospheric conditions and air currents in the upper atmosphere).

Without reaching extreme altitudes, already for a low altitude such as that of the renown Italian mountain resort of Cortina d'Ampezzo (approximately 1,210 m AMSL), the standard barometric pressure is reduced to approximately 665 mmHg (890 hPa), i.e. to a value corresponding to approximately 85% of the pressure found at sea level.

[i]These values are valid in 'standard conditions', i.e. at an altitude of 0 m above sea level, at a temperature of 0 °C, and at 45° latitude. The mBar (milliBar) is equivalent to the hPa (hectoPascal, i.e. 100 Pascal).

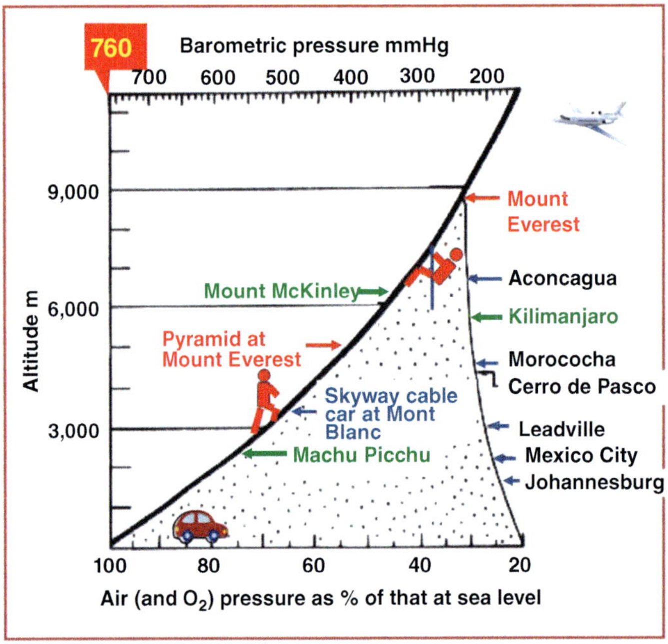

FIGURE 4.1 Variation of barometric pressure at different mountain altitudes and simultaneous variation of oxygen pressure expressed as a percentage of that found at sea level.

At an altitude of 2,000m AMSL, the barometric pressure is approximately 596mmHg (795hPa), at 3,000m AMSL 526mmHg (701hPa) and at 4,000m AMSL approximately 462mmHg (616hPa) with local and seasonal variations.[2]

Just to give a few more examples, in the city of Denver, Colorado (located at an altitude of 'one mile') the average barometric pressure is 630–633mmHg (840hPa); in the popular ski resort of Snowmass at Aspen, Colorado (at an altitude of approximately 2,450m), the average atmospheric pressure is 558mmHg (744hPa). Other examples are the city of El Alto, Bolivia, located at an altitude of 4,005m, where the barometric pressure is reported to be around 471–490mmHg (628–653hPa), and the city of Addis Ababa (Ethiopia; located at an altitude of 2,355m) in which average barometric pressure is around 570mmHg (760hPa).

I would like to point out that the altitudes reported above are those that many travellers and tourists, even of fairly advanced age and even in 'less than splendid' physical conditions, often reach: in the Italian Alps, for instance, the Auronzo refuge at the Tre Cime di Lavaredo (Drei Zinnen) is located at 2,333m AMSL and it is the starting point for walks; the Tofana peak with the arrival of the cable car is located at 3,244m AMSL; and the Skyway cable car on Mont Blanc takes tourists up to Punta Helbronner at 3,466m AMSL. Currently, the highest mountain resort reachable by cable car is Pico Espejo, in the Sierra Nevada National Park of the Venezuelan Andes: the 'Teleférico de Mérida' cable car has its arrival station at 4,765m above sea level. (The calculation of the barometric pressure for these altitudes can be approximately obtained from formulas).[3]

These are therefore altitudes that even elderly people or people with more or less known cardiovascular diseases can reach! Obviously, higher altitudes require walking uphill or climbing to be reached and therefore are the prerogative of younger people (but not always adequately trained!) and athletes.

Atmospheric Pressure and Partial Oxygen Pressure

With the reduction of the atmospheric pressure due to altitude, the partial pressure of oxygen in the inspired air (PiO_2) also progressively reduces. The partial pressure of oxygen in inspired air can be calculated using a formula:

$$PiO_2 = FiO_2 \; x \; (P_B - P_{H_2O})$$

where PiO_2 is the partial pressure of oxygen in the inspired air (the parameter we are looking for), which turns out to be directly proportional to the FiO_2 (i.e. the fraction of O_2 in the inspired air) and to the barometric pressure (P_B) subtracted by the partial pressure of water vapour (P_{H_2O}; in addition to the humidity already present in the air, the air is humidified as it passes through the respiratory tract). The FiO_2 is always, at all altitudes, equal to approximately 0.21 (exactly 0.2093; this indicates that the percentage of O_2 in the inspired air is 21%) (Figure 4.2). We have already talked about P_B, and we can measure it; P_{H_2O} is considered to be equal to 47 mmHg at the body temperature of 37 °C, on average (although at high altitudes it is sometimes significantly reduced).

Therefore, with the fraction of O_2 in the inspired air (FiO_2) and the partial pressure of water vapour (P_{H_2O}) practically constant, it can be deduced that the partial pressure of O_2 in the inspired air (PiO_2) is directly proportional to the barometric pressure (P_B). The more P_B is reduced, the more PiO_2 is reduced (Figure 4.3).

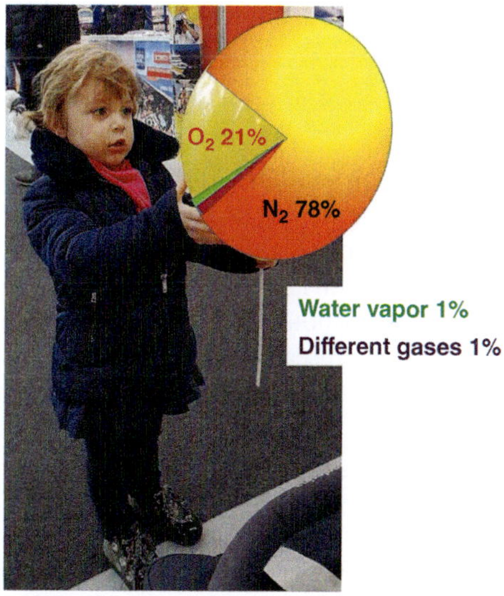

FIGURE 4.2 Composition of atmospheric air. (in the picture: my granddaughter at the age of two and a half).

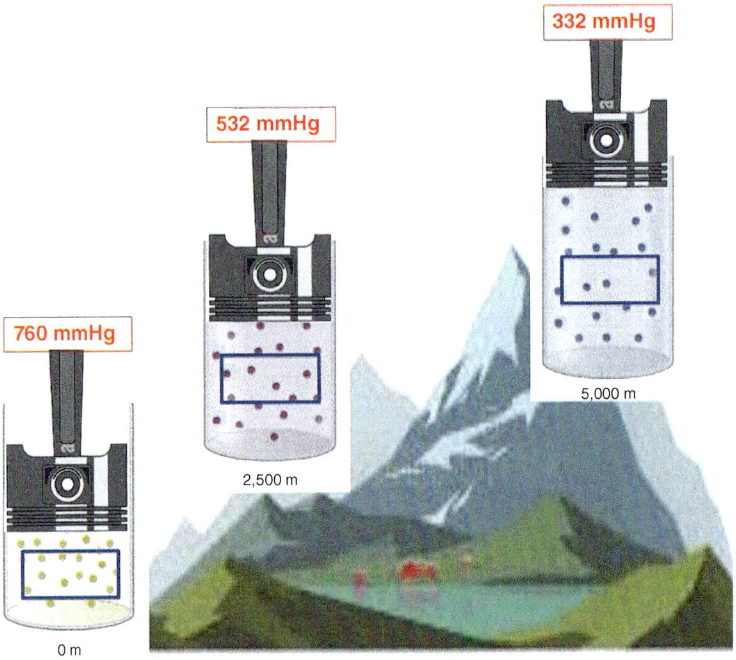

FIGURE 4.3 As altitude increases, the **percentage** of O_2 molecules in the air remains constant, but – since the air is less 'dense' due to the reduction in atmospheric pressure – the **absolute number** of O_2 molecules in the unit of volume of inspired air decreases.

For the various altitudes, the calculations can easily be performed with medical calculators, such as MediCalc.[4]

At sea level (with P_B 760 mmHg), the PiO_2 is therefore approximately 150 mmHg; on the summit of Everest, where P_B is around 253 mmHg, PiO_2 drops enormously, to around 43 mmHg.

But, to return to the most common examples cited above, in Cortina d'Ampezzo the Pi O_2 would be around 130 mmHg; at the arrival of the Tofana cable car it would be around 99 mmHg, and at Punta Helbronner of Mont Blanc it would drop to values around 93–94 mmHg. In Denver, PiO_2 is approximately 125 mmHg; at Snowmass, PiO_2 is around 109 mmHg, and almost the same PiO_2 may be found in Addis Ababa; in El Alto, PiO_2 drops to 89–94 mmHg, less than two-thirds of the values found at sea level!

Alveolar Oxygen Pressure

So far we have discussed the partial pressure of oxygen in inspired air. But at the level of the alveoli, will it be the same? And how much oxygen is able to cross the alveolar barrier and reach the pulmonary capillaries and consequently the arterial circulation?

We must take into account that in the pulmonary alveoli, in addition to oxygen and nitrogen, carbon dioxide (CO_2) is present; its quantity depends on the respiratory rate and its depth, as well as on the type of metabolism of the subject (mainly lipid, carbohydrate or mixed). On average the partial pressure of CO_2 in the alveoli corresponds to approximately 40–50 mmHg.[ii]

In ambient air, at sea level, a healthy subject has an O_2 pressure at the alveolar level (called PAO_2) of 100 mmHg (i.e. approximately, the partial pressure of O_2 in inspired air, subtracted by the partial pressure of the CO_2 found in the alveoli).

Then the oxygen must pass through the thin wall of the alveoli to reach the blood that circulates in the capillaries in contact with this wall; oxygen passes from the alveoli to the blood of the capillaries by simple diffusion, because its partial pressure in the alveolar air is higher than the partial pressure of O_2 that exists in the blood reaching the lungs from the periphery of the body (about 40 mmHg). In the pulmonary capillaries and then in the arterial blood, the value of the partial pressure of O_2 (what is called PaO_2) drops to 85–90 mmHg, therefore with an 'Alveolar-arterial gradient' equal to 15–10 mmHg.

Oxygen saturation of Haemoglobin

The oxygen absorbed through breathing then saturates the haemoglobin; we are used to evaluating the percentage of oxygen saturation of the peripheral blood using common oximeters. The oxygen absorbed in the conditions described above saturates on average 95–98% of the haemoglobin.

In summary (Figure 4.4), **at sea level**:

- Atmospheric pressure, barometric pressure (P_B): 760 mmHg
- Partial pressure of O_2 in inspired air (PiO_2): 150 mmHg
- Partial pressure of O_2 in alveolar air (PAO_2): 100 mmHg
- Partial pressure of O_2 in arterial blood (PaO_2): 85–90 mmHg
- Arterial oxygen saturation (SaO_2): 95–98%

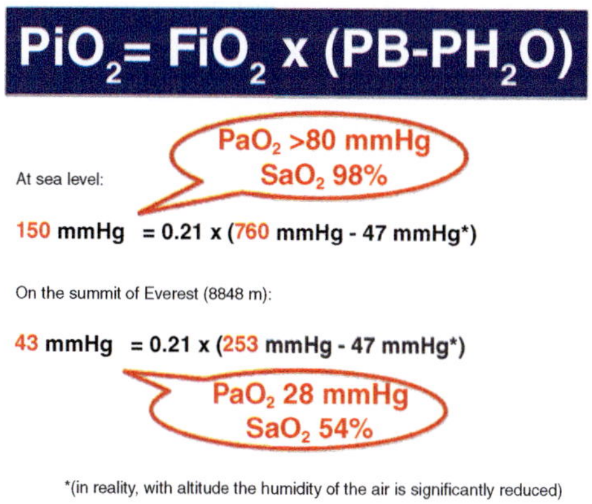

FIGURE 4.4 Atmospheric pressure and blood oxygen parameters at sea level and at extreme altitudes; see text.

[ii]Variable values depending on the Respiratory Quotient (R), which is 1 for a metabolism exclusively based on carbohydrates, or 0.7 for exclusively lipid metabolism; on average it is considered around 0.82 for a mixed diet.

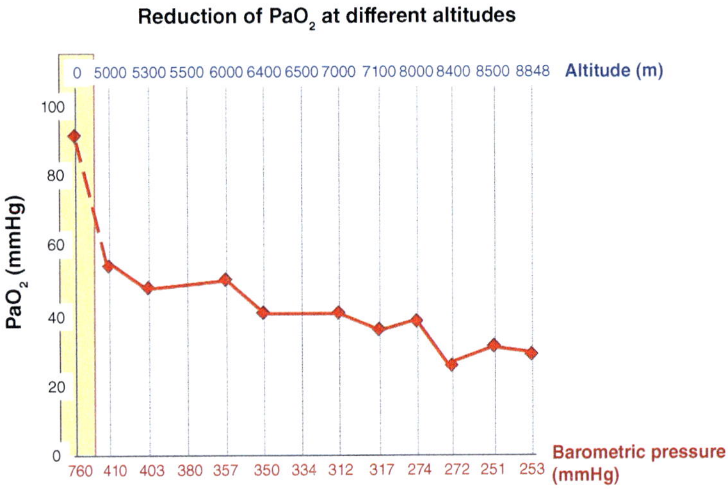

FIGURE 4.5 Modifications of PaO_2 in the altonauts studied during the Operation Everest III. Modified from Refs. [6, 7].

We have just seen that, as altitude increases, barometric pressure and PiO_2 progressively decrease; what do those reductions mean?

At an **extreme altitude of 8,400 m** AMSL (on the 'balcony of Everest', almost at the top, which is at 8,849 m AMSL) (Figure 4.5).[5]

- Atmospheric pressure, barometric pressure (P_B): 253 mmHg
- Partial pressure of O_2 in inspired air (PiO_2): 43 mmHg
- Partial pressure of O_2 in alveolar air (PAO_2): theoretically it would be around 0 mmHg, i.e. incompatible with life; in reality it is slightly higher than expected, because hypoxia stimulates the chemoreceptors, with a consequent increase in the respiratory frequency (up to 86 breaths per minute!) and increased elimination of CO_2 (the partial pressure of which in the alveoli is therefore around 12–26 mmHg, instead of 40 mmHg; values as low as 7–8 mmHg have been reported by JB West in one climber!);[1] furthermore, at such high altitudes the humidity of the inhaled air is also lower. In Everest climbers, PAO_2 was calculated to be between 26.9 and 33.2 mmHg, with an average of 30 mmHg.
- Partial pressure of O_2 in arterial blood (PaO_2): it was found to be between 19.1 and 29.5 mmHg (average 24.6 mmHg), again in the study on Everest climbers.
- Peripheral blood O_2 saturation (SaO_2): on Everest it was found to be extremely low, between 34.4 and 69.7%, with an average of 54%.

These data show us the critical situation reached by the climbers at that altitude.[iii]

[iii]To have a 'visual' representation of what it means to stay and do physical activity at those altitudes, you can see a clip relating to the historical films taken during the conquest of K2 (altitude 8,609 m AMSL) carried out by the Italian climbers Compagnoni and Lacedelli in 1952; see at minute 31:50 and following: https://youtu.be/diws6kvtTYo.

Oxygen Saturation of Haemoglobin at Altitude

If we now consider more 'human' altitudes, we can see how these parameters vary and therefore deduce what the consequences may be for healthy subjects and for subjects suffering from heart or lung diseases.

At an altitude, for example, of 2,120m AMSL, such as **on Faloria** (in Italian Dolomites):

- Atmospheric pressure, barometric pressure (P_B): 596 mmHg
- Partial pressure of O_2 in inspired air (PiO_2): 115 mmHg
- Partial pressure of O_2 in alveolar air (PAO_2): 65 mmHg
- Partial pressure of O_2 in arterial blood (PaO_2): approximately 50–55 mmHg
- Arterial oxygen saturation (SaO_2): 90–92% or less, which already indicates a slight oxygenation deficit.

At a higher altitude, for example, 3,244m AMSL of **Tofana de Rozes** (also in the Dolomites) we expect the values to be approximately:

- Atmospheric pressure, barometric pressure (P_B): 510 mmHg
- Partial pressure of O_2 in inspired air (PiO_2): 99 mmHg
- Partial pressure of O_2 in alveolar air (PAO_2): approximately 50 mmHg
- Partial pressure of O_2 in arterial blood (PaO_2): approximately 40 mmHg
- Arterial oxygen saturation (SaO_2): <80%.

To cite just a few other examples of high altitudes that are more or less easily reachable (see also Table 4.1), let us recall, for example, that the airport of La Paz (Bolivia) is located in **El Alto**, at 4,000m a.s.l; there,

- The mean barometric pressure is around 471–490 mmHg (65% that of sea level),
- The PiO_2 is reported to be 89–94 mmHg (one-third less than at sea level),
- Mean PaO_2 is as low as 60 mmHg and $PaCO_2$ is 30 mmHg (respectively, one-third and one-fourth less than at sea level).[8]

The town of **Leadville** (Colorado, USA) has North America's highest public use airport, located at an altitude of 3,097m AMSL; it offers access to nearby ski resorts and vacation resources. In Leadville,

- Atmospheric pressure is around 535 mmHg,
- PiO_2 is around 102 mmHg;
- Mean PaO_2 has been reported to be around 51 mmHg and $PaCO_2$ around 30 mmHg (with a SaO_2 of 87–88%).[11]

Such levels of significant reduction in PaO_2 and SaO_2, if found in a patient on the plains, would push us to urgently administer oxygen, or even to proceed with intubation and assisted ventilation!

TABLE 4.1 **Examples of variation of respiratory parameters at some different mountain altitudes (mean approximate data; partly derived from Refs. [9, 10]).**

	Altitude	PA	PiO_2	PAO_2	PaO_2	SaO_2	PCO_2
Sea level	0	760	150	100	85–90	95–98	—
Katmandu (Nepal)	≈1,400	656	—	78–82	—	95–96	36–39
Denver (Colorado)	1,610	630	125	73–77	—	95	34–36
Faloria (Italian Dolomites)	2,120	596	115	65	50–55	90–92	
Addis Ababa (Ethiopia)	2,355	570	[109]	—	—	—	—
Snowmass at Aspen (Colorado)	2,450	558	109	—	—	—	—
Leadville (Colorado)	3,097	535	102	—	51–57	87–88	30
Too-Ashu (Kyrgyz Republic)	3,100	[515]	—	—	58	88	36
Tofana de Rozes (Italian Dolomites)	3,244	510	99	50	40	<80	
Namche (Nepal)	3,440	509	107	—	48–49	85	30–31
Punta Helbronner, Mt. Blanc (Italian Alps)	3,466	[490]	93–94	—	—	—	—
Barcroft Station, Sierra Nevada (California)	3,800	487	92	—	50	86	34
Deboche (Nepal)	3,820	486	102	—	52–54	88–89	29–30
Kunde (Nepal)	3,840	495	—	—	54	90	24

TABLE 4.1 (continued)

	Altitude	PA	PiO_2	PAO_2	PaO_2	SaO_2	PCO_2
El Alto (Bolivia)	4,005	490	89–94	—	60	—	30
Pheriche (Nepal)	4,240	454	95	—	48	85	29
Cerro de Pasco (Peru)	4,267–4,350	465–472	—	—	41–51	81	28–33
Pikes Peak (Colorado)	4,300	463	—	—	40–50	77–87	25–33
Regina Margherita Hut, Mt. Rosa (Italian Alps)	4,559	430	—	—	39–44	70–77	26–32
Mt. Everest Pyramid Int. Lab. (Nepal)	5,050	418	—	—	43–50	76–80	26–30
Gorak Shep (Nepal)	5,160	411	86	—	36	73	26
Mt. Everest base camp (Nepal)	5,400	401	—	—	43	75	24
Mt. McKinley (Alaska)	6,190	356	—	—	35	65–75	20–26
Aconcagua (Argentine Andes)	6,962	[325]	60–70	—	—	60	—
Mt. Himlung Himal (Nepal)	7,050	[314]			30	66–69	14
Balcony of Everest (Nepal)	8,400	253–272	43	30	24.6 (19–29)	54	13.3 (10–16)
Operation Everest III, altonauts	8,848	—	—	—	30.6	58–68	11.9

Altitude AMSL = altitude above sea level, in meters; PA: atmospheric pressure (mmHg); PiO_2: partial pressure of oxygen in inspired air (mmHg); PAO_2: partial pressure of oxygen in alveolar air (mmHg); PaO_2: partial pressure of oxygen in arteriolar blood (mmHg); SaO_2: oxygen saturation of arterial blood (%); PCO_2: partial pressure of CO_2 in arterial blood (mmHg)

A group of Spanish researchers[12] studied 53 mountaineers exposed to different mountain altitudes in the Alps, Himalaya, Caucasus and Andes, and managed to extrapolate a formula capable of predicting arterial oxygen saturation at the different altitudes:

Blood Oxygen Saturation = 103.3 − (altitude × 0.0047) + (Z), being $Z = 0.7$ in men and 1.4 in women.

Physiological Definition of High Altitude

At this point, we can introduce a *physiological* concept of high altitude; that is, a definition not linked to absolute altitude, but to the effects that this has on the exchange of O_2 in our organism.

From a physiological point of view, therefore, **high altitude means a terrestrial elevation at which the O_2 saturation of haemoglobin (SaO_2) drops below 90%.**[13]

It is therefore clear that this percentage will practically be very different from individual to individual, depending on their general health conditions, their age, the use of drugs and the possible presence of lung or heart diseases.[iv]

For people in normal health, at our latitudes this altitude corresponds approximately to 2,500 m above sea level.

Above these altitudes (or – better – when SaO_2 drops, especially below 90%), hypoxia triggers and increases a series of cardiovascular and pulmonary adjustments, aimed at maintaining adequate oxygenation of the various organs and systems.

PaO_2 and PCO_2 in the Altonauts of the Operation Everest III

So far we have extrapolated theoretical data and observed some field measurements obtained on Everest climbers.

More data to understand what happens to the cardiovascular system at various levels of altitude were obtained with Operation Everest III (COMEX '97), the results of which were published in 1999.[6,7] A small number of male volunteers, eight in all (nicknamed 'altonauts'), after a period of acclimatisation at 4,350 m AMSL, were 'locked up' in a decompression chamber for 31 days, during which the atmospheric pressure was progressively reduced until it reached that existing on the summit of Everest, i.e. 253 mmHg. During this period, they were submitted

[iv]Note that the clinical oximeters we commonly use may have a measurement error of approximately ±3% between measurements; the measurements become unreliable for SpO_2 values around 80%. At low temperatures, such as those found at altitude, they may not provide correct values, especially if the subject has cold tremors or is in a very bright environment or has drumstick fingers, or nail polish or dirt on the nails, or haemoglobin abnormalities. Caution must therefore be taken in assessments carried out with an oximeter when SpO_2 values tend to be low: the situation could be worse than what is measured.[14–16]

to a series of tests that could not have been carried out in the reality of extreme altitude. Factors that could limit their physical and psychological performance, as well as those factors that could influence the appearance of acute mountain sickness, were explored.

In the five altonauts who reached barometric pressure equivalent to 8,848m AMSL, the PaO_2 dropped to 30.6 ± 1.4mmHg (Figure 4.5), i.e. similar (although a little higher) to what would have been measured a decade later in the reality of an Everest expedition by Grocott et al.[5] The PCO_2 was low (11.9 ± 1.4mmHg), indicating hyperventilation, also associated with an increase in blood pH (pH 7.58 ± 0.02). Meanwhile, the blood haemoglobin concentration also increased from 14.8 ± 1.4 to 18.4 ± 1.5g/dL.

After returning to barometric pressure corresponding to sea level, the parameters normalised in approximately 4–5 days.

Starting from an initial SaO_2 of around 96–98%, it was observed that SaO_2 actually decreased progressively with altitude: at 5,000m it was around 86–88%, at 6,000m it was 82–84%, at 7,000m it was approximately 78%, at 8,000m approximately 72–74% and was further reduced to values of approximately 66–68% at barometric pressure corresponding to the summit of Everest.

At a pressure corresponding to an altitude of approximately 7,000m AMSL, the ability of the altonauts to sustain physical effort (measured by the maximum consumption of O_2 during an exercise test) was significantly reduced, reaching less than half of their physical prowess (reduction of VO_2Max of 59%). What is extremely relevant is to observe how – in the altonauts of the study – at the altitude corresponding to 7,000m AMSL even the SaO_2 measured during exercise dropped significantly and steeply, reaching levels that could be measured at rest at an altitude of 8,800m (Figure 4.6).

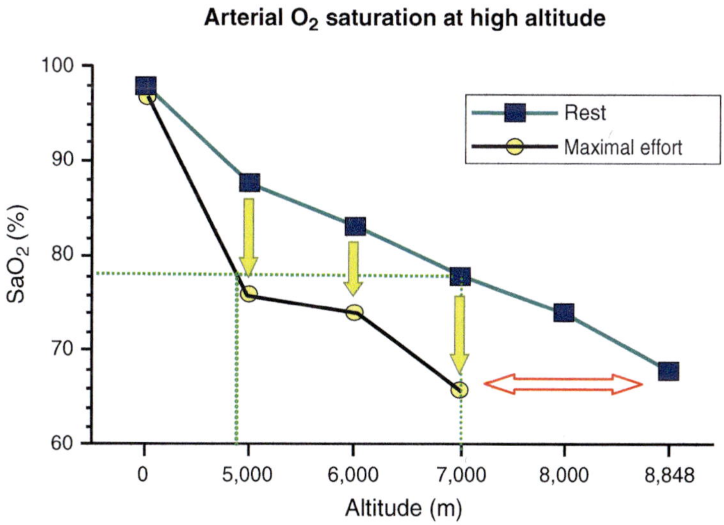

FIGURE 4.6 Arterial oxygen saturation at rest and during physical effort, at various simulated altitudes. Modified from: Richalet J-P, Herry J-P. Médecine de Montagne. 5ème éd. Elsevier Masson, 2017, page 52; graphic kindly provided by the Author.

Maximum O_2 Consumption (= Maximum Sustainable Effort) at High Altitudes

Since the ability to uptake oxygen at extreme altitudes is greatly limited by its ability to cross the alveolar-capillary membrane, it follows that a climber's maximum O_2 consumption (i.e. oxygen uptake) at the summit of Everest is very close to his basal requirements of oxygen;[17] that is, the climber at these altitudes has an extremely small functional 'reserve'.

Other studies have confirmed that athletes' maximum O_2 consumption (that means their ability to carry out physical effort) progressively reduces with altitude, approximately by an amount equal to 10% every 1,000m of altitude above 1,500m AMSL.[18]

In the small number of observed altonauts, the cardiac contractility measurements demonstrated normal values; however, changes were highlighted in the diastolic phase, with a slightly compromised relaxation phase.[19]

Cerebral circulation was also partially compromised at the simulated altitude of 8,000m above sea level.

Compensatory Mechanisms to Acute Hypoxia

These observations on acute hypoxia were accompanied by evidence of the establishment of compensatory cardiovascular mechanisms. Hypoxia, with the activation of the adrenergic system, induced tachycardia, which was inversely proportional – in an almost linear way – with the reduction of PaO_2. (In chronic exposure to altitude, however, sympathetic activation is reduced and thus tachycardia is also reduced, as we will see later).[20]

Hypoxia has been seen to induce peripheral vasodilation that is contrasted by adrenergic vasoconstriction, and pulmonary vasoconstriction. In the cited studies, the systemic arterial pressure changed little, while the pressure values in the pulmonary circulation increased (pulmonary hypertension); these pulmonary modifications can contribute to the possible appearance of high-altitude pulmonary oedema (see Chapter 6).[21]

Already from these data we can therefore deduce that patients with heart disease must take special precautions when they wish to reach high altitudes: all heart diseases can be aggravated due to sympathetic stimulation and pulmonary hypertension. In particular, patients suffering from ischaemic heart disease would notice that the threshold of physical effort at which angina appears will be lower, due to increased sympathetic activity, tachycardia and hypoxaemia.

Hyperventilation

The stimulation that hypoxia exerts on the peripheral chemoreceptors (aortic and carotid bodies) leads to an increase in the activity of the breathing centre and therefore to hyperventilation, which can even be four times the values recorded in the lowlands (Figure 4.7).[20] With exposure to hypoxia, activation of the breathing centre appears quickly, within a few minutes, and persists for the duration of stay at altitude.

Ventilation increases at rest and also for each level of exercise; the increased ventilation is achieved first by increasing the tidal volume (at least up to 3,500m altitude) and afterwards also by increasing the respiratory rate.[22] However, with each increase in altitude the curve of the relationship between O_2 consumption (= uptake) and ventilation/minute is increasingly steeper (Figure 4.8); this means that to provide a certain quantity of O_2 needed for allowing a certain physical activity, it is necessary to greatly increase ventilation.[23] For example, for an O_2 consumption of 1.5l/minute, at sea level the subject must ventilate approximately 30l/minute; for the same O_2 consumption at 5,800m AMSL this subject will have to ventilate approximately 70l/minute; at an altitude of 7,400m AMSL ventilation further rises to more than 120l/minute (in spite of a very small increase in O_2 uptake).

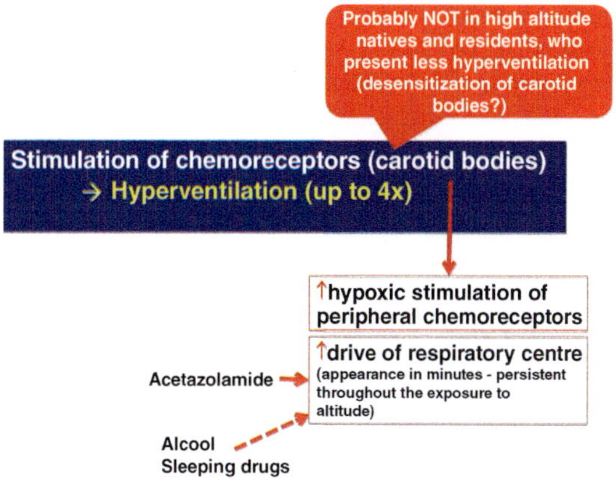

FIGURE 4.7 Hypoxia-induced hyperventilation.

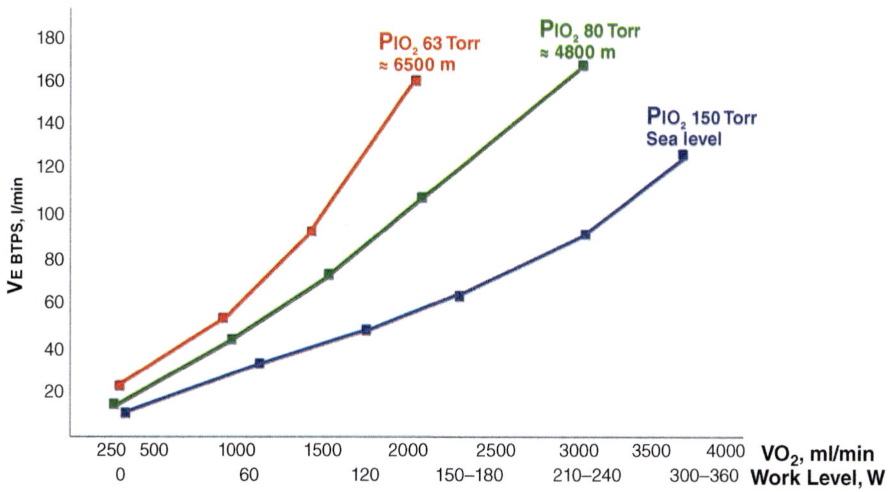

FIGURE 4.8 As altitude increases, there is a progressive reduction in PiO_2; for each sustained level of physical activity, there is a steep increase of ventilation. Graphic elaboration from data of Sutton et al (Ref. [23]).

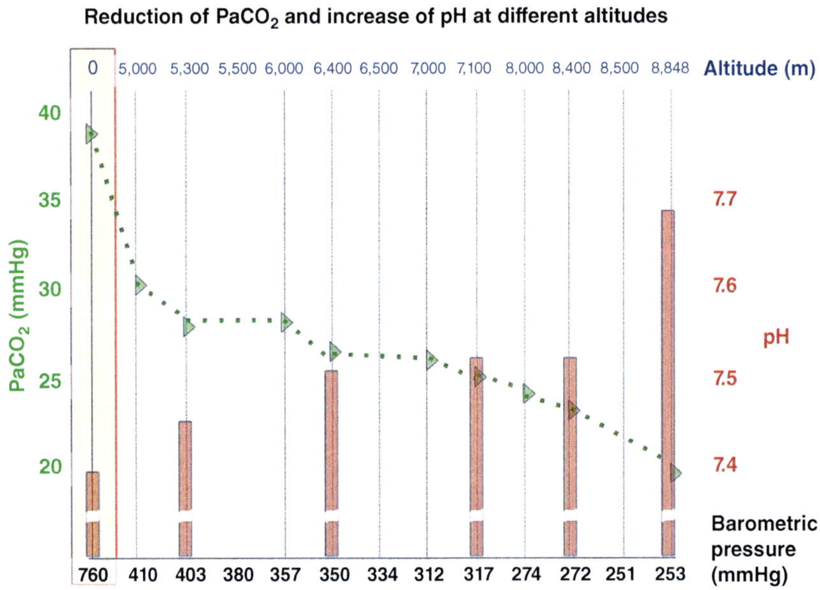

FIGURE 4.9 Hyperventilation-induced hypocapnia in altonauts at progressively increasing altitudes, during Operation Everest III. Graphic elaboration from Refs. [6, 7] and others.

Such high ventilation leads to a progressive reduction of CO_2 in the blood, i.e. hypocapnia, and therefore induces a progressive increase in blood pH (Figures 4.9 and 4.10). Acute high-altitude exposure results in a hyperventilation-induced respiratory alkalosis (pH >7.4), which appears to be of a different degree between acclimatised lowlanders and Andean and Sherpa highlanders.[24] However, from 10 to 30 minutes after exposure to hypoxia, a physiological control mechanism takes over, the 'hypoxic ventilatory depression', which varies greatly from subject to subject.[5] Over the next few hours or days, the ventilatory depression disappears and ventilation increases again (it stabilises later when ventilatory acclimatisation occurs).

Respiratory Alkalosis

The consequences of respiratory alkalosis can be very important: they range from cerebral hypo-perfusion (with consequent nausea, dizziness, impairment of consciousness and confusion, seizures even leading to coma), to electrolyte alterations with hypocalcaemia (and consequent circumoral numbness and peripheral paraesthesia, laryngospasm, muscle spasms and cramps) but above all to the possible appearance of cardiac arrhythmias linked to electrolyte disturbances combined to sympathetic activation.[25] However, the data available so far are not conclusive regarding the incidence or severity of arrhythmias linked to altitude-induced alkalosis (and sympathetic activation).[26]

Within a few days, fortunately, kidneys are mostly able to compensate for the respiratory alkalosis by increasing the excretion of bicarbonates (bicarbonaturia). Ventilation at rest, however, continues to increase slightly, until it reaches a maximum within about a week

(Figure 4.11); it constitutes the main mechanism for increasing the oxygen supply to the cells. Hyperventilation persists for years at high altitude and is a characteristic of a fully developed ventilatory acclimatisation (a fall in ventilation sometimes occurs after decades of residence at high altitude and has been called 'hypoxic desensitization').

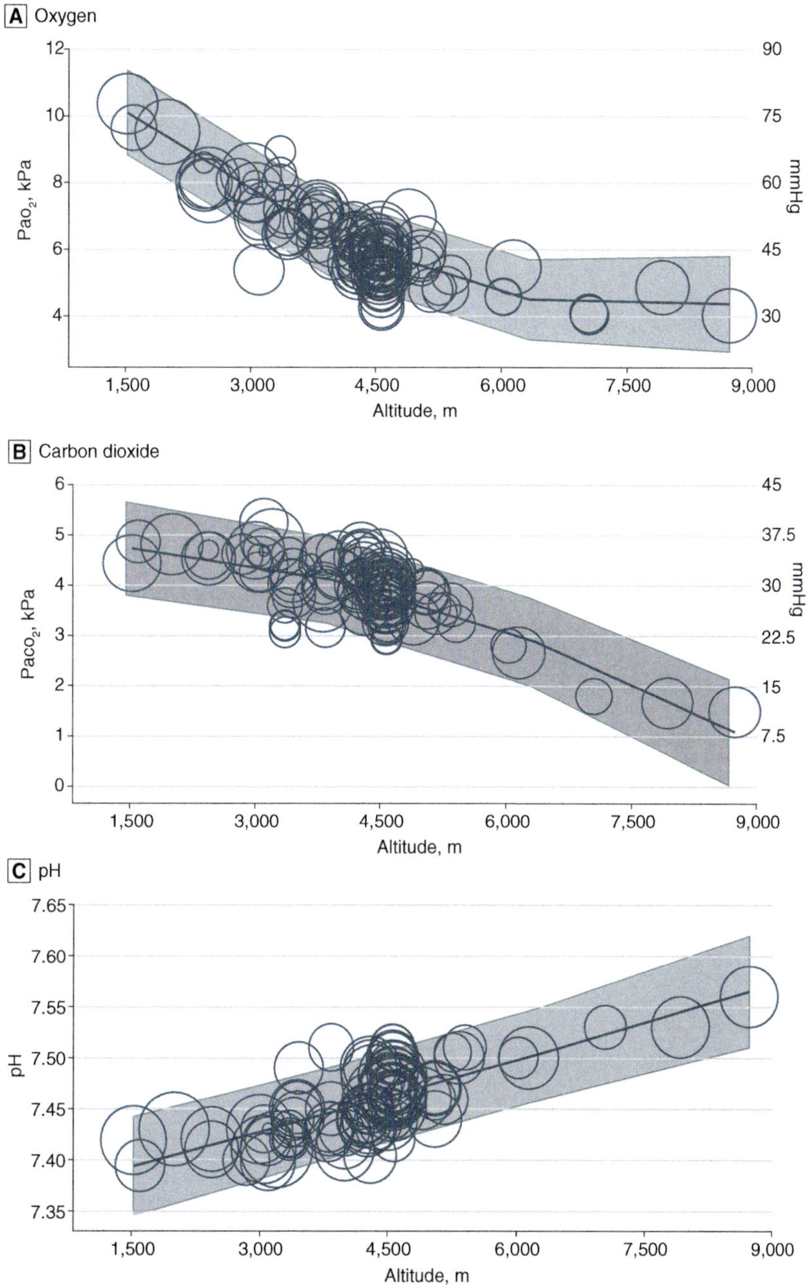

FIGURE 4.10 Arterial blood gas values by altitude, based on aggregated data; from Ref. [10]/ American Medical Association/CC BY 4.0.

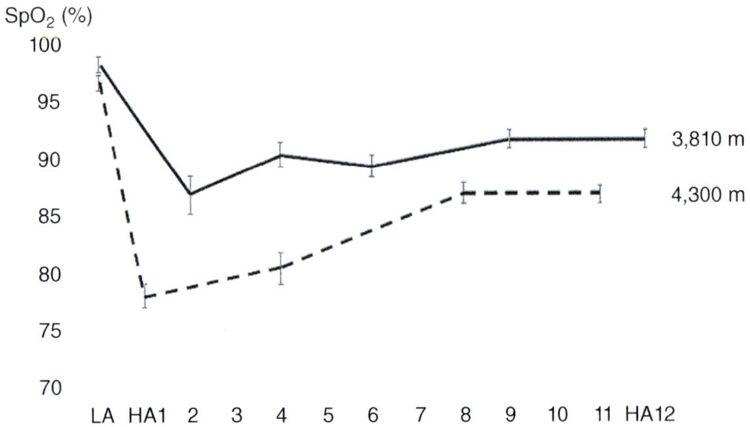

FIGURE 4.11 SpO_2 modifications as the days pass at high altitude (at two different altitudes); LA: lower altitude; HA: higher altitude; HA1 and following numbers indicate the days at high altitude. From: Ref. [9]/ MDPI / CC BY 4.0.

After the initial sharp descent, the SpO_2 tends to progressively rise modestly while remaining at altitude, until it reaches a stabilisation towards the eighth-tenth day, although still remaining at values definitely and even considerably lower than those detectable at sea level.[27]

Everest without bottled Oxygen. A 'fair' ascent, for exceptional persons.

'Is it really possible to climb the highest mountain in the world without any help from oxygen apparatus? That is the question'. Before attempting the final ascent to the summit of Mt Everest, **Reinhold Messner** and **Peter Habeler** (Figure 4.12) made themselves this question. And the rational answer should have been: no. Instead, Messner and Habeler's answer was a statement: *'a 'fair' ascent still remained, to storm the summit without masks'.*

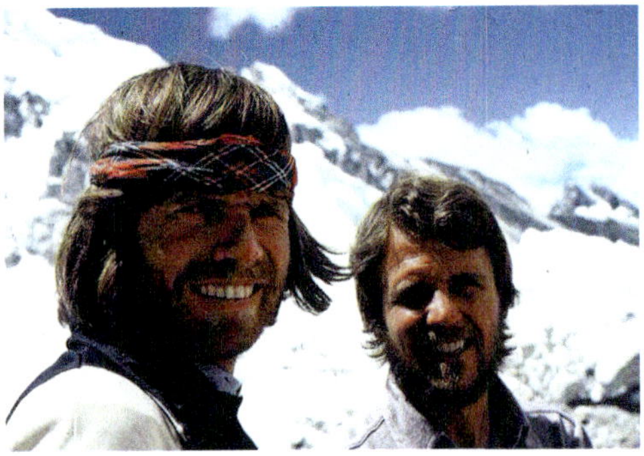

FIGURE 4.12 Reinhold Messner (b. 1944) and Peter Habeler (b. 1942) at Mount Everest in 1978; Courtesy of Mr. Reinhold Messner / https://reinholdmessner.de/en/messner-panorama/the-mountaineer/ / last accessed Feb. 20, 2026.

A 'fair' approach to the highest mountain in the world, *'by fair means'. 'My expeditions have enabled me to draw closer to myself, to see into myself more clearly'*, Messner said. Thus, any *'technical gadgets'* between him and the mountain would have distorted the relationship with the mountain.

Anyway, the undertaking was not at all easy for none of the participants of the expedition; one of the Sherpas suffered a stroke at Camp II (6,400 m) and three were badly injured, one of them with a skull fracture.

The extreme altitude hypoxia, above all, was so severe that Messner almost considered abandoning the attempt. This is the description he gives: *'Everything you do, like sitting up for instance, it makes me so, so tired'*. On the day of the final attack, as they climbed the mountain Messner and Habeler could *'... no longer keep on our feet while we rest. We crumple to our knees ... Breathing becomes such a strenuous business that we scarcely have strength left to go on. Every ten or fifteen steps we collapse into the snow to rest ... My mind seems almost to have ceased to function'*.

Despite all the enormous difficulties, Messner and Habeler attempted and succeeded in reaching the summit of Everest on May 8, 1978, without additional oxygen supply throughout the expedition, not even using it during their night's rest. *'Now, ... when I have nothing more to do than breathing ... I breath like someone who has run the race of his life ...'. '... I experience suddenly a feeling of completeness ... I am immediately shaken with sobs ... There is no sense of triumph, no feeling of potency, only of being ... Peter and I don't speak'*.

(from: Messner R. Everest: Expedition to the Ultimate. Mountaineers Books, Seattle, 1999. English translation by Audrey Salkeld of the original: Everest Expedition zum Endpunkt, BLV Verlagsgfesellschaft München, 1978).

Messner's description of extreme dyspnoea from a small effort recalls that given one hundred and twenty years earlier by John Tindall during his ascent to Mt. Bianco in 1857: *'... at the end of every twenty [steps], sometimes at the end of fifteen, we were compelled to pause. ... the heart throbbed audibly ... breathing was quick'*.

(Tindall J. The Glaciers of the Alps: Being a Narrative of Excursions and Ascents, an Account of the Origin ... Murray J, London, 1860).

Today we know that the level of hypoxia suffered by Tindall was much less profound than that of Messner and Habeler: during his ascent of Mt. Bianco, Tindall may have reached a barometric pressure around 400 mmHg and a PaO_2 of 40 mmHg. These values are very different from those experienced by Messner and Habeler: at the 'Balcony of Everest' (8,849 m; atmospheric pressure 253 mmHg), the PaO_2 has been measured on average at 24.6 mmHg, a value usually considered incompatible with life. Let alone the possibility of sustaining physical effort!

The physiology of those who have managed to reach the summit of Everest without supplemental oxygen is therefore exceptional. Only a small number of climbers have succeeded. Messner succeeded in climbing Everest without oxygen for a second time on August 20, 1980, also setting the record for the first solo ascent. **Lidia Bradley** from New Zealand is recorded as the first woman to climb Mt Everest without supplemental oxygen, in October 1988; it was reported that the first woman to climb Everest twice without supplemental oxygen was **Santosh Yadav**, an Indian mountaineer, in 1992 and 1993.

But, a place of honour goes to **Ang Rita Sherpa** (27 Jul 1948 – 21 Sept 2020), who climbed Everest 10 times between 1983 and 1996 without oxygen support; he is also the only person to have successfully climbed this peak during the winter period, always without supplementary oxygen.

References

1 West JB. American medical research expedition to Everest. High Alt Med Biol. 2010; 11(2):103–10. https://doi.org/10.1089/ham.2009.1089.

2 Samuels MP. The effects of flight and altitude. Arch Dis Child 2004; 89(5):448–455. https://doi.org/10.1136/adc.2003.031708.

3 Air Pressure at Altitude Calculator: https://www.mide.com/air-pressure-at-altitude-calculator.

4 MediCalc: Inspired Oxygen Tension. https://www.scymed.com/en/smnxpr/prdmb243.htm.

5 Grocott MP, Martin DS, Levett DZ, McMorrow R, Windsor J, Montgomery HE; Caudwell Xtreme Everest Research Group. Arterial blood gases and oxygen content in climbers on Mount Everest. N Engl J Med. 2009; 360(2):140–149. https://doi.org/10.1056/NEJMoa0801581.

6 Richalet JP, Robach P, Jarrot S, Schneider JC, Mason NP, Cauchy E, Herry JP, Bienvenu A, Gardette B, Gortan C. Operation Everest III (COMEX '97). Effects of prolonged and progressive hypoxia on humans during a simulated ascent to 8,848 M in a hypobaric chamber. Adv Exp Med Biol 1999; 474:297–317.

7 Richalet JP. Operation Everest III: COMEX '97. High Alt Med Biol. 2010; 11(2):121–132. https://doi.org/10.1089/ham.2009.1099.

8 Zubieta-Calleja G. Human Adaptation to high altitude and to sea level. Acid-Base Equilibrium, Ventilation and Circulation in Chronic Hypoxia. Dissertation, Copenhagen, 2007. VDM Verlag Dr. Müller, 2010. ISBN: 978-3-639-25276-7. https://www.altitudeclinic.com/Copenhagen/Dissertation10b.pdf.

9 Forrer A, Gaisl T, Sevik A, Meyer M, Senteler L, Lichtblau M, Bloch KE, Ulrich S, Furian M. Partial pressure of arterial oxygen in healthy adults at high altitudes: a systematic review and meta-analysis. JAMA Netw Open. 2023;6(6):e2318036. https://doi.org/10.1001/jamanetworkopen.2023.18036

10 Prosperi P, Verratti V, Taverna A, Rua R, Bonan S, Rapacchiale G, Bondi D, Di Giulio C, Lorkowski J, Spacone A. Ventilatory function and oxygen delivery at high altitude in the Himalayas. Respir Physiol Neurobiol. 2023; 314:104086. https://doi.org/10.1016/j.resp.2023.104086.

11 Hultgren HN, Grover RF, Hartley LH. Abnormal circulatory responses to high altitude in subjects with a previous history of high-altitude pulmonary oedema. Circulation 1971; 44(5):759–770. https://doi.org/10.1161/01.cir.44.5.759.

12 Lorente-Aznar T, Perez-Aguilar G, García-Espot A, Benabarre-Ciria S, Mendia-Gorostidi JL, Dols-Alonso D, Blasco-Romero J. Estimación de la saturación arterial de oxígeno en función de la altitud [Estimation of arterial oxygen saturation in relation to altitude]. Med Clin (Barc) 2016; 147(10):435–440. https://doi.org/10.1016/j.medcli.2016.07.025.

13 Rimoldi SF, Sartori C, Seiler C, Delacrétaz E, Mattle HP, Scherrer U, Alemann Y. High-altitude exposure in patients with cardiovascular disease: risk assessment and practical recommendations. Prog Cardiovasc Dis 2010; 52(6):512–524. https://doi.org/10.1016/j.pcad.2010.03.005.

14 Luks AM, Swenson ER. Pulse oximetry at high altitude. High Alt Med Biol 2011; 12(2):109–219. https://doi.org/10.1089/ham.2011.0013.

15 Windsor JS, Rodway GW. Con: pulse oximetry is useful in predicting acute mountain sickness. High Alt Med Biol 2014; 15(4):442–443. https://doi.org/10.1089/ham.2013.1140.

16 Basnyat B. Rebuttal to the con statement. High Alt Med Biol 2014; 15(4):444. https://doi.org/10.1089/ham.2014.1074.

17 Donegani E, Paal P, Küpper T, Hefti U, Basnyat B, Carceller A, Bouzat P, van der Spek R, Hillebrandt D. Drug use and misuse in the mountains: a UIAA MedCom consensus guide for medical professionals. High Alt Med Biol 2016; 17(3): 157–184.https://doi.org/10.1089/ham.2016.0080.

18 Roach RC, Lawley JS, Hackett PH. High-altitude physiology (part 1, mountain medicine, chapter 1). In: Auerbach PS (Ed). Wilderness Medicine, 7th ed.Philadelphia: Elsevier, 2017.

19 Boussuges A, Molenat F, Burnet H, Cauchy E, Gardette B, Sainty JM, Jammes Y, Richalet JP. Operation Everest III (Comex '97): modifications of cardiac function secondary to altitude-induced hypoxia. An echocardiographic and Doppler study. Am J Respir Crit Care Med 2000; 161(1): 264–270. https://doi.org/10.1164/ajrccm.161.1.9902096.

20 Severinghaus JW, Bainton CR, Carcelen A. Respiratory insensitivity to hypoxia in chronically hypoxic man. Respir Physiol 1966;1(3):308–334. https://doi.org/10.1016/0034-5687(66)90049-1.

21 Richalet JP. Altitude et système cardiovasculaire. Presse Med 2012; 41(6 Pt 1):638–643. https://doi.org/10.1016/j.lpm.2012.02.003.

22 Cogo A. The lung at high altitude. Multidiscip Respir Med. 2011; 6(1):14–15. https://doi.org/10.1186/2049-6958-6-1-14.

23 Sutton JR, Reeves JT, Wagner PD, Groves BM, Cymerman A, Malconian MK, Rock PB, Young PM, Walter SD, Houston CS. Operation Everest II: oxygen transport during exercise at extreme simulated altitude. J Appl Physiol 1988; 64(4):1309–1321. https://doi.org/10.1152/jappl.1988.64.4.1309.

24 Tymko MM, Willie CK, Howe CA, Hoiland RL, Stone RM, Tymko K, Tymko C, MacLeod D, Anholm JD, Gasho C, Villafuerte F, Vizcardo-Galindo G, Figueroa-Mujica R, Day TA, Bird JD, Foster GE, Steinback CD, Brugniaux JV, Champigneulle B, Stauffer E, Doutreleau S, Verges S, Swenson ER, Ainslie PN. Acid-base balance at high altitude in lowlanders and indigenous highlanders. J Appl Physiol. 2022; 132(2):575–580. https://doi.org/10.1152/japplphysiol.00757.2021.

25 Foster GT, Vaziri ND, Sassoon CS. Respiratory alkalosis. Respir Care 2001; 46(4): 384–391.

26 Parati G, Agostoni P, Basnyat B, Bilo G, Brugger H, Coca A, Festi L, Giardini G, Lironcurti A, Luks AM, Maggiorini M, Modesti PA, Swenson ER, Williams B, Bärtsch P, Torlasco C. Clinical recommendations for high altitude exposure of individuals with pre-existing cardiovascular conditions: a joint statement by the European Society of Cardiology, the Council on Hypertension of the European Society of Cardiology, the European Society of Hypertension, the International Society of Mountain Medicine, the Italian Society of Hypertension and the Italian Society of Mountain Medicine. Eur Heart J 2018; 39(17):1546–1554. https://doi.org/10.1093/eurheartj/ehx720.

27 Dünnwald T, Kienast R, Niederseer D, Burtscher M. The use of pulse oximetry in the assessment of acclimatization to high altitude. Sensors (Basel) 2021; 21(4):1263. https://doi.org/10.3390/s21041263.

CHAPTER 5

Sympathetic Activation at Altitude and the Cardiovascular System

As we have already seen, the progressive reduction of the barometric pressure with the increase in altitude leads to a reduction in the partial pressure of O_2 in the inspired air; the related reduction in O_2 availability at the alveolar level leads to hypoxaemia. This in turn stimulates peripheral chemoreceptors in the carotid and aortic bodies, which stimulate the brain stem breathing centre and the autonomic nervous system in its sympathetic component, along with a partial parasympathetic withdrawal.[1]

Among the effects linked to the activation of the sympathetic system, we are particularly interested in the changes induced on the cardiovascular system both at rest and during physical effort: increase in heart rate, possible increase in systemic arterial pressure and increase in pulmonary artery pressure, stimulation of production of adrenaline and noradrenaline by the adrenal glands, changes in cardiac contractility.

Effects on Heart Rate and on Blood Pressure

During Operation Everest III, which we have already talked about, the effects induced by hypobaric hypoxia in healthy volunteers exposed to simulated, increasing altitudes in a hypobaric chamber were analysed and quantified in practice.[2, 3] In these subjects, an inverse linear correlation was actually observed between the progressive reduction in SaO_2 (linked to the increase in simulated altitude) and an increase in heart rate (Figure 5.1): that is, as a higher altitude was simulated, SaO_2 became progressively reduced and at the same time heart rate progressively increased. When these volunteers returned to lower simulated altitudes for a couple of days, SaO_2 increased and heart rate decreased; both parameters began to vary again upon returning to higher altitudes, with the heart rate that progressively increased in relation to the

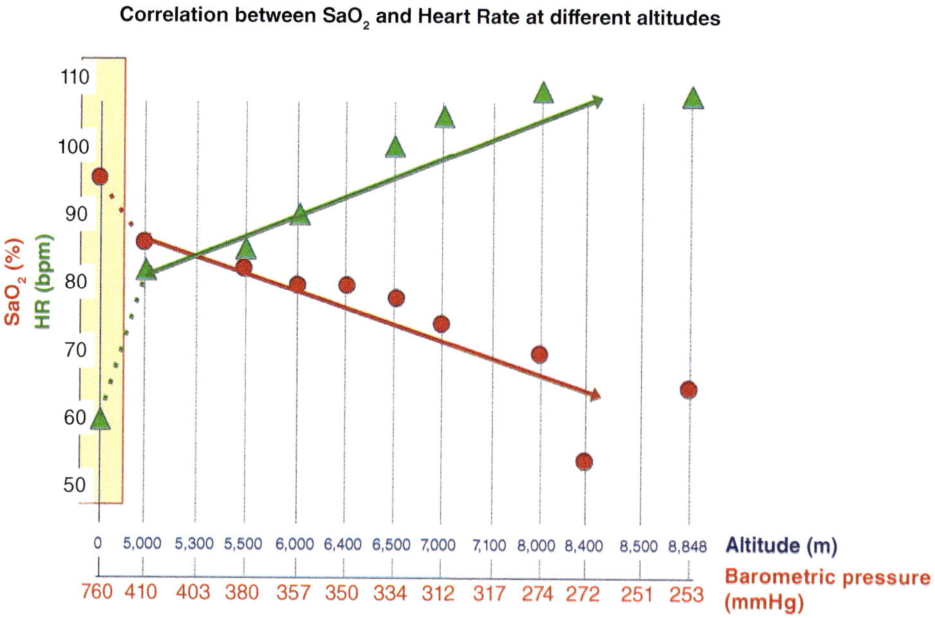

FIGURE 5.1 Correlation between SaO_2 and heart rate at high altitudes; data from Refs. [2, 3].

progressive reduction in SaO_2. The described modifications are the result of modifications of the sympathetic activity, triggered by stimulation of the peripheral chemoreceptors contained within the carotid bodies. The described heart rate behaviour had already been observed in 1975 during the Chinese Scientific Survey Expedition to Mt. Everest: even in well-acclimatised mountaineers resting heart rate increased from a mean of about 61 bpm at sea level to 86 bpm at 6,500 m and 110 bpm at 8,200 m above sea level.[4]

Similar results have also been found in individuals subjected to frequent and rapid changes of altitude, such as residents who commute daily between higher and lower mountain areas; the periodic variations in hypoxia levels induced by altitude shifts lead to significant periodic increases and decreases in heart rate.[5]

Another study[6] evaluated adrenergic activation with a different method: the discharge frequency of the sympathetic nerves at the peroneal level was directly studied via microneurography. After exposure to an altitude of 5,260 m AMSL, in 8 healthy volunteers a much higher discharge frequency of adrenergic fibres was detected compared to what was observed at sea level (high sympathetic discharge towards the vascular bed of the skeletal muscles). At the same time, an increase in mean arterial pressure of approximately 10 mmHg was also observed; however, this last data was not confirmed during the Operation Everest III study, in which mean arterial pressure values remained substantially stable,[7] as a result of the balance between the increase in sympathetic activity and a known vasodilation effect induced by marked hypoxia.[8]

While it is true that hypoxia produces peripheral vasodilation and should therefore lead to a reduction in blood pressure, on the other hand, an important sympathetic activation occurs, which produces phenomena that contrast with hypoxic vasodilation and can sometimes greatly exceed it: sympathetic activation causes peripheral vasoconstriction, increases heart rate and cardiac output, and increases myocardial contractility. The net end result is that systemic blood pressure tends to increase with ascent to high altitudes.[9] See also Chapter 12 for more detailed information.

Duration of the Adrenergic Activation

In the Operation Everest III study, SaO_2 and heart rate parameters were shown to normalise almost immediately after returning to sea level in subjects exposed to high altitude for a few days. In these subjects, it therefore seems that adrenergic activation switches off quite quickly.

During prolonged exposure to moderate altitudes (150 days at 1,860 m), the increased heart rate seems to decrease progressively.[10]

However, at higher altitudes (5,260 m, at Chacaltaya, Bolivian Andes), the study by Hansen et al.[6] highlighted that, if exposure to altitude is prolonged for a few weeks, adrenergic activation is prolonged and persists for some time even after returning to sea level, with heart rate and blood pressure that remain higher than initial values, despite normalisation of SaO_2 and haematocrit. These phenomena could be an integral part of the acclimatisation system at high altitude, but they could also be warning signs of possible harm or increased risk of diseases related to high altitude, such as arterial hypertension and pulmonary oedema.

In any case, the data indicate that the physiological responses of the organism (including cardiovascular ones) vary depending on the altitude reached and are different between acute/short-term exposure and prolonged/chronic exposure to high altitudes.

Adrenergic Activation and Physical Effort

The fact that a significant release of catecholamines occurs during exposure to high altitude is also confirmed by other observations, already made in years prior to those mentioned above. In 1965, during a 12-day Danish expedition to Monte Rosa at an altitude of 4,560 m AMSL, it was observed that catecholamines (norepinephrine) increased and doubled compared to sea level in both the blood and urine of the participants, reaching a maximum at the end of the stay at altitude.[11] Another study conducted in 1995 confirmed that norepinephrine levels increased with acute exposure at an altitude of 4,300 m AMSL, but were even higher with prolonged exposure (21 days), reaching values that were 84% higher than those measured at sea level.[12]

In the Operation Everest III study, plasma norepinephrine concentration increased up to 400% of baseline with exposure to simulated high altitude;[7] there was a further significant increase in norepinephrine levels, up to 174% more than sea level values, with physical activity (e.g. 45 minutes of sub-maximal physical exercise. Let's think about what could happen in mountaineers during climbing, or in high altitude trekkers, who may often reach sub-maximal efforts).[12]

The increase in circulating norepinephrine was not prevented by beta-blocking treatment.

At high altitudes, although a high sympathetic tone continues to prevail, a significant level of parasympathetic activity also exists. Indeed, for altitudes above 3,100 m up to 5,400 m, the maximum heart rate achievable during intense physical exertion appears to be reduced compared with at sea level, in parallel with a reduction of maximum oxygen consumption:[9] it has been estimated that maximum achievable heart rate decreases by 1 bpm for every 130 m of altitude gained above 3,100 m.[13, 14] And Lundby and van Hall observed that in two mountaineers who reached the South Summit of Mt. Everest (8,750 m) without supplemental oxygen, the maximal heart rate decreased at least up to an altitude of 5,400 m, but afterwards it remained stable at extreme altitude.[15]

The response of increased heart rate during exercise (and also at rest) appears to be less marked in subjects chronically exposed to high altitudes, due to a progressive desensitisation of the adrenergic system;[16] these people who live chronically at high altitudes have on average a lower resting heart rate than people acutely exposed to the same mountain altitudes, and during exercise they reach a lower maximum heart rate than people acutely exposed to high altitudes.

Effects of Adrenergic Activation on Heart Muscle

The increase in heart rate induced by sympathetic activation, also associated with an increase in pulmonary vascular resistances linked to altitude, leads to a modest but significant reduction in the size of the left ventricle.[16] The end-diastolic diameter of the left ventricle (LVEDD) in the volunteers studied by Boussuges et al. (again as part of Operation Everest III) decreased from about 52 mm to about 47 mm, starting from altitudes of 5,000 m AMSL and above; upon returning to sea level, LVEDD returned to normal. This lower diastolic filling of the left ventricle (and a consequently lower stroke volume) was associated with the progressive increase in heart rate with increasing altitude (heart rate increased by 41%, from around 63 beats/min to around 90 bpm in the cases studied): the result was that cardiac output remained almost constant (or showed a slight, transient and non-significant increase; in the volunteers studied by Boussuges cardiac output increased from 5.7 to 6.4 litres/min).

Another study detailed that cardiac output increased by approximately 20% in the first two days at high altitude (3,800 m AMSL) when left ventricle end-diastolic volume was still essentially unchanged but heart rate had already increased by approximately 18%; subsequently, as left ventricular volume decreased over the following days at altitude and heart rate remained constant (i.e. did not increase further), cardiac output decreased and returned to baseline values (Figure 5.2).[17]

Cardiac contractility (measured in Operation Everest III as ejection fraction and as fractional shortening of the left ventricle on echocardiogram) also remained essentially unchanged (and normal) during the volunteers' exposure to all altitudes studied. This maintenance of normal contractility occurred despite the significant reduction in PaO_2 recorded, which dropped to 37 mmHg at the simulated altitude of 8,000 m above sea level.[7]

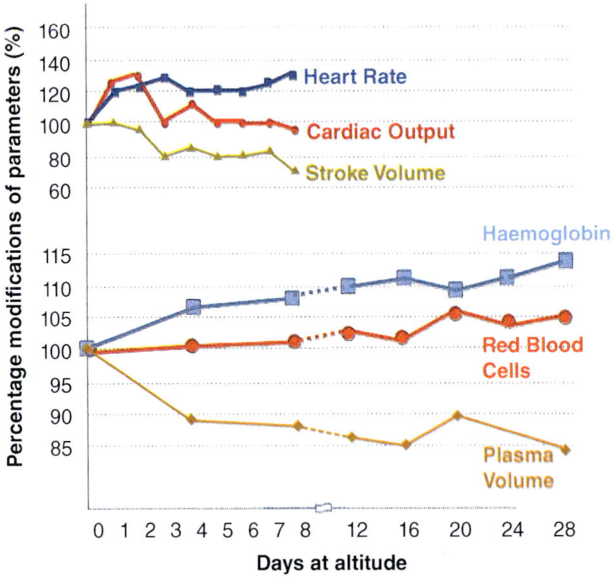

FIGURE 5.2 Percentage variations of heart rate, cardiac output and stroke volume, as well as modifications of haematological parameters, during a stay at high altitude. Data derived from Refs. [17, 18].

Diastolic Relaxation of the Left Ventricle

Diastolic relaxation of the left ventricle, that is, its ability to relax rapidly in diastole to accommodate new blood arriving from the left atrium, appeared to be reduced with exposure to high altitude and the associated hypoxia; that is, the left ventricle became, so to speak, "stiffer" in the diastolic phase.[19] However, this phenomenon was reversible upon returning to low altitudes and a normal oxygen supply.

Effects on Pulmonary Artery Systolic Pressure

It is already known since many years that, with exposure to hypoxia, the systolic pressure in the pulmonary artery increases. An increase in pressure in the pulmonary artery appears as soon as the partial pressure of O_2 in the alveoli (PAO_2) drops below 60 mmHg, which corresponds to an altitude of approximately 3,000 m above sea level. It has been calculated that pulmonary vascular resistances increase by 50% when PAO_2 drops to 50 mmHg,[7] as a result of constriction of the pre-capillary arterioles. If exposure to hypoxia is prolonged, histological changes also appear in these small vessels; high pulmonary artery pressure levels may take up to 6 weeks to subside after returning to low altitudes,[20] as positive remodelling of pulmonary arterioles may be prolonged (and certainly not completely resolved in a few days at normal PaO_2). These phenomena (increase in pulmonary vascular resistances and increase in pulmonary artery pressure) can lead, in the long term, to hypertrophy and dilation of the right ventricle, as occurs in Chronic Mountain Sickness.[21]

In conclusion, the activation of the sympathetic system that occurs with hypobaric hypoxia leads to:

1. increase in heart rate in relation to altitude (and in inverse relation to decrease of SaO_2);
2. peripheral arterial vasoconstriction, which can be more or less compensated by hypoxia-induced vasodilation, with the result that blood pressure can increase or remain substantially unchanged;
3. vasoconstriction of the pulmonary pre-capillary arterioles, which – in case of prolonged exposure to hypoxia – is followed by histological alterations of the arteriolar walls;
4. increase in pulmonary artery pressure, which reduces slowly after returning to normoxia;
5. reduction in the size of the left ventricle, whose contractility seems to be however preserved;
6. the diastolic relaxation of the left ventricle is impaired;
7. cardiac output remains substantially unchanged or increases slightly in the first days at altitude.

Patients with Heart Diseases

We can therefore deduce that patients with heart diseases who intend to travel to high altitudes must be warned that worsening may occur of:

1. all those situations that can be negatively affected by sympathetic activation (e.g. coronary artery disease, arterial hypertension, arrhythmias), and of
2. those diseases that are associated with increased pressure in the pulmonary artery (primary pulmonary hypertension, or secondary pulmonary hypertension as in COPD patients), as well as of
3. those diseases that are characterised by hypoxaemia (such as heart diseases involving a right-to-left shunt).

In particular, a common disease such as ischaemic heart disease could present signs and symptoms of myocardial ischaemia at a lower threshold (less effort) than the usual one at low altitude; in order to predict exercise tolerance at high altitude, the only reliable test is an exercise test performed in hypoxia, i.e. in an environment with a partial pressure of oxygen equivalent to that which is intended to be achieved.[22]

References

1 Zera T, Moraes DJA, da Silva MP, Fisher JP, Paton JFR. The logic of carotid body connectivity to the brain. Physiology (Bethesda). 2019; 34(4):264–282. https://doi.org/10.1152/physiol.00057.2018.

2 Richalet JP, Robach P, Jarrot S, Schneider JC, Mason NP, Cauchy E, Herry JP, Bienvenu A, Gardette B, Gortan C. Operation Everest III (COMEX '97). Effects of prolonged and progressive hypoxia on humans during a simulated ascent to 8,848 M in a hypobaric chamber. Adv Exp Med Biol 1999; 474:297–317.

3 Richalet JP. Operation Everest III: COMEX '97. High Alt Med Biol 2010; 11(2):121–132. https://doi.org/10.1089/ham.2009.1099.
4 Shi ZY, Ning XH, Zhu SC, Zhao DM, Huang PG, Yang SY, Wang Y, Dong ZS. Electrocardiogram made on ascending the Mount Qomolangma from 50 m a. s. l. Sci Sin 1980; 23(10):1316–1325.
5 Triplett JC, Zubieta-Calleja L, Zubieta-Castillo G, Zubieta-Calleja GR. Physiological changes related to rapid altitude shifts in La Paz, Bolivia. Acta Andina 1996; 5:19–22. https://www.researchgate.net/publication/257306516_PHYSIOLOGICAL_CHANGES_RELATED_TO_RAPID_ALTITUDE_SHIFTS_-_LA_PAZ.
6 Hansen J, Sander M. Sympathetic neural overactivity in healthy humans after prolonged exposure to hypobaric hypoxia. J Physiol 2003; 546(Pt 3):921–929. https://doi.org/10.1113/jphysiol.2002.031765.
7 Boussuges A, Molenat F, Burnet H, Cauchy E, Gardette B, Sainty JM, Jammes Y, Richalet JP. Operation Everest III (Comex '97): modifications of cardiac function secondary to altitude-induced hypoxia. An echocardiographic and Doppler study. Am J Respir Crit Care Med 2000; 161(1):264–70. https://doi.org/10.1164/ajrccm.161.1.9902096.
8 Heistad DD, Abboud FM. Circulatory adjustments to hypoxia. Circulation 1980; 61:463–470.
9 Bärtsch P, Gibbs JS. Effect of altitude on the heart and the lungs. Circulation. 2007; 116(19):2191–2202. https://doi.org/10.1161/CIRCULATIONAHA.106.650796.
10 Sizlan A, Ogur R, Ozer M, Irmak MK. Blood pressure changes in young male subjects exposed to a median altitude. Clin Auton Res 2008; 18(2):84–89. https://doi.org/10.1007/s10286-008-0459-y.
11 Cunningham WL, Becker EJ, Kreuzer F. Catecholamines in plasma and urine at high altitude. J Appl Physiol 1965; 20(4):607–610. https://doi.org/10.1152/jappl.1965.20.4.607.
12 Mazzeo RS, Brooks GA, Butterfield GE, Podolin DA, Wolfel EE, Reeves JT. Acclimatization to high altitude increase muscle sympathetic activity both at rest and during exercise. Am J Physiol 1995; 269(1 Pt 2):R201–R207. https://doi.org/10.1152/ajpregu.1995.269.1.R201.
13 Boushel R, Calbet JA, Rådegran G, Sondergaard H, Wagner PD, Saltin B. Parasympathetic neural activity accounts for the lowering of exercise heart rate at high altitude. Circulation 2001; 104(15):1785–1791. https://doi.org/10.1161/hc4001.097040.
14 Coustet B, Lhuissier FJ, Vincent R, Richalet JP. Electrocardiographic changes during exercise in acute hypoxia and susceptibility to severe high-altitude illnesses. Circulation 2015; 131(9):786–794. https://doi.org/10.1161/CIRCULATIONAHA.114.013144.
15 Lundby C, van Hall G. Peak heart rates at extreme altitudes. High Alt Med Biol 2001; 2(1):41–45. https://doi.org/10.1089/152702901750067909.
16 Richalet JP. Altitude et système cardiovasculaire. La Presse Médicale 2012; 41(6, Part 1):638–643. https://doi.org/10.1016/j.lpm.2012.02.003.
17 Naeije R. Physiological adaptation of the cardiovascular system to high altitude. Prog Cardiovasc Dis 2010; 52(6):456–466. https://doi.org/10.1016/j.pcad.2010.03.004.
18 Siebenmann C, Cathomen A, Hug M, Keiser S, Lundby AK, Hilty MP, Goetze JP, Rasmussen P, Lundby C. Hemoglobin mass and intravascular volume kinetics during and after exposure to 3,454-m altitude. J Appl Physiol (1985). 2015; 119(10):1194–1201. https://doi.org/10.1152/japplphysiol.01121.2014.
19 Gomez A, Mink S. Interaction between effects of hypoxia and hypercapnia on altering left ventricular relaxation and chamber stiffness in dogs. Am Rev Respir Dis 1992; 146:313–320.

20 Sime F, Peñaloza D, Ruiz L. Bradycardia, increased cardiac output, and reversal of pulmonary hypertension in altitude natives living at sea level. Br Heart J 1971; 33(5):647–657. https://doi.org/10.1136/hrt.33.5.647.

21 Peñaloza D, Sime F. Chronic cor pulmonale due to loss of altitude acclimatization (chronic mountain sickness). Am J Med 1971; 50(6):728–743. https://doi.org/10.1016/0002-9343(71)90181-1.

22 Georges T, Menu P, Le Blanc C, Ferreol S, Dauty M, Fouasson-Chailloux A. Contribution of hypoxic exercise testing to predict high-altitude pathology: a systematic review. Life (Basel) 2022; 12(3):377. https://doi.org/10.3390/life12030377.

CHAPTER 6

The Heart at High Altitude

We have already seen in previous chapters how the cardiac muscle can be affected in various ways during exposure to hypobaric hypoxia, during an ascent to altitude. The reported studies were essentially based on observations on healthy volunteers, submitted to decreasing atmospheric pressures in decompression chambers, to simulate what might happen at the different altitudes reached during mountain ascents. In these studies, it was observed that the systolic function of the left ventricle was not altered, while diastolic function appeared to be somewhat compromised; furthermore, it has been observed that the right ventricle is subjected to an increase in systolic load due to the increase in PAP.

Left Ventricle and Systemic Circulation

An effect of living on high mountains was observed in 2015 by Stembridge and Colleagues:[1] these authors reported that in Sherpas (chronically residing at high altitudes), the absolute and relative volume of the left ventricle (left ventricle end-diastolic volume) was significantly smaller than that of low-altitude residents. In persons who habitually live at low altitudes, the volume of the left ventricle decreases with the ascent to higher locations, although continuing to be larger than that of Sherpas. Parameters of diastolic relaxation of the left ventricle were also impaired in lowlanders exposed to high altitudes as well as in Sherpas.[1, 2] The cited modifications in Sherpas can be explained by a chronic remodelling of the ventricular wall in an attempt to improve myocardial efficiency; the decrease in left ventricular volume of lowlanders ascending to high altitudes has been explained by a reduction in plasma volume and a reduced return to the left ventricle, as will be presented in Chapter 8.

There is at least one other study, this time experimental, that I would like to mention because it helps shed light on the effects of high altitude on the heart muscle.

Back in 1976, Tucker et al.[3] wanted to study in experimental animals (six goats) the effects on the myocardium induced by 2-week ascent from an altitude of 1,600 m above mean sea level (AMSL) to approximately 4,300 m AMSL, where the PaO_2 dropped to 44 mmHg. But why were goats studied and not human volunteers? Because the animals were subjected to implantation of a series of various instruments and transducers, a thing that is clearly not ethical to be done in humans: a silicone rubber catheter was inserted into the descending aorta to measure the pressure in the aorta; an electromagnetic flow transducer was placed around the ascending aorta to measure systolic volume and cardiac output; electro-catheters were fixed on the left atrial appendage to perform cardiac pacing; a miniature pressure transducer was inserted into the left ventricle through the cardiac apex to obtain precise pressure curves; piezoelectric crystals were sutured to the epicardial surface of left ventricle to act as sonomicrometres.

In these goats, it was observed that the maximum speed of contraction of the left ventricle (in other words, the 'dp/dt', i.e. the ability to increase the internal pressure of the left ventricle in a unit of time) was significantly reduced in all the animals during exposure to the altitude of 4,300 m; it then returned to the initial values when the goats returned to the starting altitude of 1,600 m above sea level. These findings indicate that systolic function was transiently impaired during exposure to hypobaric hypoxia.

Afterwards, when these goats were rapidly infused with saline, the left ventricular end-diastolic pressure (pressure at the end of diastole in the left ventricle) increased much more sharply and significantly during the stay at altitude, thus indicating reduced compliance of the left ventricle, i.e. a reduced distensibility when subjected to a sudden increase in circulating volume: a diastolic dysfunction, as we have seen, has also been observed in human volunteers.

Therefore: depression of the systolic function of the left ventricle (modest, but significant, and reversible) and impaired diastolic relaxation.

It remains to be verified whether and to what extent these phenomena (especially the depression of systolic function) may occur also in humans, and what their practical relevance may be (in athletes and in heart patients) and their duration over time after returning to low altitudes.

Regarding the depression of the systolic function of the left ventricle, the data available in humans still remain controversial, while there seems to be greater consensus regarding the appearance of transient diastolic dysfunction.[4–6]

Reduced Compliance of Human Left Ventricle

The presence of diastolic dysfunction of the left ventricle, in addition to the studies by Richalet and Boussuges already cited in previous chapters, was also confirmed by observations conducted in Bolivia, in La Paz (at 3,750 m AMSL) and on Mount Huayna Potosi (4,850 m AMSL) by Huez et al., using echocardiographic methods.[7] The presence of diastolic dysfunction of both the left and the right ventricles was confirmed; such diastolic dysfunction appeared rapidly (within the first 24 hours after arriving in La Paz) in people who usually lived at sea level and persisted even after acclimatisation and after climbing to 4,850 m (when, moreover, pulmonary hypertension further increased). Bolivians native of high altitudes seem to have a lower level of pulmonary hypertension but more pronounced alterations of diastolic dysfunction.

Other studies, however, seem to have highlighted the presence of diastolic dysfunction of the left ventricle only in chronic residents at high altitudes, but not in inhabitants of low altitudes when they climb high mountains;[2] this would indicate that exposure to hypoxia for a short period of time would not lead to a significant alteration of diastolic relaxation.

It must be remembered here that the diastolic relaxation of the ventricles is not just a passive phenomenon (a container that fills up because some amount of liquid falls into it): at least during isovolumetric relaxation, and – less so – during rapid ventricular relaxation, it is an active phenomenon, which requires energy expenditure by the muscle cells of the cardiac walls to remove Ca^{++} ions from the cytoplasm and allow the dissociation of the actin–myosin contractile complex.[8] These phases can, therefore, be influenced by the availability of energy and adequate oxygen supply.

However, there seems to be a prevailing consensus on the appearance of ventricular diastolic dysfunction, as a consequence of the combined effects of hypoxia (which leads to the reduction of ventricular relaxation), tachycardia, reduced preload of the left ventricle (caused by reduced venous return due to pulmonary vasoconstriction) and the interdependence of the two ventricles (we will see later what happens to the right ventricle and how this can negatively influence the left ventricle).

Coronary Blood Flow at Altitude: At Rest and During Effort

Another aspect to consider is what the behaviour of coronary flow may be during the exposure to moderate or high altitudes. This means trying to understand whether a person with known **coronary artery disease (CAD)** (and those many with unknown CAD!) can face a climb to high altitude and possibly carry out physical activity.

As far as is known today, again on very small numbers of volunteers studied,[8] the myocardial blood flow at rest appears to increase by approximately 24% both in healthy subjects and in CAD patients when they climb to up to 2,500 m altitude. But when these individuals are submitted to physical effort, the behaviour of CAD patients is very different from that of healthy subjects (Figure 6.1): while in healthy subjects, the coronary reserve (i.e. the ability to increase the perfusion of the coronary arteries during physical effort) increases at 4,500 m AMSL by approximately 10% (not statistically significant increase), in CAD patients, the coronary reserve decreases by 18% (significant decrease) already at a lower altitude (2,500 m AMSL). These data indicate that the compensatory mechanisms responsible for increasing coronary flow during physical effort are exhausted in CAD patients already at moderate altitudes, probably due to the fixed stenoses that are present in the coronary tree.

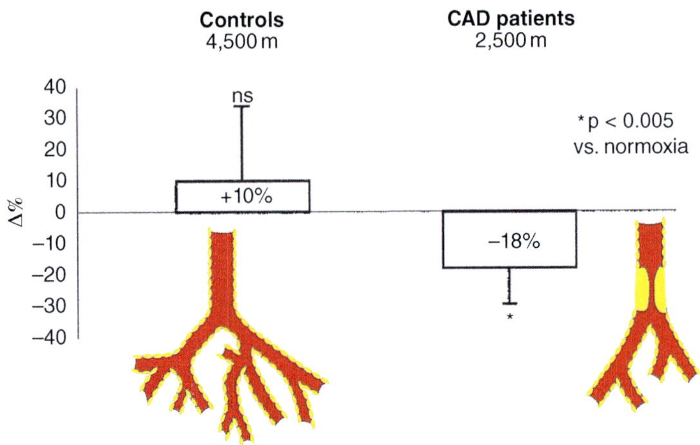

FIGURE 6.1 In conditions of hypobaric hypoxia, coronary reserve during exercise tends to increase in healthy subjects (up to 4,500 m AMSL), while it turns out to be significantly reduced in coronary heart disease patients already at lower altitudes (2,500 m AMSL). Adapted from [9].

For this reason, patients suffering from **coronary artery disease** (especially if a reduced coronary reserve has already been highlighted in them, for example, with ultrasound techniques) should be very cautious when they want to carry out physical activity at even moderate altitudes, due to the combined effects of various concomitant factors: physical exercise per se (increased cardiac work and increased O_2 demands) in a person with coronary flow limited by the presence of fixed stenoses, environmental hypoxia, increased heart rate, cold (possible reflex coronary vasoconstriction), hyperventilation resulting in hypocapnia and possible vasoconstriction, sympathetic activation.

These same problems that arise with altitude, namely increased myocardial oxygen consumption and increased heart rate (HR) and cardiac work, are also extremely relevant for people suffering from **heart failure**.

Retrograde Pulmonary Capillary Hypertension in Heart Failure and Cardiogenic Pulmonary Oedema

In a failing heart (and we are essentially referring to the left ventricle when it demonstrates a reduced contractile capacity), the phenomena that arise with the ascent to moderate or high altitudes lead to a progressive increase in left ventricular end-diastolic pressure. We have already seen that end-diastolic pressure tends to increase with climbing to altitude even in healthy subjects, due to the altered diastolic relaxation capacity of the left ventricle.

The increase in the end-diastolic pressure of the left ventricle has a backward impact on the pulmonary veins and pulmonary capillaries. When the (retrograde) pressure on the pulmonary capillaries, let's say their 'congestion', increases so much as to exceed the sum of plasma oncotic and osmotic pressures (which retain the liquids inside the capillaries), transudation of liquids from the capillaries to the pulmonary alveoli begins: this means the appearance of **acute cardiogenic pulmonary oedema** (NB – this is different from high-altitude pulmonary oedema [HAPE], which can also appear in subjects with heart failure, although – to tell the truth – it is unusual for them to reach such high altitudes). Clinically fine rales can be heard, which then progressively become coarser, resembling a 'rising tide', in a patient who presents progressive dyspnoea and orthopnoea, with shortness of breath, cough (and sometimes pink-tinged foamy sputum), cyanosis of the mucous membranes, cold sweating. From a radiological point of view (Figure 6.2a), the picture is initially characterised by 'pulmonary clouding', i.e. a marked accentuation of the broncho-vascular structure, and then – with the progressive flooding of the alveoli – by a flaky or ground glass appearance, which rises from the dependent areas of the lungs and progressively extends towards the apexes. This radiological picture is different from that which can be found in HAPE (see Figure 6.2).

Obviously, the onset of pulmonary oedema, whatever its cause, worsens the hypoxia picture we have seen present during an ascent to altitude.

The treatment of acute cardiogenic pulmonary oedema is classically based on the reduction of left ventricular preload (with diuretics and nitrates), reduction of left ventricular afterload (with vasodilators and again nitrates) and improvement of ventricular inotropism (with dopamine or other inotropes); the administration of O_2 can also be useful, but not sufficient, and sometimes positive pressure ventilation should be needed.

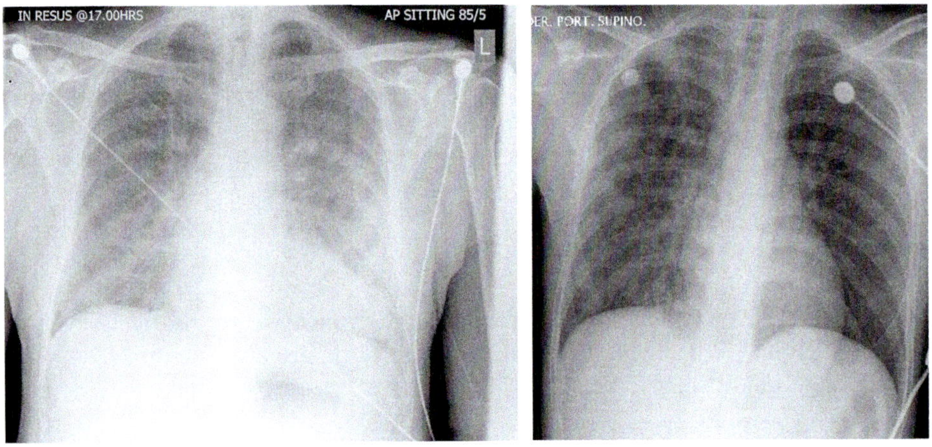

(a) (b)

FIGURE 6.2 (a) A typical chest X-Ray in a patient with acute cardiogenic pulmonary oedema. (b) Chest X-Ray of a patient admitted with high-altitude pulmonary oedema (HAPE) (progressive respiratory distress 24 hours after arriving at a town at 2,700 m above sea level), showing right greater than left indistinct airspace opacity; [10, 11]. Radiopaedia.org / https://radiopaedia.org/cases/high-altitude-pulmonary-oedema?lang=us / last accessed Dec. 27, 2025.

High-altitude Pulmonary Oedema (HAPE) in Predisposed Subjects

By the other side, the pathophysiology of **HAPE** is markedly different.

HAPE is fortunately an uncommon, albeit potentially fatal, altitude illness that usually develops 2–5 days after arrival at moderate and high altitudes. Its incidence at 2,500 m is estimated to be approximately 0.01%, increasing to 1.9% at 3,600 m and 2.5–5% at 4,300 m,[12] especially in the case of rapid ascents to these altitudes. It has been reported by Bärtsch et al. that, when ascending to 4,559 m within 24 hours, the prevalence increases in climbers without a history of HAPE to 6% and in those with a history of HAPE to a worrying 62%.[13]

People with viral upper respiratory infections and individuals with a blunted ventilatory response to altitude appear to be more predisposed to developing HAPE; genetic factors may also be responsible for an altered ability of the epithelial lining of the alveoli to reabsorb alveolar fluids.[14]

We have seen how, with climbing to altitude, the reduction in barometric pressure is accompanied by a progressive reduction in the partial pressure of O_2 in the inspired air and in the alveolar air, and consequently a lower partial pressure of O_2 in the blood. High-altitude hypobaric hypoxia causes hypoxic constriction of the pulmonary arterioles and an increase in PAP; in HAPE-susceptible individuals, systolic PAP reaches elevated levels (as high as 53 ± 16 mmHg) as early as 12–24 hours before the onset of clinical manifestations of HAPE,[15] while pulmonary wedge pressures (an indicator of left ventricular end-diastolic pressure) remain normal.

According to the theory of Hultgren,[16] in some subjects, pulmonary vasoconstriction occurs 'in patches': some arterioles constrict, while others remain unchanged in size (Figure 6.3). (I want to draw attention to the fact that here we are talking about the behaviour of the arterioles,

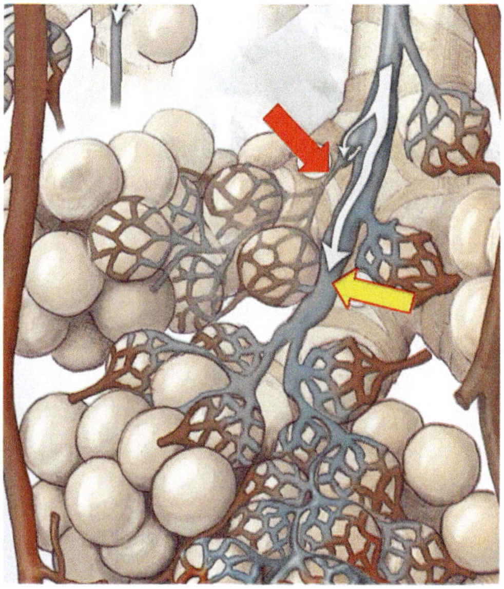

FIGURE 6.3 Graphic representation of the behaviour of the precapillary arterioles in a subject susceptible to HAPE exposed to high altitude: some arterioles constrict (red arrow), while others remain unconstricted (yellow arrow). Artpiece by © Melissa Cory; courtesy of the Author.

while in acute cardiogenic pulmonary oedema, the problem starts to occur on the venous side and then – backwards – on the pulmonary capillaries.) The fact that some arterioles constrict leads to a further increase of pressure in the pulmonary artery, even more than what happens in other individuals not predisposed to HAPE. But, alongside these arterioles that constrict, there are arterioles that do not change their calibre, that is, they do not constrict (or present a limited constriction). So it happens that the increase in pressure in the pulmonary tree spills over onto these non-constricted arterioles, somehow 'flooding' them with blood, while the part of the alveoli supplied by arterioles that have constricted remains substantially protected against the increase of pressure. In non-vasoconstricted areas, therefore, the high hydrostatic pressure leads to the loss of integrity of the endothelial lining of the small blood vessels; furthermore, the elevated pressure in these non-constricted vessels exceeds the colloid-osmotic pressure of the blood, and the exudation of liquid from the capillaries to the alveoli begins. Other pathophysiologic factors have also been considered as possible contributors to HAPE, such as hypoxia-induced inflammation and impaired alveolar fluid clearance.[17]

Often, an early symptom of HAPE is represented by exertional dyspnoea, different from past experience at that altitude and worse than that of trekking companions, along with chest tightness;[18] approximately two-thirds of patients experience a nocturnal worsening of symptoms, attributable to irregular breathing patterns during sleep. With progression of HAPE, the most frequent symptoms reported[19] are dyspnoea (75.0%), dry cough (66.7%), fatigue (62.5%), headache (62.5%), cough with phlegm (41.7%) and nausea and vomiting (33.3%). Physical examination reveals cyanosis, tachycardia and elevated body temperature (78.3%; not exceeding 38.5 °C); but the most distinctive sign of HAPE is the finding of moist rales in both lungs. The rales are often diffuse and distributed with an asymmetric pattern, due to the patchy distribution of the alveolar 'flooding'. The extension of the pulmonary rales is reported to be closely linked to disease progression and exhibits high sensitivity and specificity for severity of disease; sputum production, elevated HR and decline in SpO_2 are other reliable predictors of HAPE severity.[20]

Peripheral oxygen saturation is usually very low (SpO_2 is reported to be around 75% or even lower) with a PaO_2 on average around 40 mmHg (and as low as 29 mmHg).[19]

Approximately half of the patients may exhibit also neurological symptoms and signs of high-altitude cerebral oedema (HACE).

A marked increase in pulmonary pressure may be inferred by the auscultation of a loud second heart sound on the second left intercostal space.[21]

The radiological picture of HAPE is usually characterised by 'patches' of ground-glass opacification (Figure 6.2b), alternating with patches of normal transparency, which are typically mixed and not characterised by that gradient base → apex that is usually seen in cardiogenic pulmonary oedema.[22] In the few cases in which there was the possibility to perform a CT Scan, nodular and ground-glass opacities have been found together with patchy areas of consolidation.[19]

In cases in which an electrocardiogram (ECG) has been made in HAPE patients, it showed sinus tachycardia and high-pointed P waves (P-pulmonale, generally associated with pulmonary hypertension), along with right axis deviation of QRS and a modified T wave in leads V1 to V5 reflecting right ventricular overload and enlargement; echocardiographic and pulmonary artery catheterisation studies at high altitude have always shown marked pulmonary hypertension.[23]

As in all altitude illnesses, the primary predisposing factor to developing HAPE is a rapid ascent that does not allow 'enough' time for acclimatisation; but how much time is 'enough' depends a lot on enormous individual variability. Although no studies have prospectively assessed the preventive effects of gradual ascent, it is recommended to reduce the risk of HAPE, with level of evidence 1C. A pharmacological measure to prevent HAPE in HAPE-susceptible patients is to take nifedipine upon and during their stay at high altitude (Evidence: 1B).

The treatment of HAPE[23] is also markedly different from that of acute cardiogenic pulmonary oedema; if not treated properly, HAPE could have a mortality rate of up to 50%, most often between 4 and 11%, depending primarily on the speed of treatment initiation or descent to lower altitudes.[19] First of all, in a case of HAPE, it is precisely the administration of O_2 (4–6 L/min) that reduces the symptoms and improves the clinical picture; the goal is to increase SpO_2 to over 90% (Evidence: 1A). However, first of all, the descent to lower altitudes is fundamental and, above all, decisive! (Evidence: 1A).

Along with this, especially when descent is impossible or is delayed, or oxygen is not available, the administration of an arteriolar vasodilator is essential, such as slow-release nifedipine (20 mg every 8 hours, or 30 mg every 12 hours; Evidence: 1C) or sildenafil or tadalafil (Sildenafil: 50 mg every 8 hours; Tadalafil: 10 mg every 12 hours; Evidence: 2C), which have the power to dilate even the arterioles that had remained constricted, and, therefore, allow a redistribution of the flow and a reduction in PAP.

Diuretics have no role in the treatment of HAPE (Evidence: 1C); acetazolamide should not be used in treatment of HAPE (Evidence: 1C). All diuretics might provoke hypotension in a patient with intravascular bed already depleted.

Portable systems have also been put on the market to make HAPE patients breathe under high pressure (therefore, partially simulating a descent to lower altitudes); they are

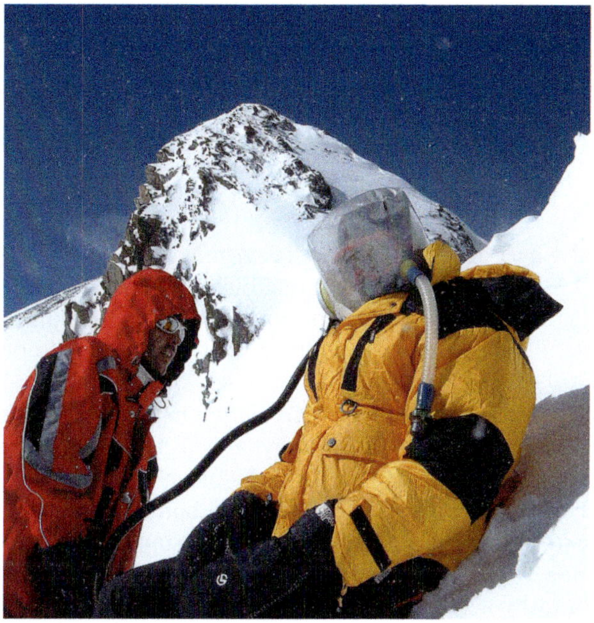

FIGURE 6.4 Portable helmet used by Koch et al. to treat HAPE in high altitude rescue operations [24]; Photo courtesy of Prof. Robert Koch.

characterised by a helmet (or a kind of diving suit)[24] or by sealed face masks into which air (and possibly – if available – oxygen)[25] is introduced, maintaining a high pressure in the system by means of a hand pump (Figure 6.4). This is a system substantially similar to the one we have recently seen being used in non-invasive ventilation in patients suffering from respiratory failure due to Covid (in which pressures were maintained automatically and mechanically). The cost of these portable systems seems to be quite reasonable, and their weight and volume are quite low. When descent is not feasible or is delayed, or supplemental oxygen is not available, the use of a portable hyperbaric chamber may be a solution (Evidence: 1C).

In addition to traditional oxygen cylinders, heavy and difficult to carry at high altitudes, portable O_2 canisters have also been made commercially available (they can also be found on online retailers, at prices ranging from around 15 to 20 Euros), with a content of around 6–10 L of O_2 (weight 90 g), with an ergonomically designed mask already connected, to facilitate correct inhalation. However, as the total O_2 content of this canister usually does not exceed 10 L, while in case of HAPE, we have to administer 4–6 L every minute, this dispenser runs out in approximately 60–90 seconds!

Right Ventricle and Pulmonary Circulation

So far, we have considered what affects us most closely, that is, what happens to the hearts of those who generally live at sea level or at low mountain altitudes when they face an ascent to high altitude.

But what will be the behaviour of the heart muscle in **natives of high-altitude** areas? What adaptations appear, and what short- or long-term consequences can these adaptations have?

Postnatal Changes of the Right Heart in High-altitude Natives and at Sea Level

A study was conducted by Dante Peñaloza and Javier Arias-Stella in 2007;[26] we are largely indebted to their work. They reviewed the existing literature on what happens in the Andean populations, which – as a whole – constitute the largest number of people in the world residing at altitudes above 3,500 m AMSL, comparing them with what occurs in other populations on the planet.

It emerged that the heart and pulmonary circulation in healthy people living at high altitudes have different characteristics compared to what is usually found in people living at sea level. To be more precise, at the moment of birth the morphology of the heart cavities is the same both in those born at high altitude and in those born at sea level: the right ventricle appears hypertrophic in both populations (due to having supported relatively high pressures during intrauterine life). Those that diverge are the postnatal changes, i.e. those that occur as the months pass. In healthy newborns at sea level, the right ventricle presents a progressive involution, with reduction in its thickness, already evident after 3 months of life, linked to the low levels of pressure in the pulmonary circulation. This involution does not occur in newborns at high altitudes, who maintain high thickness of the right ventricle wall throughout childhood, with further evolution and remodelling even in subsequent years, due to persistently high pressures in the pulmonary arterial circulation.[27]

How are these behaviours of the right ventricle explained?

It has been observed how at the moment of birth the levels of mean pressure in the pulmonary artery (PAPm) are substantially similar in newborns at high altitude as in newborns at sea level, being around (approximately) 60 mmHg. It is the subsequent behaviour that is clearly different between the two groups of newborns: in newborns at sea level, PAPm drops very rapidly, and already within the first 48–72 hours, it reaches those low levels, which it will maintain almost unchanged until the end of adulthood (generally around or less than 20 mmHg). In newborns at high altitudes (e.g. those born at 4,500 m AMSL), PAPm decreases very slowly, remaining for years at around 40–50 mmHg, and then stabilising at a young age at values around 30 or more mmHg, which will be maintained throughout life (Figure 6.5).

Remodelling of Distal Pulmonary Arterioles

Why? Because the remodelling of the walls of distal pulmonary arterioles occurs rapidly in newborns at sea level, while in newborns at high altitudes, it does not occur except to a minimal extent: the walls of the arterioles are characterised – in residents at high altitudes – by persistence of a high amount of smooth muscle cells (which instead disappear in residents at sea level); the significant muscular component in the walls leads to an increased thickness of

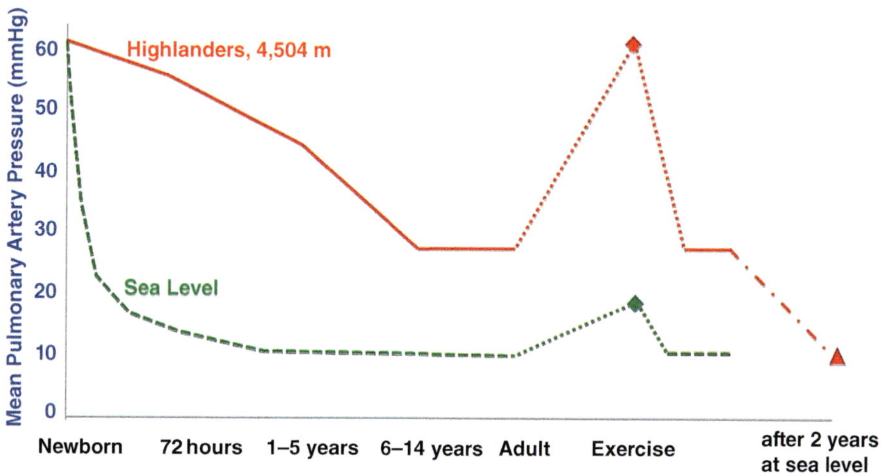

FIGURE 6.5 Pulmonary hypertension was found at birth in both high-altitude newborns (solid line) and lowland newborns (dotted line) with average values of around 60 mmHg; after birth, however, the situation diverges rapidly between the two groups, and the difference remains throughout adulthood. During physical effort, mean pulmonary artery pressure (PAPm) increases significantly in high-altitude residents and only slightly in normal sea-level residents. When highlanders move to sea level, PAPm decreases within 2 years to values similar to that of sea level residents. Modified from Ref. [26].

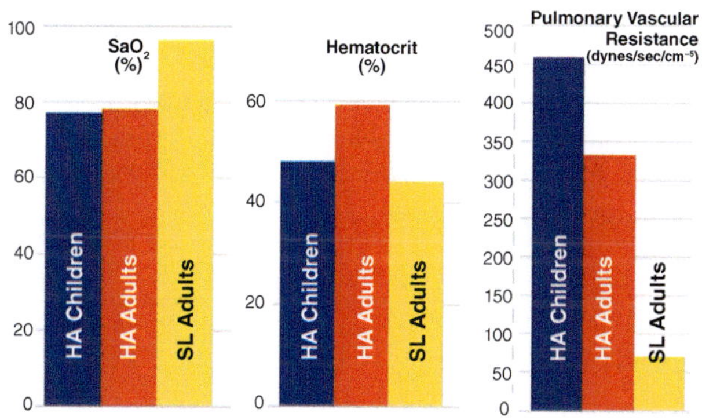

FIGURE 6.6 Pulmonary artery resistances (mean values) in healthy high-altitude (HA) residents compared with subjects residing at sea level (SL), together with values of O_2 saturation (SaO_2) and Haemotocrit. The persistence of high values of pulmonary resistance in HA residents is evident, from childhood to adulthood. [26] / with permission of the American Heart Association, Inc.

the walls of the arterioles,[28] a reduction in their lumen and, therefore, an increase in vascular resistance and hydrostatic pressure in the pulmonary system (Figure 6.6).

Even in adulthood, residents at high altitudes have, on average, pulmonary resistances equal to approximately 5–7 times compared to those of residents at sea level, and pressure levels in the pulmonary artery are approximately double or triple those of residents at sea level.

Pulmonary Vascular Resistances at Rest and During Effort

Then, when these two groups of people (sea-level residents and high-altitude residents) undergo **physical exertion**, what happens? What will their haemodynamic responses be like?

1. As is known, with physical effort carried out at sea level in residents at sea level or at low altitudes, HR increases, as does blood pressure and cardiac output, despite there being a modest reduction in systolic volume. To obtain these results, pulmonary vascular resistance decreases, allowing – so to speak – easier crossing of the pulmonary vascular tree and, therefore, greater availability of blood to the left ventricle. Systolic pressure in the pulmonary artery increases, but only slightly (about 50% more than baseline values), precisely because of the aforementioned reduction in pulmonary resistance (Figure 6.5).
2. We have already seen that in subjects who usually live on the plains or at low altitudes, carrying out physical activity at altitude leads to a greater increase in HR compared to what would occur on the plains, due to the reduced availability of O_2. At the same time, systemic arterial pressure also increases, as does the pressure in the pulmonary artery, to a greater (albeit slightly) extent compared to the plain, due to hypoxia-induced pulmonary vasoconstriction. The maximum O_2 consumption (indicator of the total work carried out by the cardiopulmonary-muscular system) is reduced to a variable extent depending on the altitudes at which the physical effort is carried out (see Chapter 4).
3. People who live chronically at high altitudes, when they carry out physical activity at altitude, show a considerable increase in systolic pressure levels in the pulmonary artery (which reaches levels at least double compared to basal ones) due to the increased cardiac output in the presence of a 'stiff' pulmonary vascular bed: the pulmonary vascular resistance is not able to reduce, but rather shows a modest increase (this behaviour is opposite to what happens in residents at sea level who carry out physical effort at sea level). These variations lead to a further increase in the overload (already chronically present) of the right ventricle and pulmonary circulation.

The Electrocardiogram (ECG) at High Altitude

As regards the ECG of volunteers exposed to simulated altitudes of 3,000–3,600 m, it has been often observed that a significant decrease in T wave amplitude in the precordial leads occurs in more than half of them, correlated to a greater increase of HR in these subjects.[29, 30] No significant differences have been found in various pulmonary function parameters between subjects with or without T wave reduction. Another study[31] conducted on individuals acutely exposed to higher altitudes (4,500–7,000 m) has reported a reduction in T wave amplitude in a greater percentage of individuals (up to 85%), likely due to the greater reduction in O_2 saturation (SaO_2) at higher altitudes. Extensive and prolonged T wave inversion can also be seen in mountaineers, especially in those suffering from HAPE, with no proven cardiac diseases.[19, 32] In a study in which 103 male, young patients with ECG abnormalities (mainly T wave inversion) at high altitude (between 2,700 and 6,700 m) have been submitted to coronary angiography, it was found that ECG changes at high altitude were not significantly associated with obstructive CAD.[33]

Due to the known increase in PAP, other morphological changes on the ECG have also been observed in sea-level residents who ascend to high altitudes: right axis deviation, right bundle branch block and changes in P wave amplitude. During the American Medical Research Expedition to Mt. Everest in 1982, 3 out of 12 American mountaineers exhibited right bundle branch conduction disturbances, and 3 others showed changes consistent with right ventricular hypertrophy within days of arriving at extreme altitude.[34] In the same group of mountaineers, an increase in P wave amplitude (>1 mm) was observed in a percentage of subjects that increased with increasing altitude, reaching 75% at an altitude of 6,300 m. During exercise, it has been reported a further increase in P wave amplitude,[34] which – in a group of Chinese mountaineers – has been described to be even 4–5 times higher than at sea level.[35] Other studies report only insignificant changes in P wave amplitude, duration or morphology.

The described modifications resolve after returning to low altitude, usually in 2–6 weeks.[30]

Depression of the ST segment in inferior and left precordial leads at high altitude has been reported rarely among middle-aged[36, 37] or mildly hypertensive climbers;[38] no residual changes were apparent after returning to sea level.

In people chronically exposed to high altitudes, right axis deviation appears to be up to 4 times more common than in people living at sea level,[39–41] often being associated with signs of right ventricular hypertrophy; chronic high-altitude residents present also a more prevalent T wave inversion in the right precordial leads and a prolonged QTc compared to sea-level residents, although within normal limits.[42] In those high-altitude natives who basally do not present right axis deviation, this modification can appear when exposed acutely to higher altitudes (such as in Sherpas who climbed from about 3,600 to 5,800 m during the British Sola Khumbu Expedition of 1959).[37]

Important genetic differences have been highlighted: in Lhasa (3,658 m), ECGs of Tibetan natives showed the presence of right ventricular hypertrophy in 17% of them, while this prevalence was much higher (29%) in Han Chinese immigrants and even more elevated (50%) in those people who presented signs of chronic mountain sickness.[43, 44] A similar difference was found also in ECG recordings between the Mustang (Tibetan origin) and the Humla (Indo-Aryans) populations living at high altitude in Nepal.[45]

Genetic Factors

So far, we have seen how there is an inverse correlation between altitude and levels of arterial SaO_2 and a direct correlation between altitude and an increase in arterial pressure in the pulmonary artery (PAP): that is, as the altitude progressively increases, SaO_2 decreases and the PAP increases (in a non-linear, but parabolic manner).

But there are important exceptions to the general 'rule': not always a decrease in SaO_2 corresponds to an increase in PAP (Figure 6.7). In Leadville (Colorado, USA), located at an altitude of 3,100 m, a markedly elevated PAP was found in adolescents of European origin and in new immigrants; in the capital of Tibet, Lhasa, located at an even higher altitude (3,600–4,200 m AMSL), unexpectedly normal PAP values were detected in natives descending from populations of ancient local origin. The PAP values in residents in these two cities, therefore, appear partly independent of the recorded SaO_2 values. These findings indicate that, in addition to the altitude levels and the associated degree of hypoxia, there are genetic

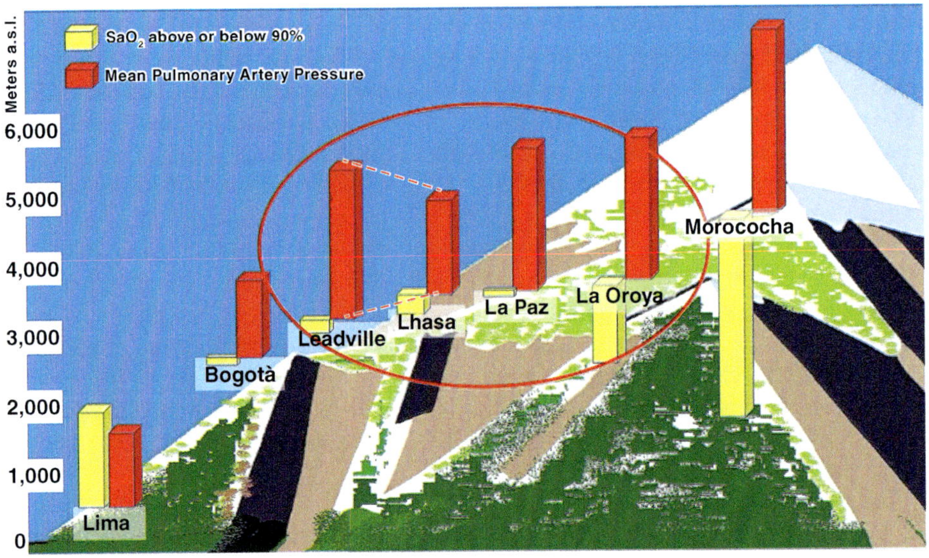

FIGURE 6.7 Different pulmonary artery pressure (PAP) values between different populations at the same altitude of residence: possible genetic differences in the response to chronic hypobaric hypoxia. Data from Ref. [26].

factors that influence the response to altitude/hypoxia.[46] The countless generations and millennia of life that the Tibetans of Lhasa have spent at high altitude have led to a genetic selection, which has made it possible to modify their response in terms of pulmonary hypertension to altitude.

In addition to genetic determinants, individual variations in pulmonary vascular reactivity to altitude hypoxia are also hypothesised, as evidenced by the finding of wide variability in PAP levels between single individuals within the two populations indicated above: some subjects are hyper-reactive to hypoxia (especially newborns) and others hypo-reactive.

Indirect confirmation of the existence of genetic factors capable of influencing the body's response to hypoxia comes from some studies conducted on people belonging to two different populations residing in Tibet. 'Native' Tibetans have been studied, as well as subjects belonging to the Han population, who immigrated to Tibet after the Chinese occupation, i.e. after 1950–1951. Individuals belonging to these two ethnic groups were submitted to stress testing (Figure 6.8).[47] Both groups developed (on average) a fair workload when they sustained the effort at an altitude of 3,417 m AMSL; but when the effort was repeated at a higher altitude (4,300 m AMSL), the Tibetans developed a significantly higher workload and maximum oxygen consumption in comparison to the results recorded in the Han individuals, as well as a smaller reduction in SaO_2 with the climb to altitude and with effort. In native Tibetans, it was also found – in another study[48] – a smaller increase in pulmonary pressure during exercise compared to the Han immigrant population.

Another observation was made in 2017 on a large group of native Tibetans and Han Chinese students, who had been living at low altitudes for 7 years. Upon returning to high

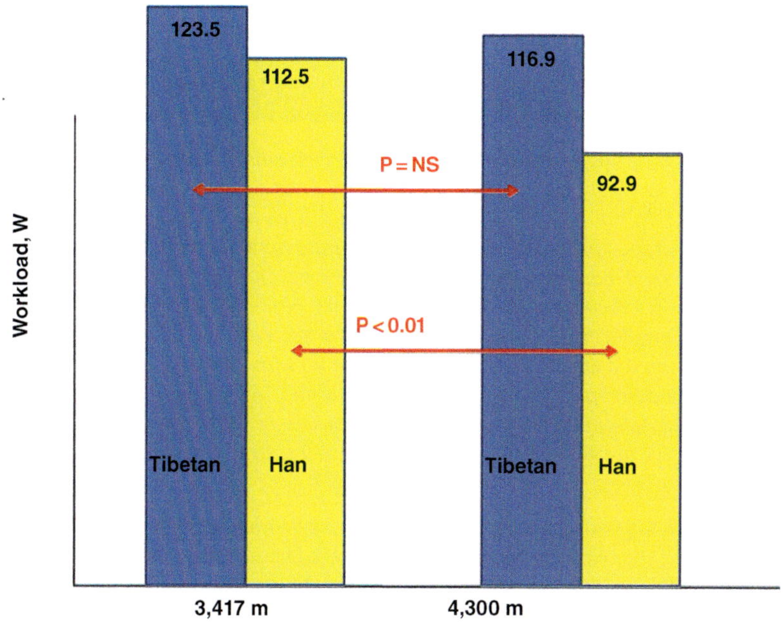

FIGURE 6.8 Workloads sustained by Tibetan and Han persons during stress tests conducted at 3,417 and 4,300 m AMSL. Adapted from Ref. [47].

altitudes (3,658 m above sea level), it is known that a certain percentage of these people may suffer from acute mountain sickness (AMS). However, new cases of AMS occurred with a highly different incidence between the two groups: only 1.2% of native Tibetans suffered from AMS in comparison to 32.7% of Han Chinese students. After reascending to Lhasa after 7 years at low altitude, the Tibetan students demonstrated also a smaller reduction in peripheral oxygen saturation and a smaller increase in HR in comparison to the group of Han students.

All these data confirm the existence of genetic factors that influence the body's cardiovascular responses to hypobaric hypoxia.[49]

High-altitude Pulmonary Oedema (HAPE), a case report from the past

'An Englishman, Mr. V., visited the district in February, 1911. The weather was snowy and damp. He arrived in the usual way, by train - forty-two hours' journey from sea-level. Three years before he had lived at the same mine for a period of three months, had not been ill on arrival, and had been in good health the whole time. For some time previous to this latter visit he had been in the altitudes of Peru, attaining a height of 17,000 ft., and had not been affected.

(continued)

High-altitude Pulmonary Oedema (HAPE), a case report from the past *(continued)*

He seemed in good health on arrival, and said that he felt quite well, but nevertheless he kept quiet, ate sparingly, and went to bed early. He woke next morning feeling ill, with symptoms of the normal type of puna. As the day drew on he began to feel very ill indeed. In the afternoon his pulse-rate was 144, respirations 40. Later in the evening he became very cyanosed, had acute dyspnoea, and evident air hunger, all the extraordinary muscles of respiration being called into play. The heart sounds were very faint, the pulse irregular and of small tension. He seemed to present a typical picture of a failing heart. This condition persisted during the night; he coughed up with difficulty. He vomited at intervals. This condition persisted during the night; he had several inhalations of oxygen; strychnine and digitalis also were given. Towards morning he recovered slightly, and as there was luckily a train going down to Antofagasta in the early morning, he was sent straight down.*

I heard that when he got down to 12,000 ft. he was considerably better, and at 7000 ft. he was nearly well. It seemed to me that he would have died had he stayed in the altitudes for another day.

...

I had a third case of this nature on July 19, 1911. I was called to see a young Turk aged 23 a well-made man, with no previous history of illness, and had lived in the district for some months before. He had been below in the port for some weeks, and arrived again in the district on July 14 late in the day. On the 15th he was getting about, though he had a slight headache; on the 16th his headache had increased considerably. The next day he was really ill, according to his friends' account, and gradually got worse till the 19th, when I was called to see him. On examination he was profoundly dyspnoic, respirations being 60, pulse 144, and hardly perceptible. Air hunger was extreme, he had frequent shivering fits, and the extremities were icy-cold. The face was pallid save for the lips and ears, which were cyanosed. The tongue was very dry, and covered with a white fur. The heart sounds were all weak. There were a few râles to be heard at both bases. During the night he became unconscious while making several efforts to get out of bed, and in the morning he was obviously dying. Death occurred about 2 p.m.'

(*From:* Ref. [50].)

The observations of Dr. Thomas Holmes Ravenhill (1881–1952) were made during the two years (from August 1909 to August 1911) in which he worked as a doctor in the Collahuasi and Poderosa mines in northern Chile, near the borders with Bolivia, at altitudes between 4,690 and 4,940 m AMSL.

Among the 38 clinical cases collected by Ravenhill, the first case reported here is interesting above all for the description of the clinical picture and its evolution and rapid improvement with the descent to lower mountain altitudes: the best treatment of all is to descend to a lower altitude. This patient has also been given Oxygen, an intervention that should have improved the clinical picture. In this specific case, however, Oxygen appeared to have very limited or no effect; this was probably due to the fact that it was a poorly concentrated oxygen therapy, since at that time O_2 had to be obtained locally by heating a mixture of potassium chloride and manganese dioxide.

High-altitude Pulmonary Oedema (HAPE), a case report from the past (*continued*)

The second dramatic case of the young Turk reminds us that even in people previously acclimatised to altitude, a descent to the plains for a few weeks followed by return to high altitude can lead to the occurrence of HAPE ('re-entry HAPE'). In all individuals ascending to high altitudes, progressive acclimatisation with gradual ascent (over the course of a week) is an important preventive measure.

*The term 'puna' has been used in Bolivia by local populations to indicate symptoms of Acute Mountain Sickness (AMS). Ravenhill identified three clinical types of Puna: *'Puna of a normal type'*, which today we call AMS, *'Puna with cardiac symptoms'* (our HAPE) and *'Puna in which nervous symptoms predominate'* (like what we now call HACE).

References

1 Stembridge M, Ainslie PN, Hughes MG, Stöhr EJ, Cotter JD, Nio AQ, Shave R. Ventricular structure, function, and mechanics at high altitude: chronic remodeling in Sherpa vs. short-term lowlander adaptation. J Appl Physiol 2014; 117(3):334–343. https://doi.org/10.1152/japplphysiol.00233.2014.

2 Stembridge M, Ainslie PN, Shave R. Short-term adaptation and chronic cardiac remodelling to high altitude in lowlander natives and Himalayan Sherpa. Exp Physiol 2015; 100(11):1242–1246. https://doi.org/10.1113/expphysiol.2014.082503.

3 Tucker CE, James WE, Berry MA, Johnstone CJ, Grover RF. Depressed myocardial function in the goat at high altitude. J Appl Physiol. 1976; 41(3):356–361. doi: 10.1152/jappl.1976.41.3.356.

4 Gibbs JS. Biventricular function at high altitude: implications for regulation of stroke volume in chronic hypoxia. Adv Exp Med Biol 2007; 618:13–24. https://doi.org/10.1007/978-0-387-75434-5_2.

5 Naeije R. Physiological adaptation of the cardiovascular system to high altitude. Prog Cardiovasc Dis 2010; 52(6):456–466. https://doi.org/10.1016/j.pcad.2010.03.004.

6 Williams AM, Levine BD, Stembridge M. A change of heart: mechanisms of cardiac adaptation to acute and chronic hypoxia. J Physiol 2022; 600(18):4089–4104. https://doi.org/10.1113/JP281724.

7 Huez S, Faoro V, Guénard H, Martinot JB, Naeije R. Echocardiographic and tissue Doppler imaging of cardiac adaptation to high altitude in native highlanders versus acclimatized lowlanders. Am J Cardiol 2009; 103(11):1605–1609. https://doi.org/10.1016/j.amjcard.2009.02.006.

8 Dall'Aglio V. Studio ecocardiografico della funzione diastolica ventricolare [An echocardiographic study of diastolic dysfunction of the ventricles]. From: Nicolosi GL, Trattato di ecocardiografia clinica, cap.14. Piccin Ed., Padova, 1999. http://www.vittoriodallaglio.com/vda.asp?p=90.

9 Wyss CA, Koepfli P, Fretz G, Seebauer M, Schirlo C, Kaufmann PA. Influence of altitude exposure on coronary flow reserve. Circulation 2003; 108(10):1202–1207. https://doi.org/10.1161/01.CIR.0000087432.63671.2E.

10 Jones J. Pulmonary edema. Case study, Radiopaedia.org. https://doi.org/10.53347/rID-6463.

11 Ruales F. High altitude pulmonary edema. Case study, Radiopaedia.org. https://doi.org/10.53347/rID-16070 (accessed 14 September 2025).

12 Hall DP, Duncan K, Baillie JK. High altitude pulmonary oedema. J R Army Med Corps 2011; 157(1):68–72. https://doi.org/10.1136/jramc-157-01-12.

13 Bärtsch P, Maggiorini M, Mairbäurl H, Vock P, Swenson ER. Pulmonary extravascular fluid accumulation in climbers. Lancet 2002; 360(9332):571; author reply 571–572. https://doi.org/10.1016/S0140-6736(02)09723-4.

14 Droma Y, Ota M, Kobayashi N, Ito M, Kobayashi T, Hanaoka M. Genetic associations with the susceptibility to high-altitude pulmonary oedema in the Japanese population. High Alt Med Biol 2025; 26(2):215–226. https://doi.org/10.1089/ham.2024.0119.

15 Bärtsch P, Maggiorini M, Ritter M, Noti C, Vock P, Oelz O. Prevention of high-altitude pulmonary oedema by nifedipine. N Engl J Med 1991; 325(18):1284–1289. https://doi.org/10.1056/NEJM199110313251805.

16 Hultgren HN. High-altitude pulmonary oedema: current concepts. Annu Rev Med 1996; 47: 267–284. https://doi.org/10.1146/annurev.med.47.1.267.

17 Tetzlaff K, Swenson ER, Bärtsch P. An update on environment-induced pulmonary oedema – "When the lungs leak under water and in thin air." Front Physiol 2022; 13:1007316. https://doi.org/10.3389/fphys.2022.1007316.

18 Swenson ER. High-altitude pulmonary oedema. In: Yuan JX-J, Garcia JGN, West JB, Hales CA, Rich S, Archer SL (Eds). Textbook of Pulmonary Vascular Disease. Boston: Springer; 2010. pp. 871–888. https://doi.org/10.1007/978-0-387-87429-6_61.

19 Hanaoka M, Kobayashi T, Droma Y, Ota M, Kobayashi N, Wada Y, Kitaguchi Y, Koizumi T, Kubo K. Clinical and pathophysiological features of high-altitude pulmonary edema in the Japanese population: a review of studies on high-altitude pulmonary edema in Japan. Intern Med 2024; 63(17):2355–2366. https://doi.org/10.2169/internalmedicine.2533-23.

20 Gesang L, Suona Y, Danzeng Z, Ci B, Gesang Q, Cidan W, Dingzeng Q, Baima Z, Zhaxi Q. A machine learning-based severity stratification tool for high altitude pulmonary edema. BMC Med Inform Decis Mak 2025; 25(1):171. https://doi.org/10.1186/s12911-025-02992-y.

21 Zubieta-Calleja GR, Zubieta-Castillo G. High Altitude Pathology at 12000 ft. La Paz, Bolivia: Instituto de Patologia de la Altura, Imprenta Papiro; 1989. https://www.researchgate.net/publication/344025807_High_Altitude_Pathology_at_12000_ft.

22 Scherrer U, Vollenweider L, Delabays A, Savcic M, Eichenberger U, Kleger GR, Fikrle A, Ballmer PE, Nicod P, Bärtsch P. Inhaled nitric oxide for high-altitude pulmonary oedema. N Engl J Med 1996; 334(10):624–629. https://doi.org/10.1056/NEJM199603073341003.

23 Maggiorini M. Prevention and treatment of high-altitude pulmonary oedema. Prog Cardiovasc Dis 2010; 52(6):500–506. https://doi.org/10.1016/j.pcad.2010.03.001.

24 Koch RO, Hinterhuber L, Faulhaber M, Gatterer H, Graupner S, Muenzel K, Burtscher M. A successful therapy of high-altitude pulmonary oedema with a CPAP helmet on Lenin Peak. Clin J Sport Med 2009; 19(1):72–73. https://doi.org/10.1097/JSM.0b013e3181915cce.

25 Krassnitzer P. Endure in thin air. [Dissertation]. Umeå Institute of Design, Umeå, Sweden, 2019. https://www.diva-portal.org/smash/get/diva2:1345219/FULLTEXT01.pdf.

26 Peñaloza D, Arias-Stella J. The heart and pulmonary circulation at high altitudes: healthy highlanders and chronic mountain sickness. Circulation 2007; 115(9): 1132–1246. https://doi.org/10.1161/CIRCULATIONAHA.106.624544.

27 Peñaloza D, Arias-Stella J, Sime F, Recavarren S, Marticorena E. The heart and pulmonary circulation in children at high altitudes: physiological, anatomical, and clinical observations. Pediatrics 1964;34:568–582.

28 Arias-Stella J, Saldana M. The terminal portion of the pulmonary arterial tree in people native to high altitudes. Circulation 1963; 28:915–925. https://doi.org/10.1161/01.cir.28.5.915.

29 Hannon KR, Pendergast DR, Strauss HC. Electrocardiogram at an altitude of 3600 m with reference to T wave depression. Aviat Space Environ Med 2014; 85(6):653–657. https://doi.org/10.3357/asem.3835.2014. Available at: https://asma.kglmeridian.com/downloadpdf/view/journals/asem/85/6/article-p653.pdf

30 Ramchandani R, Zhou Z, Parodi JB, Farina JM, Liblik K, Sotomayor J, Burak C, Herman R, Baranchuk A. A systematic review of electrocardiographic changes in populations temporarily ascending to high altitudes. Curr Probl Cardiol 2023; 48(5):101630. https://doi.org/10.1016/j.cpcardiol.2023.101630.

31 Windsor JS, Rodway GW, Montgomery HE. A review of electrocardiography in the high altitude environment. High Alt Med Biol 2010; 11(1):51–60. https://doi.org/10.1089/ham.2009.1065.

32 Fiorenzano G, Papalia MA, Parravicini M, Rastelli V, Bigi R, Dottorini M. Prolonged ECG abnormalities in a subject with high altitude pulmonary edema (HAPE). J Sports Med Phys Fitness 1997; 37(4):292–296.

33 Saif M, Rahman F, Liaqat J, Sajid U, Saeed F, Khan A, Khan MN, Samore NA, Siddique MB, Arshad J. Correlation of ECG changes at high altitude with findings on coronary angiogram. Pak Armed Forces Med J 2022; 72(Suppl-3):S423–427. https://doi.org/10.51253/pafmj.v72iSUPPL-3.9525.

34 Karliner JS, Sarnquist FF, Graber DJ, Peters RM Jr, West JB. The electrocardiogram at extreme altitude: experience on Mt. Everest. Am Heart J 1985; 109(3 Pt 1):505–513. https://doi.org/10.1016/0002-8703(85)90555-1.

35 Shi ZY, Ning XH, Zhu SC, Zhao DM, Huang PG, Yang SY, Wang Y, Dong ZS. Electrocardiogram made on ascending the Mount Qomolangma from 50 m a. s. l. Sci Sin. 1980; 23(10):1316–1325.

36 Alexander JK. Cardiac arrhythmia at high altitude: the progressive effect of aging. Tex Heart Inst J 1999; 26(4):258–263.

37 Jackson F, Davies H. The electrocardiogram of the mountaineer at high altitude. Br Heart J 1960; 22(5):671–685. https://doi.org/10.1136/hrt.22.5.671.

38 Caravita S, Faini A, Bilo G, Revera M, Giuliano A, Gregorini F, Rossi J, Villafuerte FC, Salvi P, Agostoni P, Parati G. Ischemic changes in exercise ECG in a hypertensive subject acutely exposed to high altitude. Possible role of a high-altitude induced imbalance in myocardial oxygen supply-demand. Int J Cardiol 2014; 171(3):e100–e102. https://doi.org/10.1016/j.ijcard.2013.12.003.

39 Rotta A, Lopez A. Electrocardiographic patterns in man at high altitudes. Circulation 1959; 19(5):719–28. https://doi.org/10.1161/01.cir.19.5.719.

40 Pryor R, Weaver WF, Blount SG Jr. Electrocardiographic observation of 493 residents living at high altitude (10,150 feet). Am J Cardiol 1965; 16(4):494–499. https://doi.org/10.1016/0002-9149(65)90025-1.

41 Grover RF. The paradox of hypoxic pulmonary hypertension (2013 Grover Conference series). Pulm Circ 2014; 4(2):151–157. https://doi.org/10.1086/676837.

42 Parodi JB, Ramchandani R, Zhou Z, Chango DX, Acunzo R, Liblik K, Farina JM, Zaidel EJ, Ruiz-Mori E, Carreón JMA, Liprandi AS, Baranchuk A; ANDES (Altitude Non-specific Distributed ECG Screening) Project Investigators. A systematic review of electrocardiographic changes in healthy high-altitude populations. Trends Cardiovasc Med 2023; 33(5):309–315. https://doi.org/10.1016/j.tcm.2022.01.013.

43 Halperin BD, Sun S, Zhuang J, Droma T, Moore LG. ECG observations in Tibetan and Han residents of Lhasa. J Electrocardiol 1998; 31(3):237–243.

44 Kang G, Zhang H, Bu QDL, Shen Y. The Patterns and prevalence of electrocardiogram abnormalities in high-altitude populations with different ethnic backgrounds. J Racial Ethn Health Disparities 2025. https://doi.org/10.1007/s40615-025-02466-x.

45 Aryal N, Weatherall M, Bhatta YK, Mann S. Electrocardiography in people living at high altitude of Nepal. Heart Asia 2017; 9(1):48–53. https://doi.org/10.1136/heartasia-2016-010838.

46 Moore LG. Measuring high-altitude adaptation. J Appl Physiol 2017; 123(5):1371–1385. https://doi.org/10.1152/japplphysiol.00321.2017.

47 Chen QH, Ge RL, Wang XZ, Chen HX, Wu TY, Kobayashi T, Yoshimura K. Exercise performance of Tibetan and Han adolescents at altitudes of 3,417 and 4,300 m. J Appl Physiol 1997; 83(2):661–667. https://doi.org/10.1152/jappl.1997.83.2.661.

48 Yang JS, He ZQ, Zhai HY, Yan Z, Zhang HM, Qin F. A study of the pulmonary artery pressure in healthy people living at lowland and high altitude under exercise [in Chinese]. Chin J Cardiovasc Dis 1987; 15:39–41 (cited by Peñaloza D, Ref 14)

49 Gonggalanzi, Labasangzhu, Bjertness E, Wu T, Stigum H, Nafstad P. Acute mountain sickness, arterial oxygen saturation and heart rate among Tibetan students who reascend to Lhasa after 7 years at low altitude: a prospective cohort study. BMJ Open 2017; 7(7):e016460. https://doi.org/10.1136/bmjopen-2017-016460.

50 Ravenhill TH. Some experiences of mountain sickness in the Andes. J Trop Med Hyg 1913; 16(20):313–320.

CHAPTER 7

Peripheral Vasoregulation

As we have already seen, the most important responses to hypobaric hypoxia include (Figure 7.1):

- hyperventilation (triggered by the response to hypoxia), which progressively increases in the first 8–10 days at high altitude;
- haemoconcentration (due – in acute exposure – to increased diuresis[i] and to greater fluid loss with hyperpnoea; in chronic exposure, haemoconcentration is due to increased production of red blood cells);
- the transient increase in heart rate and cardiac output (as a result of hypoxia-induced sympathetic activation);
- pulmonary vasoconstriction and increased pressure in the pulmonary artery.[1]

Regarding the regulation of peripheral arterioles, hypobaric hypoxia produces compensatory vasodilation. However, this is counteracted – within a few hours – by a series of other phenomena. At the beginning of exposure to high altitude, the stimulation of peripheral chemoreceptors located in the carotid bodies leads to sympathetic activation and an increase in circulating catecholamines. At the same time, an activation of the renin–angiotensin–aldosterone system also occurs. These phenomena produce peripheral vasoconstriction, which – together with the increased heart rate induced by sympathetic hyperactivity – leads to a tendency to increase blood pressure.

Other mechanisms are also activated: circulating levels of Angiotensin-II are altered (with consequent retention of Na and H_2O),[1] the production of nitric oxide (NO) by the endothelium of the vessels is reduced,[2] Endothelin levels and the expression of the Endothelin A receptor increase and sensitivity to intracellular calcium increases. These phenomena also tend to cause vasoconstriction and, therefore, essentially reduce the possibility of vasodilation induced by hypoxia.

In addition to all this, we must not forget the exposure to cold that is associated with increasing altitude, which causes peripheral vasoconstriction.[3]

[i]Linked to the urinary excretion of bicarbonates, with the aim of compensating for respiratory alkalosis, especially in the early stages of exposure to high altitude.

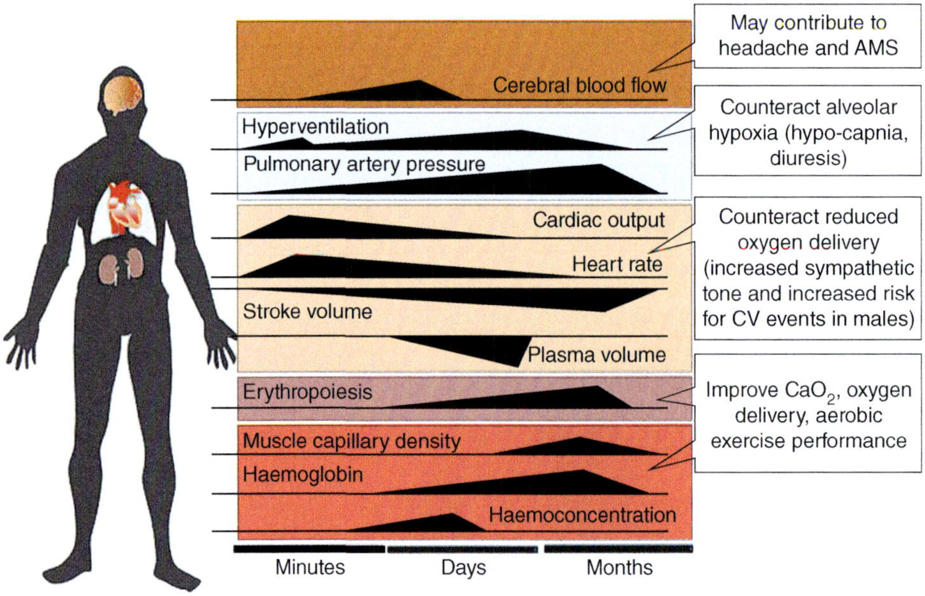

FIGURE 7.1 Main physiological responses to hypobaric hypoxia. [1] / MDPI / CC BY 4.0 with the kind permission of the author M. Burtscher.

Therefore, based on the sum of these theoretical physiopathological assumptions, we can expect that the overall outcome will lead to an increase in systemic blood pressure.

Systemic Blood Pressure at Altitude

The extent of the clinical effects of all these mechanisms may, however, be modest in healthy people (not so in untreated or poorly treated hypertensive patients!); it appears to be conditioned also by 'environmental factors' such as the level of altitude reached, as well as by large inter-individual variations linked to the individual ability to make physiological adjustments (genetic determinants), and – to a lesser extent – by effects linked to diet and physical training.

In the real world, from the limited existing studies, it appears that systemic blood pressure does not increase significantly in normal individuals with climbing to high altitudes (Figure 7.2).

Indeed, in a study published in 2000 on 8 volunteers who were subjected to simulated ascents up to 8,000 m AMSL in a hypobaric chamber, systemic blood pressure did not change significantly in both systolic and diastolic values, demonstrating – on the contrary – a tendency towards a slight decrease.[5]

Another study was conducted on 8 European climbers (healthy people, normally living at low altitudes) and 11 Nepalese during an expedition in the Himalayas.[4] In Europeans, systolic blood pressure showed a statistically significant, but still rather modest, increase with the progressive elevation from sea level up to 5,050 m AMSL, while no significant changes occurred in diastolic blood pressure. Systolic blood pressure increased progressively and reached its

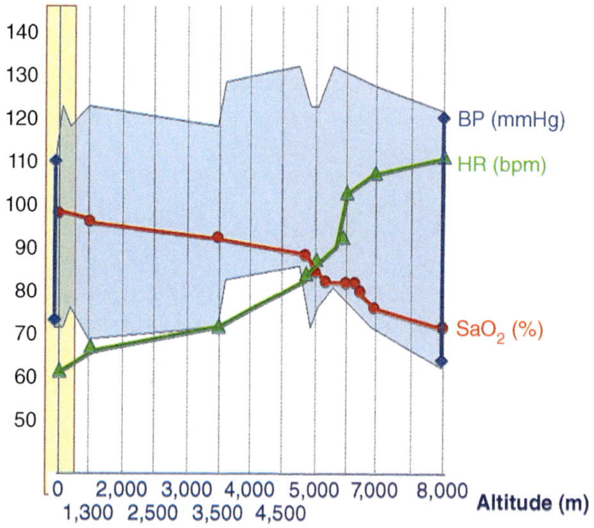

FIGURE 7.2 Trend of systolic and diastolic blood pressure (BP), heart rate (HR) and arterial Oxygen saturation (SaO_2) in European climbers when ascending to very high altitudes. Data derived from the studies by Salvi et al. [4] and Boussuges et al. [5].

maximum after 8 days of staying at altitude. No significant changes were recorded, however, in the Nepalese when they ascended from 3,400 to 5,050 m AMSL. The increase in systolic blood pressure in Europeans has been explained by increased circulating levels of norepinephrine and a transient increase in stiffness of the aorta and arterial vessels of the limbs, due to increased reactivity of the smooth muscle cells in the arterial walls.

Telmisartan for High Blood Pressure at Altitude

Taking into account the activation of the renin–angiotensin–aldosterone system that occurs with climbing to altitude, the Italian HIGHCARE-HIMALAYA study aimed to evaluate the trend of blood pressure through conventional serial checks and Holter-pressure recordings, and whether the pressure could be controlled by treatment with a drug that blocks angiotensin-II receptors, Telmisartan.[6] Unlike other studies conducted on limited numbers of volunteers, this study, in which 47 healthy volunteers were analysed, confirmed that blood pressure increases progressively and significantly with climbing to altitude, both in systolic and diastolic values, and especially that it remained high during night-time (reduction of the normal 'nocturnal dipping'); with the return to low altitudes, the pressure values returned to normal. Treatment with Telmisartan was effective in controlling the increase in blood pressure, but only up to 3,400 m AMSL, and was no longer able to maintain this control at higher altitudes (5,400 m AMSL).

From a very practical point of view, we can deduce from these studies that with ascent to high altitude, blood pressure increases in all people, even if the differences are slight in normotensive people and clinically insignificant compared to their values at low altitudes. We can also deduce that treatment with an angiotensin receptor blocker (ARB) remains effective at least up to high altitudes (but not very high altitudes). It is, therefore, important that healthy people (normotensive) or hypertensive patients ascend to moderate or high altitudes if their blood pressure values are stably normal at sea level or if they are receiving effective therapy.[7]

Attention to Blood Pressure Levels at Altitude

Despite what we have seen so far, there is a cohort study that reports that approximately 21% of even normotensive people show an increase in blood pressure of at least 10 mmHg or greater than the usual values with the climb to altitudes of 2,860, 3,400 and 4,300 m above sea level (although it must be mentioned that in 19% of the study cases the systolic pressure decreased!).[8] Therefore, appropriate attention is necessary, especially in patients whose blood pressure values are not well controlled at lower altitudes, as demonstrated by a Chinese study on 14,050 workers on a high-altitude railway[9] and by the HIGHCARE-Andes Lowlanders Study on 100 hypertensive subjects.[10] In these studies, climbing to altitude induced a significant increase in blood pressure above their usual blood pressure values, especially in people with already high blood pressure values in the plains, with a fairly marked increase during the night hours.

For low-moderate altitudes, there should be no particular problems even in hypertensive patients, provided they are well treated (i.e. with values kept steadily within the norm) and they follow the therapy regularly. This is what we can deduce from an Austrian study (Austrian Moderate Altitude Study 2000, AMAS 2000), which evaluated the blood pressure trend in 20 people with metabolic syndrome accompanied for 3 weeks to an altitude of 1,700 m AMSL, where they carried out common activities of a tourist in the mountains.[11] In these people, 24-hour ambulatory blood pressure monitoring showed a progressive reduction in values, even significant, so much so that the authors of the study concluded that exposure to moderate altitudes has favourable effects on the cardiovascular system of patients with metabolic syndrome, and a stay at moderate altitude does not entail an increased cardiovascular risk. The reduced blood pressure values then progressively returned to usual values over a period of 6 weeks after returning to low altitude (Innsbruck, 576 m AMSL). The same group of authors also confirmed these results in a second study, conducted in 2008.[12]

In another chapter (Chapter 12), we will check what the current recommendations are for hypertensive patients climbing to altitude.

References

1 Mallet RT, Burtscher J, Pialoux V, Pasha Q, Ahmad Y, Millet GP, Burtscher M. Molecular mechanisms of high-altitude acclimatization. Int J Mol Sci 2023; 24(2):1698. https://doi.org/10.3390/ijms24021698.

2 Faiss R, Pialoux V, Sartori C, Faes C, Dériaz O, Millet GP. Ventilation, oxidative stress, and nitric oxide in hypobaric versus normobaric hypoxia. Med Sci Sports Exerc 2013; 45(2):253–260. https://doi.org/10.1249/MSS.0b013e31826d5aa2.

3 Wait SO, Charkoudian N, Skinner JW, Smith CJ. Combining hypoxia with thermal stimuli in humans: physiological responses and potential sex differences. Am J Physiol Regul Integr Comp Physiol 2023. https://doi.org/10.1152/ajpregu.00244.2021.

4 Salvi P, Grillo A, Gautier S, Montaguti L, Brunacci F, Severi F, Salvi L, Pretolani E, Parati G, Benetos A. Haemodynamic adaptive mechanisms at high altitude: comparison between European lowlanders and Nepalese highlanders. J Clin Med 2022; 11(13):3843. https://doi.org/10.3390/jcm11133843.

5 Boussuges A, Molenat F, Burnet H, Cauchy E, Gardette B, Sainty JM, Jammes Y, Richalet JP. Operation Everest III (Comex '97): modifications of cardiac function secondary to altitude-induced hypoxia. An echocardiographic and Doppler study. Am J Respir Crit Care Med 2000; 161(1):264–70. https://doi.org/10.1164/ajrccm.161.1.9902096.

6 Parati G, Bilo G, Faini A, Bilo B, Revera M, Giuliano A, Lombardi C, Caldara G, Gregorini F, Styczkiewicz K, Zambon A, Piperno A, Modesti PA, Agostoni P, Mancia G. Changes in 24 h ambulatory blood pressure and effects of angiotensin II receptor blockade during acute and prolonged high-altitude exposure: a randomized clinical trial. Eur Heart J 2014; 35(44):3113–3122. https://doi.org/10.1093/eurheartj/ehu275.

7 Parati G, Agostoni P, Basnyat B, Bilo G, Brugger H, Coca A, Festi L, Giardini G, Lironcurti A, Luks AM, Maggiorini M, Modesti PA, Swenson ER, Williams B, Bärtsch P, Torlasco C. Clinical recommendations for high altitude exposure of individuals with pre-existing cardiovascular conditions: a joint statement by the European Society of Cardiology, the Council on Hypertension of the European Society of Cardiology, the European Society of Hypertension, the International Society of Mountain Medicine, the Italian Society of Hypertension and the Italian Society of Mountain Medicine. Eur Heart J 2018; 39(17):1546–1554. https://doi.org/10.1093/eurheartj/ehx720.

8 Keyes LE, Sallade TD, Duke C, Starling J, Sheets A, Pant S, Young DS, Twillman D, Regmi N, Phelan B, Paudel P, McElwee M, Mather L, Cole D, McConnell T, Basnyat B Blood pressure and altitude: an observational cohort study of hypertensive and non hypertensive Himalayan trekkers in Nepal. High Alt Med Biol 2017; 18(3):267–277. https://doi.org/10.1089/ham.2017.0001.

9 Wu T-Y, Ding SQ, Liu JL, Yu MT, Jia JH, Chai ZC, Dai RC, Zhang SL, Li BY, Pan L, Liang BZ, Zhao JZ, Qi DT, Sun YF, Kayser B. Who should not go high: chronic disease and work at altitude during construction of the Qinghai-Tibet railroad. High Alt Med Biol 2007; 8(2):88–10. https://doi.org/10.1089/ham.2007.1015.

10 Bilo G, Villafuerte FC, Faini A, Anza-Ramírez C, Revera M, Giuliano A, Caravita S, Gregorini F, Lombardi C, Salvioni E, Macarlupu JL, Ossoli D, Landaveri L, Lang M, Agostoni P, Sosa JM, Mancia G, Parati G. Ambulatory blood pressure in untreated and treated hypertensive patients at high altitude: the high altitude cardiovascular research-Andes study. Hypertension 2015; 65(6): 1266–1272. https://www.ahajournals.org/doi/epub/10.1161/HYPERTENSIONAHA.114.05003.

11 Schobersberger W, Schmid P, Lechleitner M, von Duvillard SP, Hörtnagl H, Gunga HC, Klingler A, Fries D, Kirsch K, Spiesberger R, Pokan R, Hofmann P, Hoppichler F, Riedmann G, Baumgartner H, Humpeler E. Austrian Moderate Altitude Study 2000 (AMAS 2000). The effects of moderate altitude (1,700 m) on cardiovascular and metabolic variables in patients with metabolic syndrome. Eur J Appl Physiol 2003; 88(6):506–514. https://doi.org/10.1007/s00421-002-0736-8.

12 Mair J, Hammerer-Lercher A, Mittermayr M, Klingler A, Humpeler E, Pachinger O, Schobersberger W. 3-week hiking holidays at moderate altitude do not impair cardiac function in individuals with metabolic syndrome. Int J Cardiol 2008; 123(2):186–188. https://doi.org/10.1016/j.ijcard.2006.11.127.

CHAPTER 8

Effects of Exposure to Mountain Altitudes on Haematocrit and Consequences on the Heart and Circulation

Loss of Plasma Volume at Altitude

In the first days (and already in the first 72 hours) of exposure to altitude, a reduction in intravascular liquid mass appears, which has been estimated at just under 300 ml at 2,000 m AMSL and around 600–900 ml at an altitude of 3,500 m AMSL.[1]

This happens for a number of reasons:[2, 3]

- leakage of liquids from the vascular bed into the extravascular space, probably linked to increased permeability of the capillaries to proteins (which 'drag' water with them);[4]
- loss of water, due to increased ventilation linked to hypoxia, and also due to increased perspiration and increased urinary loss of fluids (partly related to release of the atrial natriuretic peptide and increased diuresis from a reduced sodium reabsorption, caused by hypoxic stimulation of peripheral chemoreceptors);[5–7]
- reduced water intake, due to hypoxia-induced adipsia[i] (and sometimes also due to the reduced availability of drinking water).[8] The loss of plasma volume is approximately 11% on the fourth day of staying at altitude, and the plasma volume remains reduced throughout the stay at high altitudes (Figure 8.1).

[i]Adipsia = decreased or absent feeling of thirst.

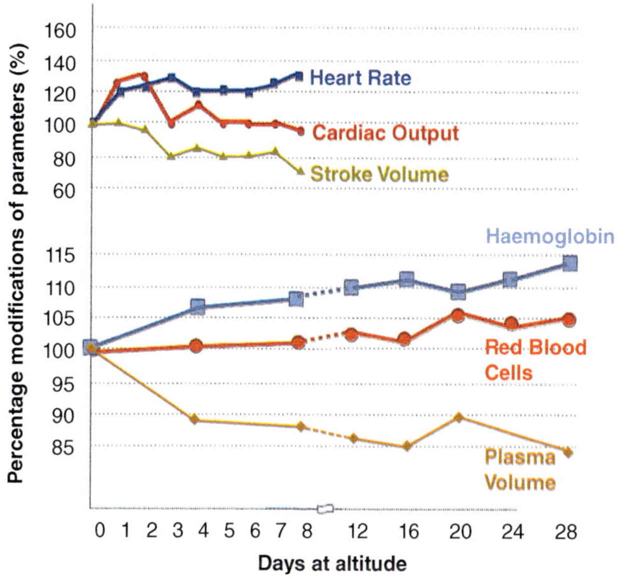

FIGURE 8.1 Reduction of plasma volume during a stay at high altitude, along with increase of Red Blood Cells count and Haemoglobin (Hb) (percentage variations). At the same time, stroke volume decreases, while heart rate increases, thus allowing cardiac output to remain substantially unchanged. Data derived from Refs. [2, 3] and other publications.

Increased Haematopoiesis

Hypobaric hypoxia also results in increased transcription of erythropoietin (EPO) in the peri-tubular cells of the renal cortex. The increased concentration of circulating EPO leads to stimulation of the haematopoietic cells of the bone marrow, with a slower progressive increase in haematocrit.

It has been observed that EPO levels increase already in the first hour of exposure to high altitude and reach 146% (±64%) already in the first day of stay at high altitude (on the Jungfraujoch, in Switzerland, 3,454 m above sea level).[2] EPO production decreases in the following days, although it remains higher than at sea level. Afterwards, with the return to sea level, the plasma concentration of EPO returns to baseline values within a week.

These oscillations in the production of EPO lead to increased production of reticulocytes (and red blood cells), which begins – like the increase in the concentration of EPO – already within the first day of exposure to high altitude.

Both phenomena, therefore, involve an increase in the mass of haemoglobin (Hb), on average of approximately 5–6% (5.26% ± 0.98%, with individual increments between 2.5 and 11%); these Hb kinetics, found on the Jungfraujoch, are similar to those found in other studies.[9]

The increase of Hb, however, takes at least 4 days (and up to 12 days) to be significantly evident, increases with the duration of the stay at altitude but then reaches a plateau around the 20th–24th day (up to the 40th day, after which it no longer increases).

For high altitudes, the Hb levels grow more than at moderate altitudes; it appears to increase in parallel with the rise in the altitude of residence (Figure 8.2).[10]

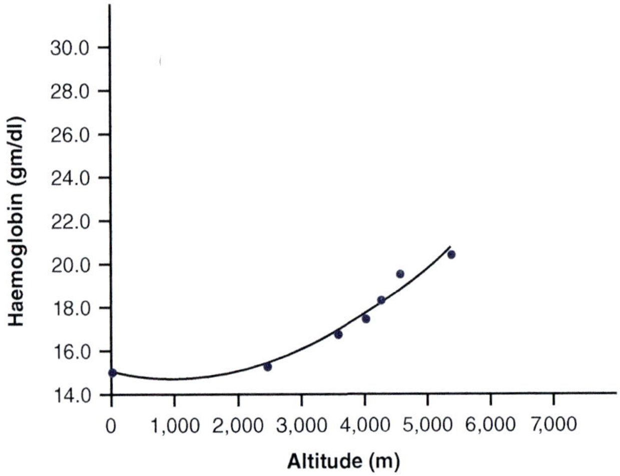

FIGURE 8.2 Hb values found at different altitudes in resident populations, by Zubieta-Calleja et al. [9]/ with permission of Gustavo R. Zubieta-Calleja.

During acute exposures, the studies by Richalet et al.[11] made evident that a 4-week stay at altitudes of approximately 5,000 m AMSL results in a further increase in Hb levels of approximately 30 g/L compared to altitudes of approximately 3,500 m AMSL. In the volunteers submitted to simulated high altitude in decompression chambers in the Everest III study, Hb values increased from baseline 148 $\pm$ 14 to 184 $\pm$ 15 g/L at an altitude of 8,000 m.

In persons chronically exposed to high altitudes, Zubieta-Castillo et al. reported values of Hb up to 254 g/L in residents at altitudes of 3,600 m AMSL (barometric pressure of 493 mmHg);[12] Champigneulle et al. observed that in dwellers in La Rinconada (5,000–5,300 m above sea level), the Hb concentration reached mean values of 203 $\pm$ 24 g/L.[13]

Obviously, for an increase in Hb to occur, the body must have iron stocks in adequate amounts. The haematopoietic response to altitude was found to be lower in women than that observed in men; in women, dietary iron supplementation improves the increase of haematocrit linked to altitude.[14] Figure 8.3, taken from a paper by Williams et al.,[15] summarises the variations in the composition of the blood mass in individuals from different geographical areas exposed to different altitudes.

Increased Blood Viscosity

What does this increase of Hb levels mean at a cardiovascular level?

We have seen that it involves an increase in the number of red blood cells from stimulation of the bone marrow and also haemoconcentration due to loss of fluids. That is, on the one hand, there is a loss of volume due to leakage of liquids from the circulatory tree towards the extravascular compartment; on the other, there is an increase in circulating mass due to an augmented production of red blood cells.

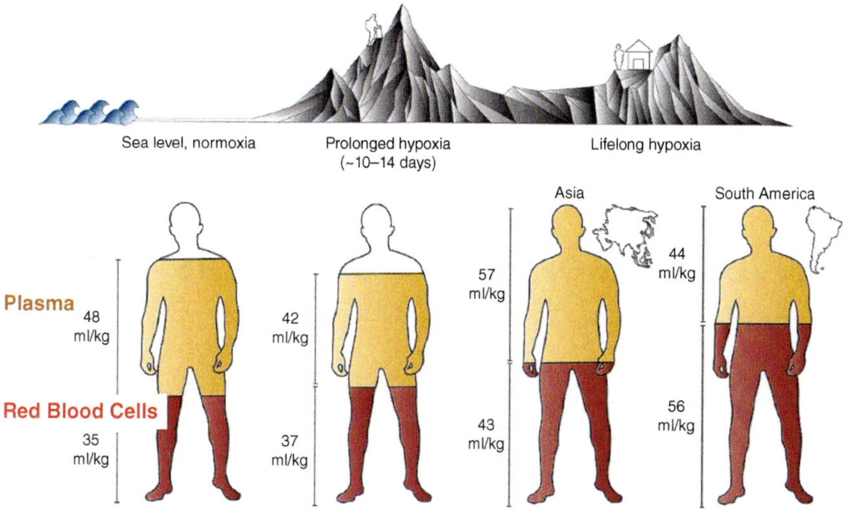

FIGURE 8.3 Composition of blood mass in individuals exposed to different altitudes. From: Ref. [14] / John Wiley & Sons / CC BY 4.0.

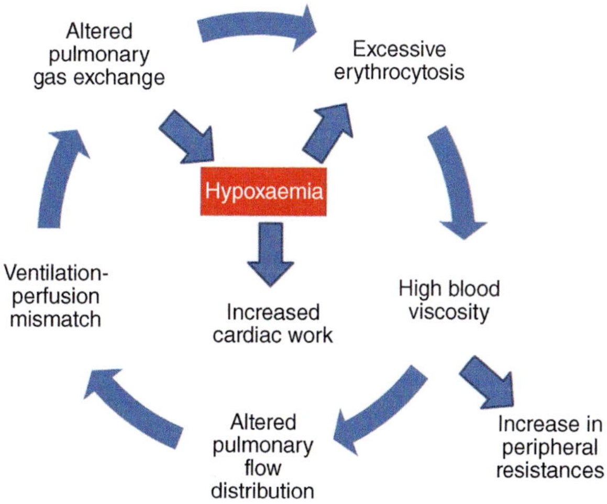

FIGURE 8.4 In 5–10% of subjects chronically exposed to high altitude, the physiological changes are 'maladaptive'.

This results in a greater blood viscosity, which has various consequences (Figure 8.4):[16]

- The higher blood viscosity would tend to reduce the venous return to the heart, but the increased overall blood mass tends to counteract this effect; consequently, cardiac output remains essentially unchanged.
- The higher blood viscosity leads to higher peripheral resistances; however, these are probably balanced by an increase in aortic elasticity and a certain degree of vasodilation, at

least in high-altitude residents. From studies conducted on experimental animals,[17] vasodilation could be due to an increased 'shear stress' on the vascular endothelium, which induces the production and release of nitric oxide (NO), which has a vasodilatory effect.

- A rise in diastolic pressure may occur (contrary to what is observed for systolic pressure), which may indicate increased venous return due to the greater blood mass.

Excessive Haemoglobin (Hb) Levels, Reduced Oxygen Extraction

It was believed for a long time that the higher Hb concentration at high altitudes constituted a beneficial factor, because it would have allowed a greater transport of O_2, capable of compensating for the reduced arterial O_2 saturation present at those high altitudes. However, it has been observed that the higher Hb concentration linked to low O_2 saturation is useful only up to a certain point: only a moderate increase in Hb concentration is useful for improving O_2 transport, while excessive increases of Hb become harmful.[14]

In 5–10% of subjects chronically exposed to high altitudes (particularly in those subjects with some associated form of lung disease, such as silicosis or chronic obstructive pulmonary disease [COPD]), the physiological mechanisms do not lead to a positive adaptation, i.e. they are 'maladaptive'.[18] Up to Hb concentration values of approximately 175 g/L (with SaO_2 of approximately 87%), the higher Hb level is useful, because it is accompanied by an increased O_2 extraction. However, when hypoxaemia becomes severe, the increased Hb concentration is no longer able to maintain efficient O_2 transport and is accompanied by a progressive reduction in O_2 extraction.[19] In people who live chronically at high altitudes and who present signs of chronic mountain sickness, the Hb concentration can reach very high values, as in some dwellers of La Rinconada in whom Hb is 231 ± 17 g/L.[13]

Ventilation–Perfusion Mismatch

The above changes are associated with a substantial increase of blood viscosity and of circulating blood volume (linked to very high levels of Hb); they lead to an altered distribution of blood flow at pulmonary level, with a mismatch in the ventilation–perfusion relationship. It follows that the exchange of gases at alveolar level is altered: this leads to further reduction of oxygenation of the blood and consequent arterial hypoxaemia, which – in turn – further stimulates erythropoiesis, contributing (in a vicious circle) to increasing circulating red blood cells and blood viscosity.[18, 20] In addition, polysomnography has demonstrated, in high-altitude residents, the presence also of nocturnal episodes of marked desaturation (with a median SpO_2 of 79% at 5,100 m vs. 84% at an altitude of 3,800 m; much lower in subjects with CMS: SpO_2 74%).[13]

Some studies have shown that the symptoms and clinical signs of these individuals improve significantly when they undergo bloodletting or haemodilution.[21]

We have seen before that modest increases in Hb concentration, circulating blood mass and blood viscosity can have limited negative effects that are compensated by the vasodilation mechanisms implemented at the arteriolar level. The situation is different when the Hb concentration increases significantly, as in the cases – just seen above – of chronic mountain sickness (characterised by **excessive erythrocytosis**, defined as a Hb concentration two standard deviations above the mean Hb concentration value of the population at the altitude of residence; consensus cut-off values: Hb $\geq$ 190 g/L in females and Hb $\geq$ 210 g/L in males).[22, 23] The first and fundamental study of the effects of a greatly increased haematocrit on cardiac activity was conducted experimentally in 1959 by physiologists Guyton and Richardson.[24] In the 14 dogs they studied, a 47% (isovolemic) increase in haematocrit led to a 51% reduction in cardiac output and a 50% increase in peripheral resistance, which were explained by the negative effects of blood viscosity on venous resistance and venous return to the heart.

It is important to keep these effects in mind, both with regard to people who live in the high mountains or who decide to visit the high mountains for sport or pleasure, but also with regard to the possible important negative effects in those athletes who use EPO for doping purposes.

Cyanosis, Breathlessness, Palpitations, Clubbing Fingers and Other Signs

From a clinical point of view, the increase of Hb concentration leads to a simultaneous increase of the amount of Hb not saturated by O_2. When this reaches values of approximately 50 g/L, cyanosis[ii] appears, precisely linked to the high levels of reduced (non-oxygenated) Hb.

Clinically, in persons suffering from chronic mountain sickness, breathlessness and palpitations may be present, as well as headache, sleep disturbances and tinnitus. Also the venous varicosities of the lower limbs that may be encountered in people living at high altitudes may be (partly) explained by the higher blood viscosity and the consequent resistance to venous flow towards the heart.

Another clinically evident sign in cases of chronic hypoxia is given by 'drumstick fingers' (or 'clubbing fingers' or 'Hippocratic fingers').[iii, 27]

In people who chronically reside at high altitudes, right heart dilation and high pulmonary artery pressure can be demonstrated by echocardiography; the left ventricle is also involved, exhibiting concentric remodelling and grade I diastolic dysfunction. The changes are more severe in high-altitude residents with chronic mountain sickness.[13]

[ii]"The term cyanosis (from the Greek κυανός, "blue") indicates the bluish, diffuse or limited colouration of the skin and mucous membranes, due to the increase in reduced haemoglobin in the capillary blood, which occurs in numerous circulatory and respiratory diseases and in some other particular conditions. ... Cyanosis occurs when the amount of reduced haemoglobin equals or exceeds 5 g/dl. ... Since the determining factor is represented by the absolute quantity of reduced haemoglobin, it follows that this appearance can be conditioned by the presence of some pathological situations, such as for example, a hypochromic anaemia (in which the haemoglobin content of the blood is reduced to a more or less marked extent) or, on the contrary, a polycythaemia (where the haemoglobin content is higher than normal).....' Translated from: Ref [25].

[iii]Clubbing fingers, also called Hippocratic or drumstick fingers: this condition consists of enlargement of the last phalanx accompanied by watch-glass nails. It is a progressive bone deformity due to a type of periostitis followed by new bone formation, thickening of the bone cortex and proliferation of adjacent connective tissue, which occurs in numerous chronic diseases. See also: Ref. [26].

The Quingay Score has been developed to assess the severity of chronic mountain sickness.[23]

In people who climb to high altitude for a short time and then return to sea level (or at least to low altitudes), the Hb concentration decreases quite rapidly. Plasma EPO concentration was seen to drop rapidly and return to baseline levels within about a week. The number of circulating reticulocytes also decreases rapidly; red blood cells have an average lifespan of approximately 120 days, so their number (and, therefore, the haematocrit and Hb concentration) progressively decreases, returning to baseline values in a few weeks.[2]

But what does it happen to a person who has lived chronically at high altitude if he/she moves to live at sea level?

From High Altitude to Sea Level

There are scanty data on this topic. It seems that the descent from high altitude to sea level can present peculiar manifestations in the acute phase (days, weeks), which differ from the chronic modifications (during prolonged residence at sea level).

Observations made by Zubieta-Calleja et al. in Bolivia have shown that – with the descent from 3,510 m AMSL to the sea level – the haematocrit values had a linear fall over 18–23 days, due to a reduction of red blood cell production and probably also to neocytolysis.[28] The minute ventilation of the observed subjects was dramatically reduced in the first day after the descent, reaching values as low as one-sixth of their usual ones and being lower than those of persons normally living at sea level. This large decrease in ventilation has been explicated as a sort of defence mechanism against a 'hyperoxic' environment; such an acute stage is generally limited to 3 days. Water retention was also observed, with possible appearance of oedema in the lower limbs.[29] The most important data on the effects of a permanent descent from high altitude to sea level were provided by Peñaloza in 2007,[30] however, on a small number of subjects studied: 11 young people aged 20 years. In these subjects (Figure 8.5), who chronically lived up to the

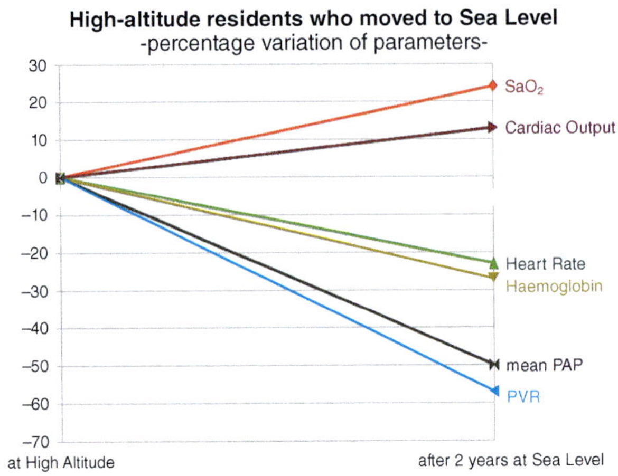

FIGURE 8.5 Changes in blood and haemodynamic parameters in persons chronically residing at high altitudes 2 years after relocation to sea level. Data derived from: Ref. [30].

age of 20 in the Andes at 4,540 m AMSL, after 2 years of living at sea level, the arterial O_2 saturation (SaO_2) was found to have increased from 78.5 ± 4.16% to the normal values of 97.3 ± 2.25%. Together with this normalisation of SaO_2, the Hb concentration decreased from 185 ± 18.1 g/L to 135 ± 8.1 g/L, i.e. falling to normal values; the haematocrit went down from 55.4 ± 5.3% to 41.9 ± 2.8%. Pulmonary vascular resistance (PVR) and mean pulmonary pressure (PAP) normalised, heart rate reduced and cardiac output improved, being all indicators of an improvement in overall cardiac performance linked to the reduction of blood viscosity.

A curious phenomenon in the high Alps: dehydration and 'evaporation'.

It has long been known that in lowlanders the ascent to high altitudes involves a series of physiological responses: within hours of arrival at high altitude, the decrease of partial pressure of Oxygen leads to an increase of heart rate and respiratory rate. The latter involves, on the one hand, a greater dispersion of water vapour through breathing (especially during physical exertion), and, on the other, a tendency towards respiratory alkalosis. To correct respiratory alkalosis, the kidneys increase diuresis (probably in response to increased levels of atrial natriuretic peptide) and bicarbonaturia. Some degree of fluid redistribution with extravascular fluid accumulation also occurs, evidenced by the appearance of subcutaneous oedema, increased intracranial pressure and B-lines in the lungs; these phenomena contribute to the reduction in plasma volume. Despite a significant decline in plasma volume, mountain climbers still experience only modest (not significant) weight loss.

This dehydration occurring in humans (and animals) at high altitude is different from the concept of evaporation from liquid surfaces, such as water reservoirs (natural or artificial). Available data on this subject are scarce: in theory, evaporation should increase with altitude, since the reduced atmospheric pressure offers fewer obstacles for water molecules to escape from a freely exposed surface of water; however, by the other side, lower temperatures counteract the effects of the decreasing barometric pressure.

What we just wrote is valid for liquids freely exposed to air, but how do liquids contained in a closed container behave?

In 1864, Edward Whymper together with his companions A. W. Moore and Horace Walker were climbing the Glacier de Bonne Pierre in the Massif des Écrins (France) at approximately 2,900 m above sea level.

During the days of the climb, Whymper noticed a strange phenomenon, never described before: some form of 'dehydration' was occurring not only in the humans but also in the reserve of liquids (particularly wine) that they had brought with them.

A special form of 'evaporation', which led to significant reductions in the volume of these liquids: was it due to the dryness of the air?

Only after days did the phenomenon receive an explanation. Here is the original description of the phenomenon, given by Whymper in his diary of the climbing:

> *'The night passed over without anything worth mention, but we had occasion to observe in the morning an instance of the curious evaporation that is frequently noticeable in the High Alps. On the previous night we had hung up on a knob of rock our mackintosh bag containing five bottles of Rodier's bad wine. In the morning, although the stopper appeared to have been in all night, about four-fifths had evaporated. It was strange;*

(continued)

A curious phenomenon in the high Alps: dehydration and 'evaporation'. *(continued)*

my friends had not taken any, neither had I, and the guides each declared that they had not seen anyone touch the bag. In fact, it was clear that there was no explanation of the phenomenon, but in the dryness of the air. Still it is remarkable that the dryness of the air (or the evaporation of wine) is always greatest when a stranger is in one's party. The dryness caused by the presence of even a single Chamounix porter is sometimes so great, that not four-fifths but the entire quantity disappears. For a time I found difficulty in combating this phenomenon, but at last discovered that if I used the wine-flask as a pillow during the night, the evaporation was completely stopped.'

(From: Ref. [31]).

Note – Drinking alcohol is not recommended during high-altitude ascents (see Chapter 21). Perhaps, what Whymper's mountain guides did was a form of protection for their clients!

References

1 Bärtsch P, Saltin B. General introduction to altitude adaptation and mountain sickness. Scand J Med Sci Sports 2008; 18 (Suppl 1):1–10. https://doi.org/10.1111/j.1600-0838.2008.00827.x.

2 Siebenmann C, Cathomen A, Hug M, Keiser S, Lundby AK, Hilty MP, Goetze JP, Rasmussen P, Lundby C. Hemoglobin mass and intravascular volume kinetics during and after exposure to 3,454-m altitude. J Appl Physiol 2015; 119(10):1194–1201. https://doi.org/10.1152/japplphysiol.01121.2014.

3 Naeije R. Physiological adaptation of the cardiovascular system to high altitude. Prog Cardiovasc Dis 2010; 52(6):456–466. https://doi.org/10.1016/j.pcad.2010.03.004.

4 Sawka MN, Young AJ, Rock PB, Lyons TP, Boushel R, Freund BJ, Muza SR, Cymerman A, Dennis RC, Pandolf KB, Valeri CR. Altitude acclimatization and blood volume: effects of exogenous erythrocyte volume expansion. J Appl Physiol 1996; 81(2):636–642. https://doi.org/10.1152/jappl.1996.81.2.636.

5 Albert TS, Tucker VL, Renkin EM. Atrial natriuretic peptide levels and plasma volume contraction in acute alveolar hypoxia. J Appl Physiol 1997; 82(1):102–110. https://doi.org/10.1152/jappl.1997.82.1.102.

6 Jain SC, Bardhan J, Swamy YV, Krishna B, Nayar HS. Body fluid compartments in humans during acute high-altitude exposure. Aviat Space Environ Med 1980; 51(3):234–236.

7 Swenson ER, Duncan TB, Goldberg SV, Ramirez G, Ahmad S, Schoene RB. Diuretic effect of acute hypoxia in humans: relationship to hypoxic ventilatory responsiveness and renal hormones. J Appl Physiol 1995; 78(2):377–383. https://doi.org/10.1152/jappl.1995.78.2.377.

8 Honig A. Peripheral arterial chemoreceptors and reflex control of sodium and water homeostasis. Am J Physiol 1989; 257(6 Pt 2):R1282–R1302. https://doi.org/10.1152/ajpregu.1989.257.6.R1282.

9 Rasmussen P, Siebenmann C, Diaz V, Lundby C. Red cell volume expansion at altitude: a meta-analysis and Monte Carlo simulation. Med Sci Sports Exerc 2013; 45:1767–1772. https://www.zora.uzh.ch/id/eprint/85258/1/Red_cell_volume.pdf.

10 Zubieta-Calleja GR, Ardaya G, Zubieta N, Paulev PE, Zubieta-Castillo G. Tolerance to hypoxia. Fiziolohichnyĭ zhurnal 2013; 59(4):65–71. https://zuniv.net/pub/TolerancetoHypoxiaFiziol.pdf.

11 Richalet JP, Robach P, Jarrot S, Schneider JC, Mason NP, Cauchy E, Herry JP, Bienvenu A, Gardette B, Gortan C. Operation Everest III (COMEX '97). Effects of prolonged and progressive hypoxia on humans during a simulated ascent to 8,848 M in a hypobaric chamber. Adv Exp Med Biol 1999; 474:297–317.

12 Zubieta-Castillo G, Zubieta-Calleja G. The triple hypoxia syndrome at altitude. Abstracts of the 1988 Annual Meeting of the American Lung Association and the American Thoracic Society. Am Rev Respir Dis 1988; 137(4):509.

13 Champigneulle B, Brugniaux JV, Stauffer E, Doutreleau S, Furian M, Perger E, Pina A, Baillieul S, Deschamps B, Hancco I, Connes P, Robach P, Pichon A, Verges S. Expedition 5300: limits of human adaptations in the highest city in the world. J Physiol 2024; 602(21):5449–5462. https://doi.org/10.1113/JP284550.

14 Hannon JP, Shields JL, Harris CW. Effects of altitude acclimatization on blood composition of women. J Appl Physiol 1969; 26(5):540–547. https://doi.org/10.1152/jappl.1969.26.5.540.

15 Williams AM, Levine BD, Stembridge M. A change of heart: mechanisms of cardiac adaptation to acute and chronic hypoxia. J Physiol 2022; 600(18):4089–4104. https://doi.org/10.1113/JP281724.

16 León-Velarde F, Villafuerte FC, Richalet JP. Chronic mountain sickness and the heart. Prog Cardiovasc Dis 2010; 52(6):540–549. https://doi.org/10.1016/j.pcad.2010.02.012.

17 Ruschitzka FT, Wenger RH, Stallmach T, Quaschning T, de Wit C, Wagner K, Labugger R, Kelm M, Noll G, Rülicke T, Shaw S, Lindberg RL, Rodenwaldt B, Lutz H, Bauer C, Lüscher TF, Gassmann M. Nitric oxide prevents cardiovascular disease and determines survival in polyglobulic mice overexpressing erythropoietin. Proc Natl Acad Sci USA 2000; 97(21):11609–11613. https://doi.org/10.1073/pnas.97.21.11609.

18 West JB. Are permanent residents of high altitude fully adapted to their hypoxic environment? High Alt Med Biol 2017; 18(2):135–139. https://doi.org/10.1089/ham.2016.0152.

19 Reeves JT, Leon-Velarde F. Chronic mountain sickness: recent studies of the relationship between hemoglobin concentration and oxygen transport. High Alt Med Biol 2004; 5(2):147–155. https://doi.org/10.1089/1527029041352090.

20 Villafuerte FC, Cárdenas R, Monge-C C. Optimal hemoglobin concentration and high altitude: a theoretical approach for Andean men at rest. J Appl Physiol 2004; 96(5):1581–1588. https://doi.org/10.1152/japplphysiol.00328.2003.

21 Winslow RM, Monge CC, Brown EG, Klein HG, Sarnquist F, Winslow NJ, McKneally SS. Effects of hemodilution on O2 transport in high-altitude polycythemia. J Appl Physiol 1985; 59(5):1495–1502. https://doi.org/10.1152/jappl.1985.59.5.1495.

22 Monge C, León-Velarde F, Arregui A. Increasing prevalence of excessive erythrocytosis with age among healthy high-altitude miners. N Engl J Med 1989; 321(18):1271. https://doi.org/10.1056/NEJM198911023211819.

23 León-Velarde F, Maggiorini M, Reeves JT, Aldashev A, Asmus I, Bernardi L, Ge RL, Hackett P, Kobayashi T, Moore LG, Penaloza D, Richalet JP, Roach R, Wu T, Vargas E, Zubieta-Castillo G, Zubieta-Calleja G. Consensus statement on chronic and subacute high altitude diseases. High Alt Med Biol 2005; 6(2):147–157. https://doi.org/10.1089/ham.2005.6.147.

24 Richardson TQ, Guyton AC: Effects of polycythemia and anemia on cardiac output and other circulatory factors. Am J Physiol 1959; 197: 1167–1170.

25 Urbinati G. Universo del Corpo. Cianosi. In: Enciclopedia Treccani. 1999. https://www.treccani.it/enciclopedia/cianosi_%28Universo-del-Corpo%29.

26 Sarkar M, Mahesh DM, Madabhavi I. Digital clubbing. Lung India 2012; 29(4):354–362. https://doi.org/10.4103/0970-2113.102824.

27 Villafuerte FC, Corante N. Chronic mountain sickness: clinical aspects, etiology, management, and treatment. High Alt Med Biol 2016; 17(2):61–69. https://doi.org/10.1089/ham.2016.0031.

28 Zubieta-Calleja GR, Paulev PE, Zubieta-Calleja L, Zubieta-Castillo G. Altitude adaptation through hematocrit changes. J Physiol Pharmacol 2007; 58(Suppl 5(Pt 2)):811–818.

29 Zubieta-Calleja G. Human adaptation to high altitude and to sea level. Acid-base equilibrium, ventilation and circulation in chronic hypoxia. Dissertation, Copenhagen, 2007. VDM Verlag Dr. Müller, 2010. ISBN: 978-3-639-25276-7. https://www.altitudeclinic.com/Copenhagen/Dissertation10b.pdf.

30 Penaloza D, Arias-Stella J. The heart and pulmonary circulation at high altitudes: healthy highlanders and chronic mountain sickness. Circulation 2007; 115(9):1132–1146. https://doi.org/10.1161/CIRCULATIONAHA.106.624544.

31 Whymper E. Scrambles Amongst the Alps in the Years 1860-69. Philadelphia: Lippincott JB; 1873, 85 p. https://archive.org/details/scramblesamongst00whymrich/page/n7/mode/2up.

PART 3

Travelling to High Altitude with Pre-existing Cardiac Diseases

CHAPTER 9

Magnitude of Cardiovascular Risk Associated with Ascent to Altitude

Increased Pulmonary Artery Pressure

We have already seen how acute hypoxia (such as that observed during climbs to high altitudes, especially if carried out in a short time and without adequate acclimatisation) directly determines a pulmonary vasoconstriction effect and therefore an increase in pulmonary artery pressure values, more evident and exaggerated in patients who already have pulmonary hypertension due to other causes; over a more or less prolonged period, this pulmonary hypertension can lead to chronic cor pulmonale and right ventricular failure.

At systemic level, if on the one hand hypoxia tends to cause systemic arteriolar vasodilation (which should lead to arterial hypotension), on the other hand, we have seen how it creates a stimulation of the sympathetic nervous system. The consequences of this stimulation have already been reported and are summarised here.[1]

Increased Activity of Sympathetic Nervous System

- Systemic vasoconstriction (which may be exaggerated in already hypertensive patients) with a consequent variable increase in systemic blood pressure values.
- Increased platelet aggregability, together with arterial hypertension this can be involved in causing a stroke.

- Increase in coronary flow due to vasodilation, but not in patients with fixed coronary stenoses, in whom – on the contrary – a vasodilation of some coronary districts could create a 'theft' to the detriment of already partially ischaemic areas.
- Increased heart rate, together with alterations in the distribution of coronary flow, increased blood pressure and systemic vasoconstriction (increased cardiac work), these factors may be involved in triggering a myocardial infarction.
- The increased heart rate and respiratory alkalosis linked to hypoxia (in addition to altered coronary flow) can favour the appearance of arrhythmias, sometimes serious.
- The stimulus to increase cardiac output and myocardial contractility induced by the increased sympathetic tone can 'send contractile-impaired hearts into crisis' (especially in coronary patients) and lead to episodes of acute heart failure.

During various expeditions to high altitudes, records were kept of adverse events that occurred to participants, in relation to the altitude reached and the time it took to get there. Campbell et al.[2] carried out a review of the literature and in 2015 they reported some case studies relating to accidents that occurred during high-altitude ascents; other recent observations are also reported in Box 9.1.[3]

Box 9.1

- Mount McKinley (Alaska, 6,190 m), in the period 1992–2011:
  - 29.6% high altitude syndrome
  - 18.8% cold damage (18.1% frostbite)
  - 8.4% lung infections
  - 7.9% musculoskeletal trauma (76% from a fall)
  - 5.3% gastrointestinal or genitourinary disorders
- Aconcagua (Argentine Andes, 6,962 m), in 2001, among tourists and mountaineers:
  - 39% acute mountain sickness
- Kilimanjaro (Tanzania, 5,895 m), climbed in 6 days, in 2010:
  - 61% acute mountain sickness
  - 14% high-altitude cerebral oedema
  - 0% high-altitude pulmonary oedema
- Kilimanjaro (Tanzania, 5,895 m), climbed in 4 days, in February 2018:
  - 30% moderate symptoms of AMS
  - 70% mild symptoms of AMS
- Everest Base Camp (Nepal, 5,300 m), ascended over 8 days, in March 2024:
  - 0% acute mountain sickness
- Colorado, ascent from 2,895 to 4,100 m in 12 hours ('adventure race'), in 2004:
  - 4.5% altitude sickness upon departure
  - 14.1% cumulative incidence altitude sickness
  - 0.81% altitude pulmonary oedema

As can be seen from these data, it seems that the incidence of cardiovascular complications is very low, while neurological complications appear to be more relevant.

To understand what can happen to those who visit the Alps, a review of the literature was carried out in 2010 by Martin Burtscher and Andrea Ponchia,[4] who described the possible cardiovascular manifestations in adult subjects who climb to altitudes >2,000 m above sea level.

Mortality

It is estimated that at least 40 million people visit the Alps every year, albeit at highly variable altitudes.[5] An epidemiological study conducted in the Italian Alps[6] calculated the occurrence of one case of sudden death every 980,000 person/day,[i] during physical activity at mountain altitudes up to approximately 3,400 m above sea level.

Previously, a study (not easily comparable with the one just mentioned) had been conducted on the Austrian Alps at altitudes up to 3,800 m above sea level;[7] in this study, it was observed that every year, every 100,000 people, a certain number of cases of death occurred; in three-quarters of cases, deaths were due to traumatic causes. The incidence was found to be very different depending on the type of physical activity performed by people: lower incidence among downhill skiers (0.76 cases/100,000 person/year), higher among hikers (3.97 cases/100,000 person/year) and even higher among rock climbers and ice climbers (6.77 cases/100,000 person/year).

In particular, it was found that 25% of this mortality was due to sudden death, which mostly affected people aged >59 years.

Non-traumatic Mortality During Winter Sport Activities

A more recent review of the literature[8] reported the incidence of mortality due to non-traumatic causes (predominantly cardiovascular mortality, which constitutes 96% of cases) occurring during winter sports activities in the mountains, and analysed the relative risks of the various disciplines carried out (Figure 9.1):

- Downhill skiing and snowboarding (Austrian Alps) was burdened by 0.35 cases of death for non-traumatic causes per 1,000,000 persons/day in the years between 2000 and 2018; the incidence was greater for males aged >34 years.
- Mortality was still relatively low among cross-country skiers (in the longest cross-country ski race, the Vasaloppet in Sweden; years 1970–2005), probably due to the younger average age and better degree of training of participants in such events: 2.6 deaths per million persons/hour (approximately 0.24 cardiac deaths per million exposure days), i.e. overall 1 case of death for every 53,700 race participants.

[i] 'person/day' means the sum of days of physical activity at altitude spent by people before a case of the event under study appears. In this case, relating to the incidence of sudden death, the number indicates that – if there are 980,000 people in the mountains every day – we can expect a case of sudden death every day. If there were 100,000 people in the mountains, we could expect a case of sudden death every about 10 days.

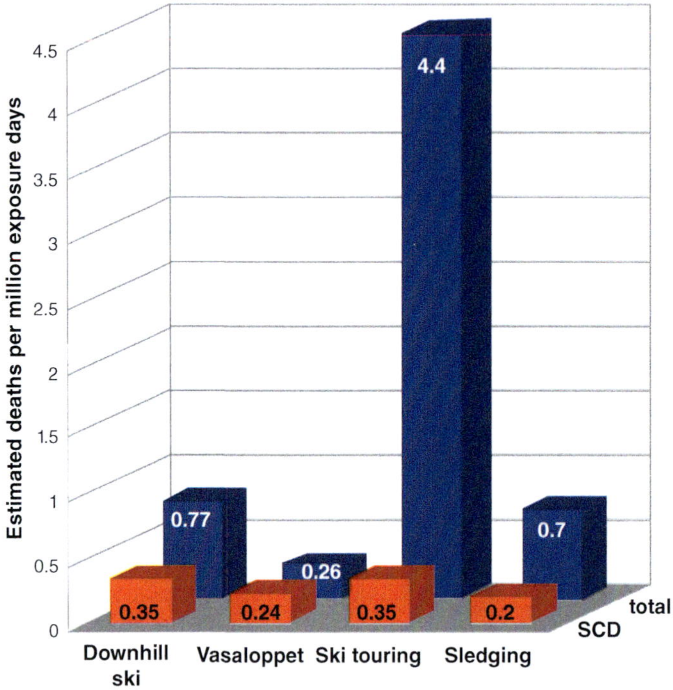

FIGURE 9.1 Estimated incidence of mortality from various causes (of which approximately 25% are cardiovascular) during different types of winter sports activities, per million exposure days; SCD: sudden cardiac death. [8] / MDPI / CC BY 4.0.

- For off-piste skiing (alpine ski touring, backcountry skiing), the risk was high due to traumatic causes (avalanches), but fairly low due to cardiovascular causes in people under 59 years of age (less than 1 case per 100,000 skiers, or less than 8% of the overall mortality); however, this risk increased significantly for ages over 59, with an incidence of 10.4 cases per 100,000 skiers, almost exclusively among males (Austrian Alps, 1986–1995).
- Sledging carried the lowest risk of cardiovascular mortality (although the risk of dragging the sled uphill was also included), with approximately 0.15–0.20 cases per million days of exposure, mainly in males aged >51 years.

Incidence of SCD During Winter Sport Activities

While a good percentage of the people who practice physical activity in the mountains are young, it must, however, be remembered that at least 58% of hikers and 43% of skiers (downhill) are over 40 years old, and that a percentage varying between 15.3 and 28% of these have a history of cardiovascular disease.[4] This is therefore a population at potential risk of cardiovascular complications. The most serious clinical manifestation of heart disease (and – so far – often fatal in mountain environments) is **sudden cardiac death (SCD)**, a death mainly caused by **ventricular fibrillation**; 90% of SCDs occur in males aged ≥35 years.[9] The risk

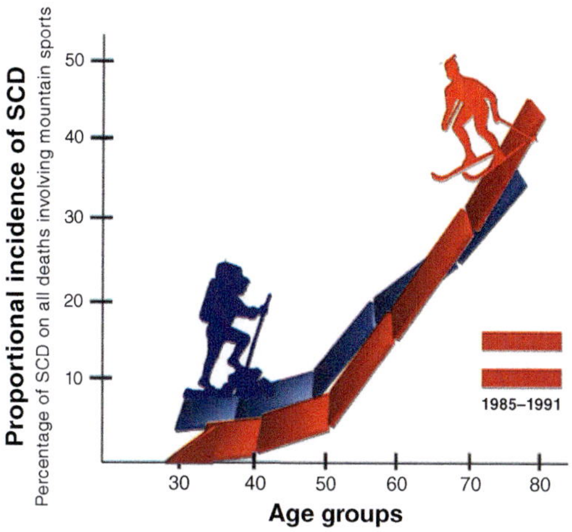

FIGURE 9.2 Proportion of sudden cardiac deaths in various age groups of hikers and skiers. Adapted from [4].

of SCD during downhill skiing or mountain hiking increases sharply with increasing age (Figure 9.2); while in younger males the incidence of SCD is very low and slightly greater in hikers, in persons aged 50 years or more the incidence grows dramatically in both hikers and skiers, with old-aged skiers being more affected. These risks have been found to be much lower for women.

It has been calculated that – in people aged >35 years – one case of SCD could occur every 780,000–802,000 hours of activity in male hikers, while the incidence seems to be lower in male downhill skiers (one case of SCD approximately every 630,000–1,500,000 hours of exposure).[9, 10]

It is interesting to analyse what were found to be the risk factors present in people who suffered sudden death during mountain activities:

- Hikers who died suddenly had a history of previous myocardial infarction 19 times more frequently than their peer control group (17 vs. 0.9%); they had a known coronary artery disease without previous heart attack 4 times more frequently (17 vs. 4%); they suffered from diabetes 6 times more than the controls (6 vs. 1%) and almost 3 times more frequently they had hypercholesterolaemia (54 vs. 20%); they carried out activities in the mountains more rarely (31 vs. 58% of the controls).
- Skiers who suffered sudden death had a history of prior myocardial infarction 27 times more frequently than controls (41 vs. 1.5%); they had arterial hypertension 3 times more frequently (50 vs. 17%), as well as known coronary artery disease without previous myocardial infarction (9 vs. 3%); they also performed physical activity in the mountains less frequently than controls (4 vs. 15%).

But, if mortality due to SCD is estimated as reported before (1 case/802,000 hours of activity in male hikers and 1 case/1,500,000 hours of activity in male skiers), what do these incidences mean?

For a proper comparison, it is estimated that in the general population between the ages of 35 and 70, one case of SCD can occur every 3,370,000 hours;[11] this therefore leads us to believe that SCD is 4.2 times more frequent in mountain hikers (and also in cross-country skiers and joggers) than in the general population, and that it is 2.2 times more frequent in downhill skiers.[4] The difference in the risk of SCD (lower in downhill skiers compared to hikers) could be linked to the type of effort performed and the degree of physical preparation.

However, it must be remembered that even in the general population, even in the lowlands, if a person not accustomed to significant efforts performs heavy physical activity, their risk of SCD increases approximately 17 times (from approximately 10.5 to 27 times!), with one case of SCD every approximately 1.51 million episodes of intense effort (i.e. similar to what happens in skiers).[12] This consideration led some authors[4] to believe that the general incidence of sudden death during recreational activities in the mountains is not significantly greater than what can happen in the plains or at low altitudes.

Non-fatal Cardiovascular Events

As regards the incidence of non-fatal cardiovascular accidents occurring during physical activity in the mountains, data are poorly available. However, it seems that even non-fatal events are more frequent in males and increase in incidence with advancing age. An incidence of one case of **acute coronary syndrome** (ACS) on average every 2,895,000 person/day has been calculated,[6] which would therefore be approximately 3 times lower than the risk of SCD. In male hikers older than 40 years, the risk of ACS would be approximately 1 case per 1,587,000 person/day; the risk of ACS would be approximately four times higher in downhill skiers (males, age >40 years), with 1 case every 410,000 person/day.

For a useful comparison, the incidence of ACS in the general population is reported to be approximately 1 case of non-fatal myocardial infarction every 2,691,000 hours in males aged 35 to 70 years. However, in this same population, the risk of ACS would increase by 1.6 to 5.7 times even at sea level when performing moderate or intense (approximately 5 and 6 METs)[ii] physical activity, respectively.[13]

It can therefore be deduced that the incidence of ACS during physical activity in the mountains is not substantially different from what happens during activities on the plains in comparable population groups. However, it is necessary to continue to collect information on the specific risk factors present in individuals who experienced the events, and on the risk factors that may have triggered these events.

Overall Risk of CV Events

Overall, the occurrence of 1 case of cardiovascular events (comprehensive of sudden deaths, myocardial infarctions, strokes and other non-traumatic events attributable to cardiovascular causes) is estimated for every 319,000 person/day of physical activity in the mountains.[6]

[ii]MET means 'metabolic equivalent of task', that is, it indicates the amount of energy required to carry out a certain job. 1 MET is equivalent to the energy spent while resting, sitting (1 Kcal/Kg/h). Moderate physical activity is equivalent to 3-6 METs (you feel your breathing 'busy' but you can still speak); above 6 METs it involves intense physical activity (difficulty in conversation). For example, watching TV on the sofa = 1.1 MET; paperwork = 1.2 MET; housework = 2-4 METs; walking on level ground for 1-2 blocks = 3 METs; cycling = 4 METs; walking slowly on hills = 4-6 METs; playing golf = 6 METs; tennis = 7 METs; climb stairs quickly = 8 METs; weightlifting = 8 METs; swim = 10 METs; cross-country skiing 11 MET; fast long distance running = 12-16 METs. An elite athlete can exceed 20 METs.

Present or Previous Diseases and Risk of Events for Activities at Altitude

Let us now analyse the phenomenon of 'cardiovascular events' from a different perspective: that is, let us evaluate the expected risk of cardiovascular events in people who already present some of the main cardiovascular risk factors and carry out hiking or skiing activities in the mountains.[4] Some variables have been shown, through logistic regression analysis, to be significantly predictive of SCD.

If a person goes hiking in the mountains and has suffered a previous myocardial infarction, he/she has 10.9 times more risk of sudden death than someone who has not had a heart attack; a person who suffers from diabetes has 7.4 times more risk of SCD; if he/she has known coronary heart disease (but without a previous myocardial infarction), he/she runs a 4.7-fold increased risk; if the person presents hypercholesterolaemia, he/she has a 3.4 times greater risk. But if he/she uses to carry out sporting activities in the mountains for more than 2 weeks a year, his/her risk is reduced by 77%.

On the other hand, if a male subject practices downhill skiing and has suffered from a previous myocardial infarction, his adjusted risk of SCD is 92.9 times greater; if he is hypertensive, he has a 9.0 times greater risk; if he has known coronary artery disease but without a previous myocardial infarction, the risk is increased by 4.8 times. However, if such a person practices intense physical exercise more than once a week, the risk is reduced by 83%.[4]

These differences in SCD risk between hikers and skiers can be explained by the type of effort performed:

- Usually, hikers make a prolonged and relatively uniform effort, whose intensity is lower than the anaerobic threshold, mostly during the spring–summer periods, with progressive ascent and descent.
- Downhill skiers perform intermittent effort, which at times can be intense, with sudden variations between static and dynamic effort, of short duration (1–3 minutes), carried out in winter, in a cold environment, and undergoing rapid changes in altitude.

What are the moments in which cardiovascular problems most frequently appear in people who frequent the mountains for tourism? Or rather, what are the factors triggering cardiovascular events?

Triggering Factors for CV Events

It has been observed that cardiovascular events occur more frequently during the first day in the mountains (Figure 9.3); 50% of SCDs occur in the first 24 hours at altitude. They happen most frequently during physical activity, particularly during the first hour of activity (in 75% of cases) or in the late morning, away from a meal and after little fluid intake. Males are affected approximately 15–20 times more than women; the age at which cardiovascular problems most frequently occur is the broad range over 34 years of age.[4]

In fact, we have already seen how climbing to altitude involves an increase in sympathetic activity, which sometimes presents an abrupt and significant peak of up to 60–80% more in the

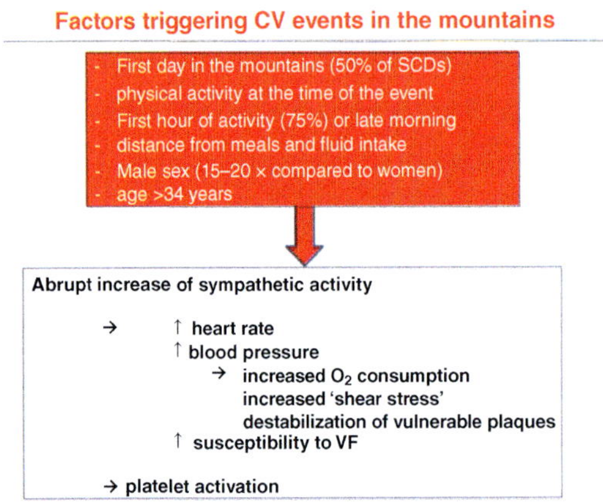

FIGURE 9.3 Factors triggering cardiovascular events in the mountains.

first 24–48 hours (for altitudes of 3,800–4,550 m AMSL, compared to values recorded at sea level).[1] Sympathetic hyperactivity, in turn, leads to increased myocardial O_2 consumption due to higher heart rate (up to +40%) and blood pressure.

Furthermore, the latter factors lead to an increase in 'shear stress'[iii], i.e. the damage caused by the sliding of the blood flow along the internal walls of the arteries, which can cause 'destabilisation' of unstable coronary plaques. These, in turn, can break, triggering a coronary occlusion and consequent myocardial infarction or ventricular fibrillation (with sudden death).

Propensity to ventricular arrhythmias is likely to be exacerbated in the first 2–3 days at altitude; the susceptibility to ventricular fibrillation is also increased, due to the increased 'excitability' of the myocardium caused by the increased sympathetic tone and possible appearance of myocardial ischaemia (as a result of hypoxaemia, hyperventilation and alkalosis).[14]

The higher level of circulating catecholamines also leads to platelet activation, resulting in greater ease of intravascular thrombosis.

Deep Vein Thrombosis and Pulmonary Embolism

At this point, it must be remembered that there is a risk not only of vascular thrombosis in the arterial tree but also in the venous tree, especially affecting the venous circulation of the lower limbs (Figure 9.4)[15]. Hypercoagulability is favoured by the relative dehydration that people can experience in the mountains, especially at high altitudes, linked to haemoconcentration, cold and use of tight clothing and – in certain situations – due to venous stasis (e.g. in cases

[iii]'Shear stress' or 'shear force' is determined by the blood flow and is a traction force [on the walls of the vessel] that acts according to a vector parallel to the axis of the vessel.

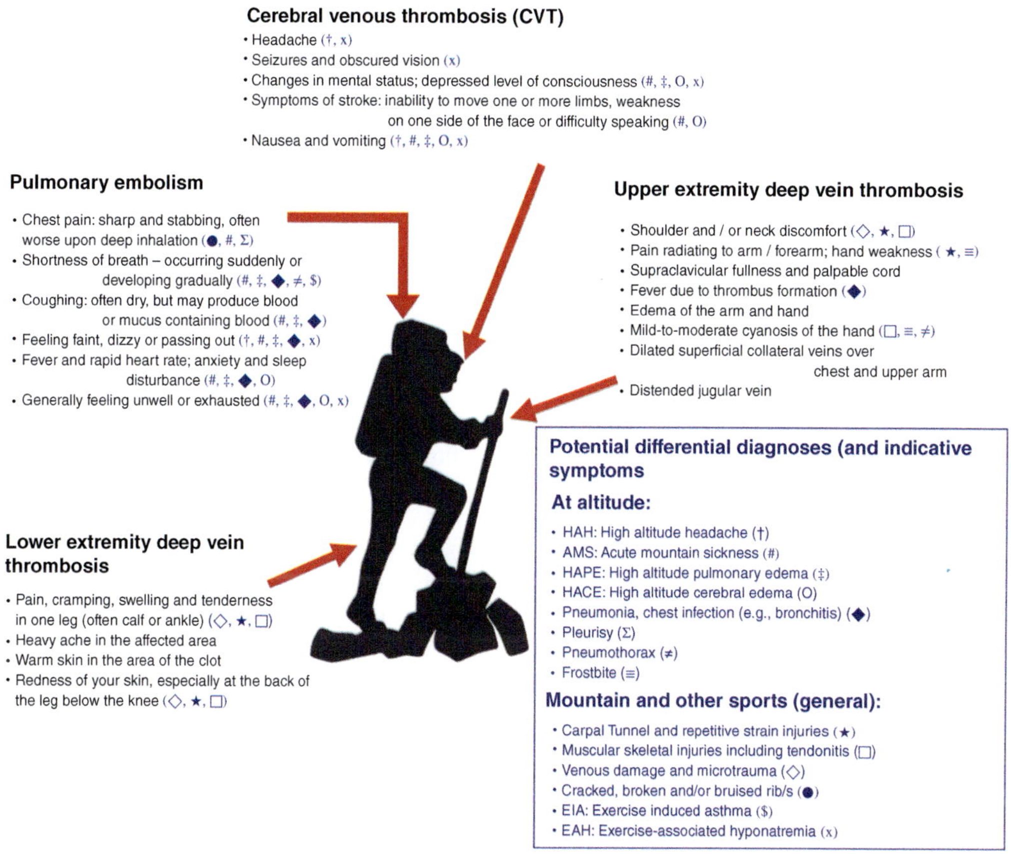

FIGURE 9.4 Risk of Deep Vein Thrombosis (DVT) and Pulmonary Embolism (PE) in persons going to high altitudes. [5] / Wilderness Medical Society / Public domain.

of prolonged immobility due to bad weather conditions). Any trauma that the person may suffer further favours the possibility of (deep) **venous thrombosis** and the appearance of **pulmonary embolism**. Studies conducted in India and Pakistan on soldiers, residents at low altitudes and transported to high altitudes for duty, have shown in the long term an incidence of deep vein thrombosis 24 – 30 times higher than at sea level.[16]

However, it has been observed that even in people with known thrombophilia, acute exposure to altitudes <4,000 m above sea level appears to be safe.[17]

However, no unequivocal data are available for prolonged exposure to high and extreme altitudes, where it seems that both an activation of coagulation and a simultaneous stimulation of fibrinolysis and decreased platelet activation may occur.[18]

In all individuals without known heart or pulmonary disease who present sudden onset of progressive dyspnoea, the possibility of pulmonary embolism must be considered; these people should be referred to a health centre where further diagnostic procedures can be performed.

Prevention of Events

What can be done to prevent cardiovascular events, and particularly sudden death, during high-altitude recreational activities, especially in high-risk males?

Once pre-existing cardiovascular diseases and the triggers of acute events are understood, the deductions regarding prevention are quite obvious.

Before patients with previous myocardial infarction venture into physical activity at altitude, it is necessary to carry out a cardiological assessment of their risk of developing malignant arrhythmias and – consequently – to evaluate any indication for implantation of a pacemaker-defibrillator (ICD).

The medical therapy to which these patients are subjected must be 'optimal', that is, it must include all the drugs indicated to reduce myocardial oxygen consumption (essentially reduction of cardiac pre- and after-load, heart rate, and adrenergic stimulus = beta-blockers, ACE inhibitors, nitro-derivatives), to promote blood flow in the coronary arteries reducing the risk of thrombosis (= antiplatelet drugs), and to reduce the risk of destabilisation of coronary plaques (= statins).

The use of 'optimal' medical therapy is obviously also indicated in patients who are aware of being affected by coronary artery disease (without having suffered a heart attack), or who suffer from systemic hypertension, or diabetes mellitus, or hypercholesterolaemia.

In all people who present cardiovascular risk factors and usually practice little physical activity, an evaluation of their tolerance to effort is indicated through a stress test (or better – if possible – a Cardiopulmonary test), best if conducted in hypoxia comparable with that of the altitudes that the individual wishes to reach. If the tolerated level of effort is deemed unsatisfactory, the affected individuals should undergo a cycle of physical training appropriate in terms of intensity and duration.

People who do not usually reside at altitude or are not accustomed to frequenting moderate or high altitudes should rest or perform light physical activity during the first day of arrival in the mountains; afterwards, they should acclimatise and begin physical activity gradually (Evidence: 1C).

Anyone intending to engage in physical activity at altitude must refrain from fasting or fluid restriction and must – instead – periodically introduce nutrients and liquids in adequate quantities (every half hour – every hour).

References

1 Rimoldi SF, Sartori C, Seiler C, Delacrétaz E, Mattle HP, Scherrer U, Allemann Y. High-altitude exposure in patients with cardiovascular disease: risk assessment and practical recommendations. Prog Cardiovasc Dis 2010; 52(6):512–524. https://doi.org/10.1016/j.pcad.2010.03.005.

2 Campbell AD, McIntosh SE, Nyberg A, Powell AP, Schoene RB, Hackett P. Risk stratification for athletes and adventurers in high-altitude environments: recommendations for preparticipation evaluation. Clin J Sport Med 2015; 25(5):404–411. https://doi.org/10.1097/JSM.0000000000000231. Erratum in: Clin J Sport Med 2015; 25(6):553. https://doi.org/10.1097/01.jsm.0000473552.59434.45.

3 Kelly C, Saxena S, Kelly KN. Degree of hypoxia and physiological differences between fast and slow ascents to very high altitude. Oxygen 2025; 5(3):13. https://doi.org/10.20944/preprints202505.1780.v1.https://www.mdpi.com/2673-9801/5/3/13

4 Burtscher M, Ponchia A. The risk of cardiovascular events during leisure time activities at altitude. Prog Cardiovasc Dis 2010; 52(6):507–511. https://doi.org/10.1016/j.pcad.2010.02.008.

5 Burtscher M, Bachmann O, Hatzl T, Hotter B, Likar R, Philadelphy M, Nachbauer W. Cardiopulmonary and metabolic responses in healthy elderly humans during a 1-week hiking programme at high altitude. Eur J Appl Physiol 2001; 84(5):379–386. https://doi.org/10.1007/s004210100393.

6 Ponchia A, Biasin R, Tempesta T, Thiene M, Dalla Volta S. Cardiovascular risk during physical activity in the mountains. J Cardiovasc Med (Hagerstown) 2006; 7(2):129–135. https://doi.org/10.2459/01.JCM.0000203853.20762.bb.

7 Burtscher M, Philadelphy M, Nachbauer W et al. Todfallrisiko im Bergsport [Risk of death in mountain sports]. In: Jenny E, Flora G (Eds). Jahrbuch 94 der Österreichischen Gesellschaft für Alpin- und Höhenmedizin. Austria: Innsbruck; 1994. pp. 145–152. https://alpinmedizin.org/at/themen/332-jahrbuch-1994.

8 Niedermeier M, Gatterer H, Pocecco E, Frühauf A, Faulhaber M, Menz V, Burtscher J, Posch M, Ruedl G, Burtscher M. Mortality in different mountain sports activities primarily practiced in the winter season-a narrative review. Int J Environ Res Public Health 2019; 17(1):259. https://doi.org/10.3390/ijerph17010259. https://www.ncbi.nlm.nih.gov/pmc/articles/PMC6981978/pdf/ijerph-17-00259.pdf

9 Burtscher M. Risk of cardiovascular events during mountain activities. Adv Exp Med Biol 2007; 618:1–11. https://doi.org/10.1007/978-0-387-75434-5_1.

10 Cornwell WK 3rd, Baggish AL, Bhatta YKD, Brosnan MJ, Dehnert C, Guseh JS, Hammer D, Levine BD, Parati G, Wolfel EE; American Heart Association Exercise, Cardiac Rehabilitation, and Secondary Prevention Committee of the Council on Clinical Cardiology; and Council on Arteriosclerosis, Thrombosis and Vascular Biology. Clinical implications for exercise at altitude among individuals with cardiovascular disease: a scientific statement from the American heart association. J Am Heart Assoc 2021; 10(19):e023225. https://doi.org/10.1161/JAHA.121.023225. https://www.ncbi.nlm.nih.gov/pmc/articles/PMC8649141/pdf/JAH3-10-e023225.pdf

11 Cupples LA, Gagnon DR, Kannel WB. Long- and short-term risk of sudden coronary death. Circulation. 1992; 85(1 Suppl):I11–I18.

12 Albert CM, Mittleman MA, Chae CU, Lee IM, Hennekens CH, Manson JE. Triggering of sudden death from cardiac causes by vigorous exertion. N Engl J Med 2000; 343(19):1355–1361. https://doi.org/10.1056/NEJM200011093431902. https://www.nejm.org/doi/pdf/10.1056/NEJM200011093431902?articleTools=true

13 von Klot S, Mittleman MA, Dockery DW, Heier M, Meisinger C, Hörmann A, Wichmann HE, Peters A. Intensity of physical exertion and triggering of myocardial infarction: a case-crossover study. Eur Heart J 2008; 29(15):1881–1888. https://doi.org/10.1093/eurheartj/ehn235.

14 Alexander JK. Coronary heart disease at altitude. Tex Heart Inst J 1994; 21(4):261–266. https://pmc.ncbi.nlm.nih.gov/articles/PMC325187/pdf/thij00039-0023.pdf

15 Hull CM, Rajendran D, Fernandez Barnes A. Deep vein thrombosis and pulmonary embolism in a mountain guide: awareness, diagnostic challenges, and management considerations at altitude. Wilderness Environ Med. 2016; 27(1):100–106. https://doi.org/10.1016/j.wem.2015.10.010.

16 Anand AC, Jha SK, Saha A, Sharma V, Adya CM. Thrombosis as a complication of extended stay at high altitude. Natl Med J India 2001; 14(4):197–201.

17 Bärtsch P. How thrombogenic is hypoxia? JAMA 2006; 295(19):2297–2299. https://doi.org/10.1001/jama.295.19.2297.

18 Treml B, Wallner B, Blank C, Fries D, Schobersberger W. The influence of environmental hypoxia on hemostasis – a systematic review. Front Cardiovasc Med 2022; 9:813550. https://doi.org/10.3389/fcvm.2022.813550. https://www.ncbi.nlm.nih.gov/pmc/articles/PMC8894865/pdf/fcvm-09-813550.pdf

CHAPTER 10

Patients with Known Ischaemic Heart Disease and Physical Activity at Altitude

To make a short summary of the mechanisms that lead to coronary atherosclerosis (Figure 10.1), let us remember that this is a progressive pathological process, triggered and supported by a series of insults (sometimes apparently modest) on the endothelium of the arteries.[1] These factors can be of the 'toxic' type, as is the case with high LDL cholesterol values, diabetes mellitus or oxidative stress, or of the 'mechanical' type, as in the case of arterial hypertension. These insults lead to endothelial damage and an inflammatory response, which induces increased platelet aggregability and hypercoagulative state, increased parietal permeability and the release of molecules that promote adhesion and chemokines. Foam cells are then formed at the level of the vascular wall, made up of macrophages filled with LDL cholesterol; these foam cells aggregate with each other (and with the T lymphocytes, which in turn support and increase the inflammatory state), macroscopically forming lipid streaks. From these, with the migration of smooth muscle cells from the tunica media of the arterial wall, fibrous plaques begin to appear, made up of a mixture of smooth muscle cells, necrotic debris, proteins and intra- and extra-cellular lipids. At a certain point, the fibrous cap covering the plaque may break or fissure; this ulceration therefore exposes the sub-endothelial components to the blood flow, which triggers the body's 'defence', initiating thrombosis on that damaged wall. The problem is that this thrombosis occurs inside a vessel... and can quickly lead to occlusion.[2]

We have already repeatedly seen, so far, how acute exposure to high altitude leads to a clear increase in heart rate, left ventricular ejection fraction, systemic blood pressure and, above all, increased pressure in the pulmonary artery. The same phenomena also occur, to a lesser extent, during chronic exposure to high altitudes.[4]

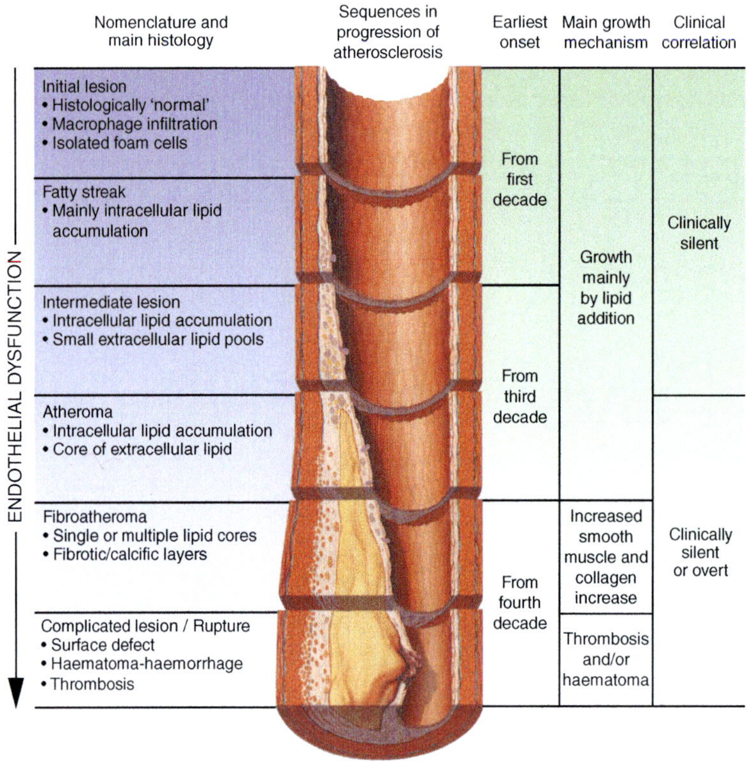

FIGURE 10.1 Scheme of possible progression of the atherosclerotic process [3]. YitzhakNat / https://commons.wikimedia.org/wiki/File:Atherosclerosis_timeline_-_endothelial_dysfunction.svg / CC BY-SA 4.0 / last accessed Dec. 27, 2025

All these phenomena involve an increase in cardiac work and O_2 consumption by the myocardium, which can only be compensated by an increase in coronary flow through a certain degree of vasodilation.

However, coronary blood flow (CBF) can only increase if the coronary arteries are free of lesions.

Coronary Blood Flow During Physical Activity: in Healthy Subjects and in Persons with Coronary Stenosis

In healthy subjects, carrying out aerobic physical activity leads to a progressive increase in coronary flow, which can reach up to approximately 5 times the flow at rest when the individual is carrying out maximal physical effort.[5] Even acute exposure to high altitudes is capable of increasing coronary flow, but only in healthy subjects.[4]

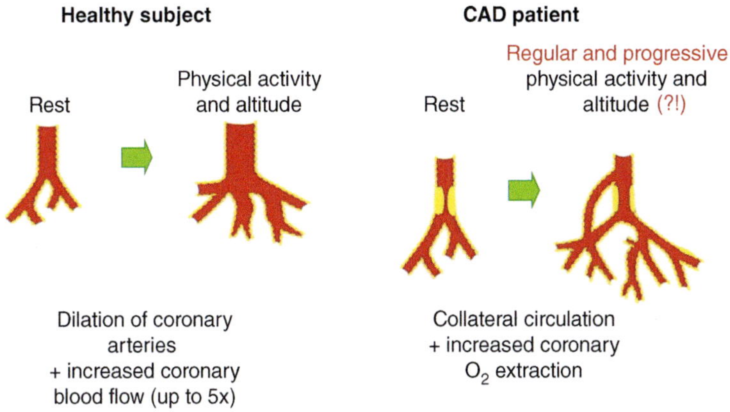

FIGURE 10.2 In healthy subjects, with physical exercise or altitude, there is a dilation of the coronary vessels and an increase in CBF. In coronary artery disease (CAD), only the progressive appearance of collateral circulation is possible.

In response to exercise in a healthy subject, a dilation of the coronary vessels occurs, through a complex series of interactions between neuro-hormonal, endothelial and myocardial factors;[5] in addition to this, adaptations of the coronary micro-vessels occur, which include an increase in the density or diameter of the arterioles (endothelium-dependent vasodilation) and the formation of new capillaries or the recruitment of previously unused capillaries (Figure 10.2).

In a subject who presents one or more coronary stenoses with consequent reduction of the vessel lumen, the perfusion pressure downstream of the stenosis is markedly reduced compared to normal (and compared to that existing upstream of the stenosis) already at rest.

A certain degree of vasodilation is already present (induced by the reduced blood flow to the myocardium downstream of the stenosis), which may be of such a degree that the endogenous reserve of vasodilation may be exhausted; that is, the vessels are already dilated so much that beyond that level they are unable to dilate further.

During physical activity (and – by analogy – also during exposure to high altitude) the coronary flow downstream of the stenosis may therefore be unable to increase as required by the metabolic needs of the myocardium. Due to this 'mismatch' between increased O_2 demands and unchanged or reduced O_2 supply, the region 'goes into crisis', that is, it undergoes ischaemia. This can be further aggravated by the fact that during physical activity there is a normal vasodilation in the part of the coronary tree not affected by stenosis; this vasodilation is capable of causing a 'theft' of blood to the detriment of the area dependent on the stenotic coronary artery (see also Chapter 6).

Physical Activity and Coronary Flow

For years, however, it has been observed that carrying out moderate and regular physical activity on the plains is associated with a reduced risk of cardiovascular mortality in the general population (Figure 10.3);[6] it is also known how physical activity can improve coronary

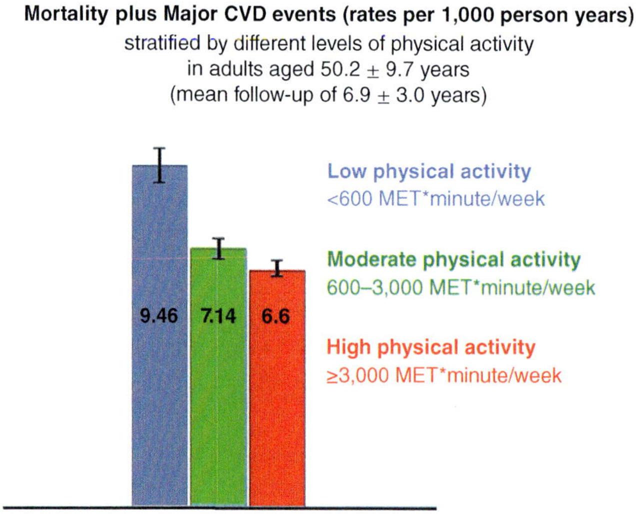

FIGURE 10.3 Incidence of mortality and major cardiovascular events per 1,000 persons/year in relation to different levels of physical activity carried out weekly. Adapted from [6].

flow and reduce ischaemic manifestations even in patients with coronary stenosis and in elderly people, by recruiting arterioles and capillaries, as happens in normal subjects.[7, 8]

Probably, even cautious and progressive exposure to a moderate altitude can exert a similar effect on the coronary circulation, at least according to a few data collected on healthy volunteers[9] and data obtained in experimental animals.[10] Some activities carried out in the mountains, such as ski mountaineering (after adequate physical preparation), have been found to lead to an improvement of the endothelial function and of the tone of peripheral arterioles, and – since they are also pleasant activities – are considered useful for promoting maintenance of regular physical activity in the population.[11]

On the contrary, sudden exposure to high altitudes seems to lead to paradoxical (and therefore potentially dangerous, in the short term) coronary vasoconstriction; this vasoconstriction; however, seems to disappear after 8–9 days of acclimatisation.[9]

CAD Patients at Altitude

To evaluate what can happen in clinical practice, we have few studies available on a limited number of subjects; these studies evaluated the incidence of electrocardiographic alterations at rest and during exercise in patients suffering from CAD, exposed to altitudes between 2,500 and 3,500 m above sea level: overall, it appears that prudent exposure to these altitudes still seems relatively safe. In fact, none of the patients observed showed accentuation of angina or the appearance of ECG alterations at rest (20 patients) or during exercise on the cycle-ergometer (85 patients) at those altitudes, while they continued to present the symptoms or signs of ischaemia at heart rates similar to those observed on the plains (but at a lower workload and at 5% lower double-product[i]).[12–15]

[i]The double product is given by the systolic blood pressure multiplied by the heart rate; it is considered as an index of myocardial oxygen consumption.

CAD Patients with Reduced EF at Altitude

One study analysed what happens to patients with stable CAD but with reduced ejection fraction when exposed to high altitude.[16] In this study, 23 patients with an average age of 51 years suffering from stable CAD and reduced left ventricular ejection fraction (average 39 ± 6%, compared to approximately 60% in healthy people) underwent a maximal stress test after being transported rapidly to an altitude of 2,500 m AMSL; none of the patients developed angina, or ischaemic ECG changes, major arrhythmias or other complications. Another study[17] confirmed that patients with stable ischaemic heart disease and reduced ejection fraction tolerated the 6-minute walk test well at an altitude of 2,000 and even at 2,970 m AMSL (even though they presented an 11 ± 3% reduction in the distance walked).

Another factor to consider is that high-altitude physical activity is often performed in a cold environment. Chapter 9 has already presented the currently available data regarding the risk of sudden cardiac death and acute coronary syndrome in people with coronary heart disease who perform physical activity at altitude. Performing vigorous physical activity at low ambient temperatures may lead to increased thrombotic tendency in CAD patients, due to pathological shear stress on the endothelial wall resulting in attenuated nitric oxide production, endothelial dysfunction and pro-coagulant microenvironments; this could contribute to an increased morbidity and mortality among these patients during cold seasons.[18] Conversely, moderate-intensity exercise, particularly lower-body exercise (such as brisk walking), does not appear to affect coagulation parameters in patients with stable CAD, even when exposed to a cold environment; therefore, the limited data available suggest that these conditions would not increase the risk for thrombosis within this population.[19]

Overall, these observations indicate that exposure to an altitude up to 2,500 m seems to be safe even in patients with stable CAD and reduced performance of the left ventricle, provided that

- they carry out an activity that must be of lower intensity (in absolute terms) compared to that sustainable on the plain, or
- they check their heart rate during exercise (e.g. by a heart-rate monitor, or a smart-watch), so that their heart rate does not exceed what was identified on the plain as the threshold for appearance of ischaemic alterations, and
- they protect themselves adequately during exposure to cold environments.

What has been described above is supported by data relating to acute cardiovascular events which occurred during commercial flights, where the aircraft cabin is pressurised to values corresponding to 1,500–2,400 m above sea level.[20] During such flights, no increased incidence of acute cardiovascular events was observed in comparison with similar populations at sea level, unless they were patients with recent (less than 2 weeks) uncomplicated myocardial infarction, or patients with complicated myocardial infarction less than 6 weeks earlier, or patients with unstable angina, as well as those who have undergone thoracic surgery less than 3 weeks earlier, or patients with heart failure or poorly controlled arrhythmias or hypertension.[21]

Some Scholars have furthermore stated that *the prevalence of cardiovascular diseases is lower in high altitude dwellers than in sea level inhabitants,*[22] and that the favourable effect of life in the mountains is not limited *to those who where born at this altitude but also seen in those who moved to high altitude later in their life,* even though *it is not known whether in patients with coronary artery diseases, long-time high-altitude exposure may have similar beneficial effects.*[4]

How to Evaluate Patients with Coronary Artery Disease Before They Undertake Mountain Activities?

As always, it is necessary to carry out an accurate medical history and evaluation of the symptoms present, and check whether the person has recently suffered from cardiovascular ischaemic events (see above). It is also important to evaluate the possible presence of the traditional risk factors and check whether the patient has recently undergone an exercise test (ideally a cardiopulmonary exercise test) or a stress echocardiogram, or other imaging procedures, in order to understand what the severity of the cardiovascular risk and possible clinical instability may be.

As regards traditional risk factors, an Austrian study observed how – in subjects who intend to carry out sporting activities in the mountains – the greatest risk factor for sudden cardiac death during physical activity in the mountains is given by the habit of being sedentary in the plains.[23, 24]

Absolute Contraindications to Exposure to High Altitudes

The following are considered absolute contraindications to exposure to high altitudes (please, see also Chapter 18 for further details):

- the presence of unstable clinical conditions, such as:
  - unstable angina,
  - signs or symptoms of myocardial ischaemia at low workload (workload ≤80 W or <5 metabolic equivalents) during a cycle-ergometer or treadmill exercise test,
  - presence of signs and symptoms attributable to decompensated heart failure,
  - atrial or ventricular arrhythmias not adequately controlled.
- a recent myocardial infarction or recent coronary revascularisation (events that occurred less than 3–6 months earlier). Due to the increased platelet aggregability observed at high altitudes together with the relative hypovolaemia, the risk of thrombosis on coronary stents or in aorto-coronary by-passes could increase, although it must be remembered that this type of patient still takes antiaggregating therapy (frequently double antiaggregation).

As we saw in Chapter 9, a certain (modest) percentage of people who frequent high altitudes may suffer an acute myocardial infarction or may manifest symptoms of angina pectoris. It was William Heberden in 1772 who gave a detailed description of the symptoms that appear in case of an **angina pectoris** episode: "*Those who are afflicted with it, are seized while they are walking (more especially if it be uphill, and soon after eating) with a painful and most disagreeable sensation in the breast, which seems as if it would extinguish life if it were to increase or to continue; but the moment they stand still, all this uneasiness vanishes. In all other respects, the patients are, at the beginning of this disorder, perfectly well, and in particular have no shortness of breath ... The pain is sometimes situated in the upper part, sometimes in the middle, sometimes in the bottom of the os. sterni, and often more inclined to the left than to the right side. It likewise very frequently extends from the breast to the middle of the left arm.*"

Typical and Atypical Symptoms of ACS at High Altitude

Also the typical symptom of an **acute coronary syndrome** is pain in the retrosternal region or in the epigastric region (Figure 10.4), mostly oppressive or burdensome, intense, sometimes radiating to the neck and jaw or to the back, occasionally radiating to the left armpit and left arm; sometimes associated with cold sweating, dyspnoea, or a sense of general malaise. This pain is prolonged and sometimes difficult to treat; it does not subside with rest, but only with the reopening of the affected coronary artery.

But at high-altitudes symptoms may sometimes be absolutely atypical.

For example, in some cases the pain may appear localised to the jaw and therefore be mistaken for a toothache.

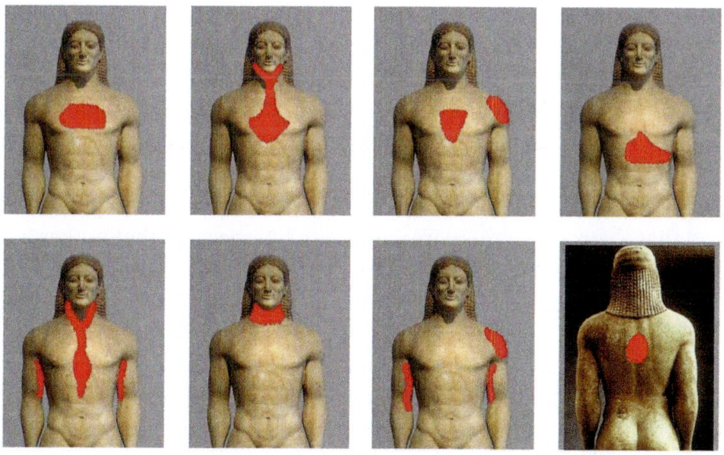

FIGURE 10.4 Most frequent areas of pain during acute coronary syndromes. (The areas are represented on the torso of the Kroisos Kouros, a marble statue from Anavyssos in Attica, Greece, dated c. 540–515 BC).

Sometimes the symptom may be a headache, or unexplained dyspnoea (with the possible appearance of acute cardiogenic pulmonary oedema), or dizziness, which – at high altitudes – can easily be confused with the symptoms of mountain sickness, or syncope (especially during exercise, while sitting or supine). Sometimes acute coronary syndrome may present with nausea, vomiting or profuse cold sweats.

Not having access to adequate tools to allow a diagnosis of acute myocardial infarction (e.g. the ECG is not easily available at high altitudes, even if some 'smartwatches' could be of help nowadays), the suggestion that can be given to healthcare professionals who accompany tourists to high altitudes or who witness dubious symptoms is to consider suspicious for myocardial ischaemia any acute pain (especially if burdensome/oppressive) that appears in the large area between the navel and the jaw. In these cases, it is advisable to alert the emergency medical service[ii] as soon as possible, carefully explaining to the operator the symptoms presented by the patient, the context in which they appeared and the clinical picture observed. The emergency service operator will therefore be able to best assess the appropriate emergency dispatch in order to allow for any reperfusion treatment to be carried out quickly and effectively (Evidence: 1B).

Worse Initial Presentation of ACS at High Altitude

When the emergency service reaches the patient at high altitude, approximately one in three cases (35%, as reported by a French study relating to the coronary emergency service, RESURCOR)[25] presents a clinical picture classifiable as Killip ≥ 2;[iii] this means that the patient presents pulmonary stasis (rales or crackles) or pulmonary oedema or cardiogenic shock, and in 7.9% of cases the patient is found in cardiac arrest. The percentage of compromised patients is therefore more than double that observed in patients with acute coronary syndrome rescued in the plains (about 15% are in Killip class ≥ 2), and the percentage of people in cardiac arrest is almost three times greater (in the plains approximately 3% of cases present cardiac arrest when the emergency service arrives).

It is therefore essential that qualified emergency services reach the patient in the shortest possible time and that a coronary emergency network is accessible that makes coronary reperfusion practicable in the shortest possible time: in the case of myocardial infarction, *time is muscle* i.e. the sooner a coronary artery is reopened, the greater the amount of cardiac muscle saved from necrosis.

In a mountain area, it is of the utmost importance to minimise as much as possible those delays that are linked to difficult or extreme geographical conditions. In the above-mentioned RESUCOR study, the average time between onset of symptoms and treatment was 165 minutes

[ii]The Emergency Medical Service can be contacted in Europe and other Countries, including India and Nepal, by calling the telephone number 112 toll-free; in the United Kingdom, 999; in the United States, 911; in Australia, 000.
[iii]Killip classification of patients with acute myocardial infarction: Killip 1 = good cardiovascular situation; Killip 2 = presence of signs of pulmonary congestion (rales or crackles at the bases when auscultating the lungs); Killip 3 = acute pulmonary oedema; Killip 4 = cardiogenic shock.

(with limits between 52 and 770 minutes). If the delay between onset of symptoms and treatment could be reduced, the short-term prognosis of patients suffering from acute myocardial infarction (with ST-segment elevation, STEMI) is also good in these contexts, with a 3.5% in-hospital mortality.

First Interventions in Case of Suspected ACS in the Mountains

If we are faced with a possible acute myocardial infarction (or acute coronary syndrome), what can we do while waiting for equipped emergency services to arrive?

As healthcare professionals, our obligation is to remain at the patient's side and keep his clinical conditions monitored (with the very few tools available). We must organise ourselves for the possibility that the patient experiences circulatory arrest (mostly due to the appearance of ventricular fibrillation); therefore, we must ask for a first aid kit and a defibrillator to be brought to us (nowadays an automatic external defibrillator is present in almost all Alpine refuges). We must prepare for possible cardiopulmonary resuscitation (external cardiac massage) and prepare for possible defibrillation (Evidence: 1B).

If available, it is indicated to assess glucose levels during the evaluation of a patient with suspected acute coronary syndrome (Evidence: 1B).

It is important to maintain an adequate body temperature (Evidence: 1B); in fact, the reduction in temperature, with the consequent chills and the release of acidic substances into the blood, predisposes to the appearance of major arrhythmias. Cold-induced vasoconstriction (with consequent increase in cardiac work) and possible hyperventilation can promote coronary spasm and also contribute to the appearance of major arrhythmias.[25]

Regarding other possible interventions, while waiting for the arrival of equipped emergency services, if the patient is conscious and cooperative, it may be useful to administer Aspirin 150–300 mg,[26] due to its anti-platelet effect (Evidence: 1A). Caution: check if the patient is taking anti-coagulants because of the associated high risk of bleeding!

Other interventions, besides being problematic from an organisational point of view, have dubious usefulness, such as, for example, the administration of oxygen (the availability of which at altitude is scarce); if available, at high altitude it could still be useful to administer O_2 to a person with suspected/possible ischaemic heart disease, to reduce the frequent high-altitude hypoxaemia and reduce hyperventilation. However, if a pulse oximeter was available, it would be important to evaluate the SpO_2 trend beforehand and during administration: oxygen is recommended in patients with hypoxaemia (SpO_2 <90%; Evidence: 1C), while in patients with SpO_2 ≥90% it is recommended not to administer O_2, as it is not associated with clinical benefits and could indeed paradoxically increase the infarct area (Evidence: 3A).[26]

The administration of nitrates (which the patient could have with him) is problematic, due to the possibility that these could induce severe hypotension if the patient is dehydrated (as can happen in the high mountains) or has a right ventricular myocardial infarction.

It may be useful to administer gastroprotectants (proton pump inhibitors; Evidence: 1A), given the risk of gastroduodenal lesions in a patient in a state of stress, who sometimes takes antiplatelet agents.

Having access to morphine to relieve pain (Evidence 2aC) or benzodiazepines in very anxious patients (Evidence 2aC) outside a hospital setting is problematic, also due to the related legal aspects as well as the possible risks.

References

1 Alabdulkarim N, Altuwaijri N, Ismael L, Alsayyari A, Alsalouli M, Al Yahya A, Alsweirki H. Atherosclerosis (PAD + carotid stenosis), Acute Limb Ischemia. King Saud University Medical Student Council. http://ksumsc.com/download_center/Archive/3rd/435/Teams/General%20Surgery/1st%20Semester/3-Atherosclerosis%20and%20Acute%20limb%20Ischemia%20.pdf.

2 Virmani R, Kolodgie FD, Burke AP, Farb A, Schwartz SM. Lessons from sudden coronary death: a comprehensive morphological classification scheme for atherosclerotic lesions. Arterioscler Thromb Vasc Biol 2000; 20(5):1262–1275. https://doi.org/10.1161/01.atv.20.5.1262. https://www.ahajournals.org/doi/epub/10.1161/01.ATV.20.5.1262

3 Yitzhak Nat. Stages of endothelial dysfunction in atherosclerosis of arteries. Wikimedia commons. August 19, 2022. https://commons.wikimedia.org/wiki/File:Atherosclerosis_timeline_-_endothelial_dysfunction.svg.

4 Rimoldi SF, Sartori C, Seiler C, Delacrétaz E, Mattle HP, Scherrer U, Allemann Y. High-altitude exposure in patients with cardiovascular disease: risk assessment and practical recommendations. Prog Cardiovasc Dis 2010; 52(6):512–524. https://doi.org/10.1016/j.pcad.2010.03.005.

5 Duncker DJ, Bache RJ. Regulation of coronary blood flow during exercise. Physiol Rev 2008; 88(3):1009–1086. https://doi.org/10.1152/physrev.00045.2006. https://journals.physiology.org/doi/pdf/10.1152/physrev.00045.2006

6 Lear SA, Hu W, Rangarajan S, Gasevic D, Leong D, Iqbal R, Casanova A, Swaminathan S, Anjana RM, Kumar R, Rosengren A, Wei L, Yang W, Chuangshi W, Huaxing L, Nair S, Diaz R, Swidon H, Gupta R, Mohammadifard N, Lopez-Jaramillo P, Oguz A, Zatonska K, Seron P, Avezum A, Poirier P, Teo K, Yusuf S. The effect of physical activity on mortality and cardiovascular disease in 130 000 people from 17 high-income, middle-income, and low-income countries: the PURE study. Lancet 2017; 390(10113):2643–2654. https://doi.org/10.1016/S0140-6736(17)31634-3. Erratum in: Lancet 2017; 390(10113):2626. https://doi.org/10.1016/S0140-6736(17)32596-5.

7 Makar O, Siabrenko G. Influence of physical activity on cardiovascular system and prevention of cardiovascular diseases (review). Georgian Med News 2018;(285):69–74.

8 Jakovljevic DG. Physical activity and cardiovascular aging: Physiological and molecular insights. Exp Gerontol 2018; 109:67–74. https://doi.org/10.1016/j.exger.2017.05.016. https://www.sciencedirect.com/science/article/pii/S0531556517301006?via%3Dihub

9 White AJ, Boulet LM, Shafer BM, Vermeulen TD, Atwater TL, Stembridge M, Ainslie PN, Wilson RJA, Day TA, Foster GE. The coronary vascular response to the metaboreflex at low altitude and during acute and prolonged high altitude in males. J Appl Physiol. 2022; 132(6):1327–1337. https://doi.org/10.1152/japplphysiol.00018.2022. https://journals.physiology.org/doi/epdf/10.1152/japplphysiol.00018.2022

10 Turek Z, Turek-Maischeider M, Claessens RA, Ringnalda BE, Kreuzer F. Coronary blood flow in rats native to simulated high altitude and in rats exposed to it later in life. Pflugers Arch 1975; 355(1):49–62. https://doi.org/10.1007/BF00584799.

11 Niederseer D, Steidle-Kloc E, Mayr M, Müller EE, Cadamuro J, Patsch W, Dela F, Müller E, Niebauer J. Effects of a 12-week alpine skiing intervention on endothelial progenitor cells, peripheral arterial tone and endothelial biomarkers in the elderly. Int J Cardiol 2016;214:343–347. https://doi.org/10.1016/j.ijcard.2016.03.229.

12 Levine BD, Zuckerman JH, deFilippi CR. Effect of high-altitude exposure in the elderly: the Tenth Mountain Division study. Circulation 1997; 96(4):1224–1232. https://doi.org/10.1161/01.cir.96.4.1224. https://www.ahajournals.org/doi/10.1161/01.cir.96.4.1224?url_ver=Z39.88-2003&rfr_id=ori:rid:crossref.org&rfr_dat=cr_pub%20%200pubmed

13 Morgan BJ, Alexander JK, Nicoli SA, Brammel HL. The patient with coronary heart disease at altitude: observations during acute exposure to 3100 meters. J Wilderness Med 1990; 1(3):147–153. https://doi.org/10.1580/0953-9859-1.3.147.

14 Schmid JP, Noveanu M, Gaillet R, Hellige G, Wahl A, Saner H. Safety and exercise tolerance of acute high altitude exposure (3454 m) among patients with coronary artery disease. Heart 2006;92(7):921–925. https://doi.org/10.1136/hrt.2005.072520. https://www.ncbi.nlm.nih.gov/pmc/articles/PMC1860700/pdf/921.pdf

15 Yaron M, Hultgren HN, Alexander JK. Low risk of myocardial ischemia in the elderly visiting moderate altitude. Wilderness Environ Med 1995; 6:20–28. https://doi.org/10.1016/S1080-6032(13)80005-1.

16 Erdmann J, Sun KT, Masar P, Niederhauser H. Effects of exposure to altitude on men with coronary artery disease and impaired left ventricular function. Am J Cardiol 1998; 81(3):266–270. https://doi.org/10.1016/s0002-9149(97)00901-6.

17 Vona M, Mazzuero G, Lupi A, Vettorato C, Bosso P, Cohen-Solal A. Effects of altitude on effort tolerance in non-acclimatized patients with ischemic left ventricular dysfunction. Eur J Cardiovasc Prev Rehabil 2006;13(4):617–624. https://doi.org/10.1097/01.hjr.0000220583.27140.9b.

18 Ikäheimo TM. Cardiovascular diseases, cold exposure and exercise. Temperature (Austin). 2018; 5(2):123–146. https://doi.org/10.1080/23328940.2017.1414014. https://www.ncbi.nlm.nih.gov/pmc/articles/PMC6204981/pdf/ktmp-05-02-1414014.pdf

19 Parkkila K, Valtonen RIP, Hiltunen L, Hintsala HE, Jaakkola JJK, Ikäheimo TM. The effects of submaximal exercise and cold exposure on blood coagulation parameters in coronary artery disease patients. BMC Cardiovasc Disord 2021; 21(1):93. https://doi.org/10.1186/s12872-021-01907-9. https://pmc.ncbi.nlm.nih.gov/articles/PMC7885551

20 Silverman D, Gendreau M. Medical issues associated with commercial flights. Lancet 2009; 373(9680):2067–2077. https://doi.org/10.1016/S0140-6736(09)60209-9. https://www.ncbi.nlm.nih.gov/pmc/articles/PMC7137984/pdf/main.pdf

21 Allemann Y, Saner H, Meier B. Höhenaufenthalte und Flüge bei koronarer Herzkrankheit [High altitude stay and air travel in coronary heart disease]. Schweiz Med Wochenschr 1998; 128(17):671–678.

22 Heath D, Williams DR: Heart and coronary circulation. In: Heath D, Williams DR (Eds). High-Altitude Medicine and Pathology. 2nd ed. London: Butterworths; 1989. pp. 186–195.

23 Campbell AD, McIntosh SE, Nyberg A, Powell AP, Schoene RB, Hackett P. Risk stratification for athletes and adventurers in high-altitude environments: recommendations for preparticipation evaluation. Clin J Sport Med 2015; 25(5):404–411. https://doi.org/10.1097/JSM.0000000000000231. Erratum in: Clin J Sport Med 2015; 25(6):553. https://doi.org/10.1097/01.jsm.0000473552.59434.45.

24 Burtscher M, Ponchia A. The risk of cardiovascular events during leisure time activities at altitude. Prog Cardiovasc Dis 2010; 52:507–511. https://doi.org/10.1016/j.pcad.2010.02.008.

25 Chacornac M, Baronne-Rochette G, Schmidt MH, Savary D, Habold D, Bouvaist H, Marliere S, Belle L, Machecourt J, Vanzetto G; REseau des URgences COROnariennes (RESURCOR). Characteristics and management of acute ST-segment elevation myocardial infarctions occurring in ski resorts in the French Alps: impact of an acute coronary care network. Arch Cardiovasc Dis 2010; 103(8–9):460–468. https://doi.org/10.1016/j.acvd.2010.09.002. https://www.sciencedirect.com/science/article/pii/S1875213610001683?via%3Dihub

26 Byrne RA, Rossello X, Coughlan JJ, Barbato E, Berry C, Chieffo A, Claeys MJ, Dan GA, Dweck MR, Galbraith M, Gilard M, Hinterbuchner L, Jankowska EA, Jüni P, Kimura T, Kunadian V, Leosdottir M, Lorusso R, Pedretti RFE, Rigopoulos AG, Rubini Gimenez M, Thiele H, Vranckx P, Wassmann S, Wenger NK, Ibanez B; ESC Scientific Document Group. 2023 ESC guidelines for the management of acute coronary syndromes. Eur Heart J 2023; 44(38):3720–3826. https://doi.org/10.1093/eurheartj/ehad191. https://academic.oup.com/eurheartj/article/44/38/3720/7243210?login=false

CHAPTER 11

Mountain Altitudes and Patients with Heart Failure

Heart failure essentially means the inability of the heart to perform the work necessary to satisfy and maintain intact the various functions of the organism.

From a speculative point of view, we can distinguish the prevalent failure of the left ventricle and that of the right ventricle; but on many occasions the causal pathology affects both ventricles at the same time, so much so that we speak of global failure.

Left Heart Failure

Let's briefly summarise the various clinical pictures.

When the left ventricle is no longer able to pump an adequate amount of blood to meet the body's needs, the patients notice that they become unable to perform those physical activities that they previously did without problems. Therefore, exertion intolerance appears, characterised by easy tiredness (exertional asthenia), reduced perfusion of peripheral tissues (exertional pallor and cold sweating at exertion) up to cyanosis and tissue hypoxia.

At the same time, the insufficient pumping capacity of the left ventricle entails that the pressures at the end of diastole within the left ventricle itself progressively increase and have repercussions backwards on the pulmonary venous tree, and then on the pulmonary capillaries, with consequent pulmonary congestion. The patient will present exertional dyspnoea, initially for major efforts, then for progressively smaller efforts, until dyspnoea at rest appears; he/she will present orthopnoea (i.e. the need to rest with the torso raised), a persistent dry cough that can become productive with frothy and blood-streaked expectoration, and episodes of paroxysmal nocturnal dyspnoea until the appearance of pulmonary oedema.

Right Heart Failure

As regards the right ventricle, if it is not able to push the normal quantity of blood forward, congestion occurs 'upstream': upstream of the right ventricle means the peripheral venous system. Signs of distension of the jugular veins then appear; distension and increase in volume of the liver, which presents with a rounded and often tender edge, and with a compromised function; increased pressure in the veins of the lower limbs, with the appearance of oedema in the dependent areas, one of the first signs that the patient observes; venous stasis also at the intestinal level, with oedema of the intestinal walls, a sense of bloating, digestive difficulties (and difficulty absorbing nutrients and even drugs!), anorexia and weight loss; appearance of ascites.

Compensated Heart Failure

Patients who frequent the mountains (even at low altitudes) rarely present signs or symptoms of very advanced heart failure.

However, they may present one or more obvious signs of heart failure, or they may suffer from a form of heart failure that is still 'compensated' by the mechanisms activated by the organism, such as activation of the sympathetic nervous system, activation of the renin–angiotensin–aldosterone system (RAAS) and cardiac remodelling.

A relevant key point in the vicious circle of heart failure is the important activation of the sympathetic nervous system (Figure 11.1), which has the aim of 'whipping' the heart, trying to make it reach a better performance.

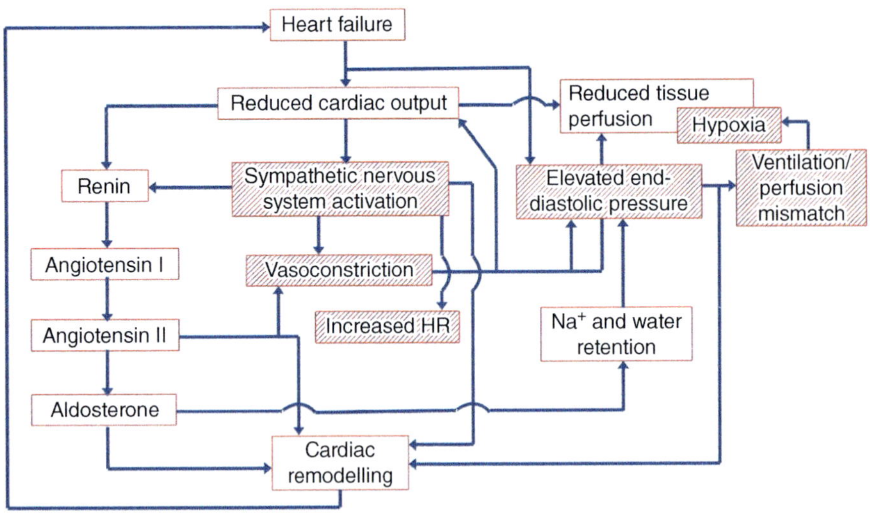

FIGURE 11.1 Main compensatory mechanisms in patients with heart failure; the components that are affected with the exposure to high altitude are highlighted on a red background.

However, we have seen that sympathetic activation already occurs in all people when they go to high altitude. In the case of a patient with heart failure, this activation may be exaggerated and therefore lead to a greater relevance of the various phenomena that we have already had the opportunity to consider: increase in heart rate, increase in peripheral resistance with cutaneous vasoconstriction and increase in blood pressure, activation of the RAA system.

All these mechanisms, when they become 'exaggerated', are no longer useful for maintenance of a haemodynamic balance (the state of 'compensation'): they become harmful as they involve a significant increase in cardiac work (in an insufficient heart, i.e. not able to bear it) and an increase in O_2 consumption, thus precipitating the patient towards frank heart failure. Even if the patient had been in apparent haemodynamic compensation on the plains, upon reaching a mountain altitude (even medium altitude), he/she could manifest the symptoms of heart failure and some (or several) clinical signs that we have just described.

However, climbing to high altitude is not absolutely precluded for all patients with 'compensated' heart failure. The extremely important factor is that patients must take optimal, continuous, regular medical therapy, such as to counteract the sympathetic hyperactivity and the effects of the activation of the RAA system and to promote the reduction of peripheral vascular resistances. Obviously, the intensity of the physical activity that these patients can perform in the mountains must be very cautiously progressive and limited to that which does not cause the onset of significant symptoms.

Heart Failure Patients with Markedly Reduced EF

To estimate how patients with heart failure might tolerate a high-altitude ascent, we have very limited literature data, based on an extremely small number of patients.

One of these studies has been performed by Agostoni et al,[1] who evaluated the behaviour of 38 patients with an average age of 61 years, with a marked reduction of the ejection fraction of the left ventricle (average EF 35%). These subjects, exposed in a hypobaric chamber to atmospheric pressures equivalent to various altitudes, up to approximately 3,000 m AMSL, demonstrated that they were able to carry out physical activity (assessed by a cardiopulmonary exercise test) of a lesser amount than that which they had tolerated in plains; the reduction in exercise tolerance was (obviously) greater in those with greater impairment of left ventricular function. However, what is important is that none of these subjects showed an increase in exercise-induced arrhythmias, nor appearance of any signs of myocardial ischaemia or of acute heart failure. The reduction in exercise tolerance has also been quantified as approximately 4–10% (up to approximately 15%) decrease for every 1,000 m of ascent (while it is approximately 2% in normal individuals);[2] this can help in providing correct suggestions to people with compensated heart failure who intend to go to the mountains.

A second study was conducted in Switzerland by Schmid et al,[3] who quickly took (by bus, in about 3.5 hours) 29 patients with an average age of 60 ± 9 years, from the city of Bern (542 m AMSL) to an altitude of 3,454 m AMSL on the Jungfraujoch. These were patients with a very reduced left ventricular ejection fraction (on average 29 ± 5%), who had demonstrated a functional capacity in an exercise test at least greater than 50% of the predicted (measured by evaluating the peak O_2 consumption during effort); clinically all were in NYHA functional class first or second (therefore in fair physical conditions)[i]. Upon arrival at altitude, two of these patients experienced mild symptoms of mountain sickness. However, all of them were submitted to a Cardiopulmonary Stress Test, which they tolerated well, highlighting, however, a reduction in working capacity: the peak O_2 consumption during exercise was reduced on average by approximately 22%, probably due to the increase in pulmonary resistances associated with the high altitude, reduced diastolic filling of the left ventricle, and diastolic dysfunction of the left ventricle itself. In addition to the finding of an increased resting heart rate of approximately nine beats compared to that found at the valley bottom, only one patient presented an episode of non-sustained ventricular tachycardia at peak effort, while in all the others no increased incidence of arrhythmias during exercise was registered.

The authors therefore concluded that this type of patient with stable chronic heart failure and in fair general conditions are able to tolerate a short period of acute exposure to high altitude and also to carry out a certain degree of physical activity without major problems; however, the authors draw attention to the fact that it cannot be excluded that some of these patients may be more susceptible to the appearance of ventricular arrhythmias, possibly linked to the increase in sympathetic tone caused by altitude and hypoxia.

In fact, an old study (Figure 11.2) performed with Holter ECG recording on a single 65-year-old person who climbed up to 5,895 m AMSL had highlighted the appearance of ventricular arrhythmias (frequent and sometimes bigeminal ventricular premature beats) even in a healthy subject, during the ascent and throughout the entire period of activity at altitude, with subsequent normalisation after returning to low altitudes.[4]

So, there are few studies in the literature that help us resolve doubts on the issue relating to the climbing of patients with compensated heart failure. But, quoting Rimoldi's deduction,[5] '*taken together, available data suggest that high-altitude exposure up to 3,000 m is not associated with a substantially increased risk of cardiovascular complications in patients with stable, compensated heart failure*'.

A particular aspect to consider is that related to the 'ascent' during commercial flights. Also in this case, little data are available so far: they indicate that even patients with stable chronic heart failure tolerate air travel well and may behave similarly to what they usually do during normal daily life.[6]

[i]NYHA Classification – The Stages of Heart Failure: Class I – No symptoms and no limitation in ordinary physical activity, e.g. shortness of breath when walking, climbing stairs etc. (the presence of heart disease is recorded, but without consequent limitations in physical activity. The patient's ordinary physical activity is not limited, but symptoms may appear for more than ordinary activities). Class II – Mild symptoms (mild shortness of breath and/or angina) and slight limitation during ordinary activity; the patient feels well at rest, but moderate physical activity (such as climbing two flights of stairs or climbing a few steps carrying light weights) causes dyspnoea or fatigue. Class III – Marked limitation in activity due to symptoms, even during less-than-ordinary activity, e.g. walking short distances (20–100 m); comfortable only at rest. Class IV – Severe limitations; experiences symptoms even while at rest; mostly bed-bound patients. See: https://manual.jointcommission.org/releases/TJC2018A/DataElem0439.html#:~:text=NYHA%20Classification%20-%20The%20Stages%20of,slight%20limitation%20during%20ordinary%20activity.

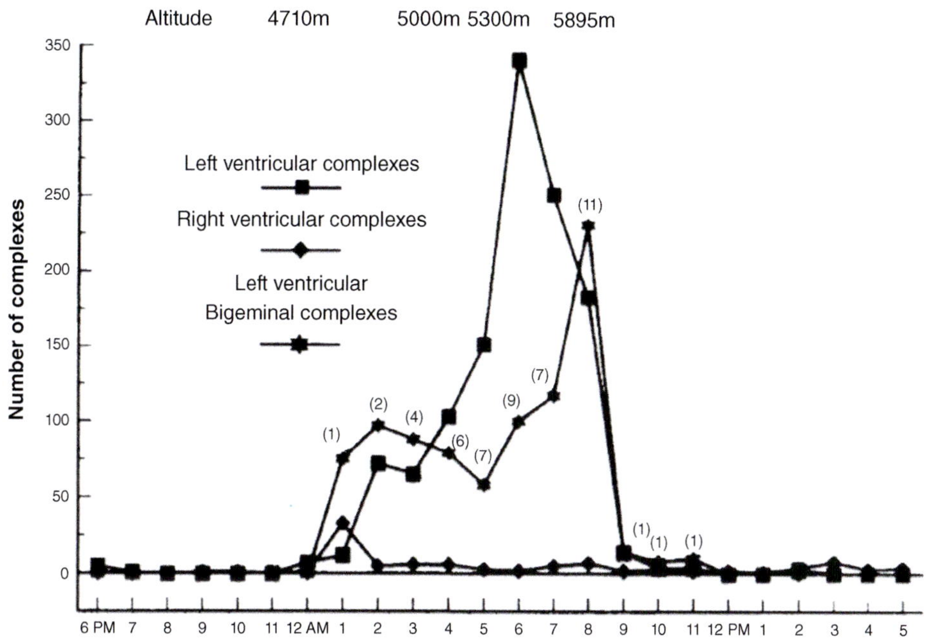

FIGURE 11.2 Incidence of ventricular arrhythmias (squares), ventricular bigeminy (asterisks) and supraventricular arrhythmias (circles) in a 65-year-old patient, in relation to climbing altitude. [4] / with permission of The Texas Heart Institute.

Progressive Exposures of Heart Failure Patients to Increasing Altitudes

There are even observations[7] that patients with chronic heart failure and left ventricular ejection fraction ≤35%, in stable clinical conditions, could benefit from progressive exposure to increasing altitudes, from 1,500 to 2,700 m AMSL, carried out in hypobaric chambers with sessions of 3–4 hours each and simulated altitude increases of approximately 300 m per session over 22 days. The benefits would be both in terms of performance during exercise, muscle tone and quality of life. Even in this study, however, the number of patients observed was very limited (12 patients) and definitive conclusions are therefore not possible.

Drugs for Heart Failure at Altitude

In patients with compensated heart failure who intend to ascend to altitude, another aspect to be considered is that of the type of medical therapy they are taking.[8, 9]

For instance, ACE inhibitors (ramipril and similar) and angiotensin-II receptor blockers (sartans), which at sea level have an undisputed positive effect, can reduce the ability of the kidneys to produce erythropoietin and therefore reduce the compensatory increase in haematocrit (and consequently O_2 transport) in response to high mountain hypoxia.

The use of the beta-blocker carvedilol (extremely important in the lowlands as it reduces the sympathetic activation present in patients with heart failure) has been shown to reduce the ventilatory response to altitude and therefore could have unfavourable effects; these phenomena, however, do not appear to occur with the β_1-selective beta-blocker nebivolol.

Patients with heart failure often take diuretics, which – at high altitudes – can contribute to worsening dehydration and electrolyte imbalances, especially if acetazolamide is added to them with the aim to prevent and treat mountain sickness (high-altitude cerebral oedema).

Pre-exposure Evaluation of HF Patients

What should we do to evaluate a patient with known or probable heart failure who intends to ascend to altitude?[10]

It is generally recommended to carry out a cardiological examination to evaluate the NYHA functional class and the presence of comorbidities (Evidence: 1C), and a trans-thoracic echocardiogram to get an idea of the anatomical-functional situation of the heart, in particular to evaluate the ejection fraction of the left ventricle and the pressure in the pulmonary artery, as well as to highlight the possible presence of valvular diseases (moderate-severe mitral insufficiency or aortic stenosis).

Performing an exercise test (preferably a cardiopulmonary exercise test) could be useful in order to evaluate exercise tolerance and any clinical-electrocardiographic symptoms and signs that may appear during exercise.

Another aspect not to be forgotten is a recommendation that must be given to these patients: to continue taking their usual therapy, without modifications or interruptions, and – it seems banal, but it is an aspect worth highlighting – to remember to bring with them all the drugs they generally use, in adequate amounts. We can also give general indications on any dosage changes that may be necessary when climbing to altitude, (see also Chapter 18 for further recommendations).

References

1 Agostoni P, Cattadori G, Guazzi M, Bussotti M, Conca C, Lomanto M, Marenzi G, Guazzi MD. Effects of simulated altitude-induced hypoxia on exercise capacity in patients with chronic heart failure. Am J Med 2000; 109(6):450–455. https://doi.org/10.1016/s0002-9343(00)00532-5.

2 Agostoni P. Considerations on safety and treatment of patients with chronic heart failure at high altitude. High Alt Med Biol 2013; 14(2):96–100. https://doi.org/10.1089/ham.2012.1117. https://air.unimi.it/handle/2434/235558.

3 Schmid JP, Nobel D, Brugger N, Novak J, Palau P, Trepp A, Wilhelm M, Saner H. Short-term high altitude exposure at 3454 m is well tolerated in patients with stable heart failure. Eur J Heart Fail 2015; 17(2):182–186. https://doi.org/10.1002/ejhf.227. https://onlinelibrary.wiley.com/doi/epdf/10.1002/ejhf.227.

4 Alexander JK. Age, altitude, and arrhythmia. Tex Heart Inst J 1995; 22(4):308–316. https://pmc.ncbi.nlm.nih.gov/articles/PMC325279/pdf/thij00035-0036.pdf.

5 Rimoldi SF, Sartori C, Seiler C, Delacrétaz E, Mattle HP, Scherrer U, Allemann Y. High-altitude exposure in patients with cardiovascular disease: risk assessment and practical recommendations. Prog Cardiovasc Dis 2010; 52(6):512–524. https://doi.org/10.1016/j.pcad.2010.03.005.

6 Koh CH. Commercial air travel for passengers with cardiovascular disease: stressors of flight and aeromedical impact. Curr Probl Cardiol. 2021; 46(3):100746. https://doi.org/10.1016/j.cpcardiol.2020.100746. https://www.ncbi.nlm.nih.gov/pmc/articles/PMC8514285/pdf/main.pdf.

7 Saeed O, Bhatia V, Formica P, Browne A, Aldrich TK, Shin JJ, Maybaum S. Improved exercise performance and skeletal muscle strength after simulated altitude exposure: a novel approach for patients with chronic heart failure. J Card Fail 2012; 18(5):387–391. https://doi.org/10.1016/j.cardfail.2012.02.003.

8 Parati G, Agostoni P, Basnyat B, Bilo G, Brugger H, Coca A, Festi L, Giardini G, Lironcurti A, Luks AM, Maggiorini M, Modesti PA, Swenson ER, Williams B, Bärtsch P, Torlasco C. Clinical recommendations for high altitude exposure of individuals with pre-existing cardiovascular conditions: a joint statement by the European Society of Cardiology, the Council on Hypertension of the European Society of Cardiology, the European Society of Hypertension, the International Society of Mountain Medicine, the Italian Society of Hypertension and the Italian Society of Mountain Medicine. Eur Heart J 2018; 39(17):1546–1554. https://doi.org/10.1093/eurheartj/ehx720. https://www.ncbi.nlm.nih.gov/pmc/articles/PMC5930248/pdf/ehx720.pdf.

9 Cornwell WK 3rd, Baggish AL, Bhatta YKD, Brosnan MJ, Dehnert C, Guseh JS, Hammer D, Levine BD, Parati G, Wolfel EE; American Heart Association Exercise, Cardiac Rehabilitation, and Secondary Prevention Committee of the Council on Clinical Cardiology; and Council on Arteriosclerosis, Thrombosis and Vascular Biology. Clinical implications for exercise at altitude among individuals with cardiovascular disease: a scientific statement from the American heart association. J Am Heart Assoc 2021;10(19):e023225. https://doi.org/10.1161/JAHA.121.023225. https://www.ncbi.nlm.nih.gov/pmc/articles/PMC8649141/pdf/JAH3-10-e023225.pdf.

10 von Haehling S, Birner C, Dworatzek E, Frantz S, Hellenkamp K, Israel CW, Kempf T, Klein HH, Knosalla C, Laufs U, Raake P, Wachter R, Hasenfuss G. Travelling with heart failure: risk assessment and practical recommendations. Nat Rev Cardiol 2022;19(5):302–313. https://doi.org/10.1038/s41569-021-00643-z. https://www.nature.com/articles/s41569-021-00643-z.

CHAPTER 12

People with High Blood Pressure Climbing to Altitude

Relevance of the Hypertension Problem

Is it worth analysing the problem of 'arterial hypertension' in the context of preventing cardiovascular diseases with mountain climbing?

Europe is reported to be heading the statistics on the prevalence of hypertension (as well as of cardiovascular diseases) among its population,[1] with an average prevalence of 44.2% among persons aged 35–74 years (Figure 12.1). Such a prevalence is 60% higher compared to that found in the United States and Canada.[2] Prevalence results are even more elevated in the countries of central and eastern Europe, affecting more than 50% of the adult population.[3]

However, the available data are partially questionable and probably incomplete. For instance, in Italy the available data on the prevalence of arterial hypertension in the adult population indicate that at least one-third of the Italians over 35 years of age have high blood pressure values,[4, 5] and that over the last 30 years a slight progressive decline in this prevalence has been observed in both males and females.[6, 7] However, some observations (e.g. those obtained during the World Hypertension Day) report much higher prevalences of arterial hypertension in the adult population, affecting more than 50% of women and 60% of males.[7]

In European and North American Countries,[2, 4, 8] the prevalence of arterial hypertension increases progressively with increasing age, especially starting from the age of 45, in both males and females; in the age groups over 65, approximately two-thirds of people are hypertensive.

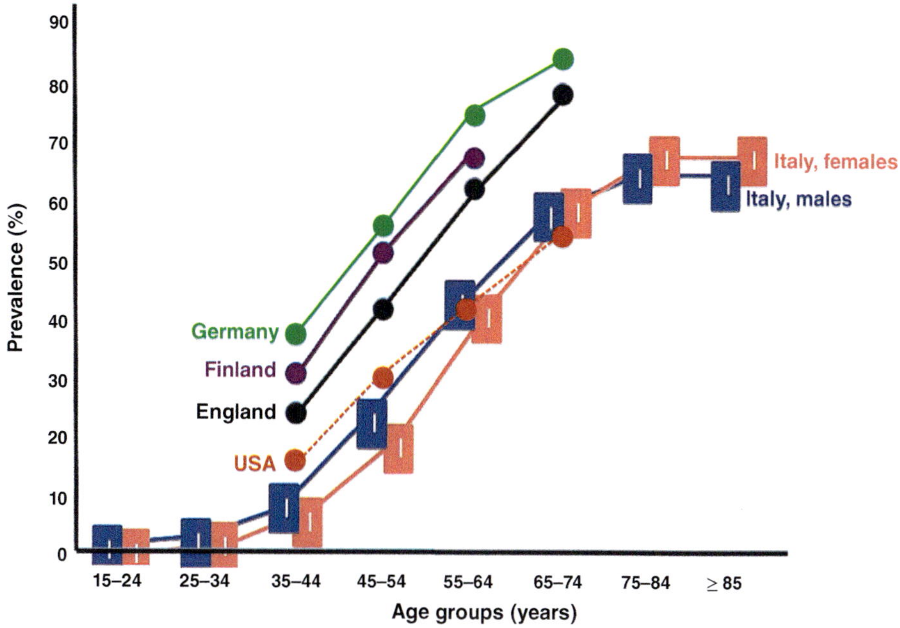

FIGURE 12.1 Increase in the prevalence of arterial hypertension with increasing age, in Italy, Germany, Finland, England and the USA. Data derived from Refs. [2, 4].

Low Awareness and Inadequate Treatment of Hypertension

A worrying fact for the prevention of complications in the mountains is that most hypertensive patients appear to be untreated or treated inadequately. It appears that in Italy, for instance, approximately 35–50% of hypertensive people are unaware of their condition, and that another percentage of approximately 13–18% are aware of having hypertension but do not take hypotensive drugs. Similar results have been reported for the European population, which is ranked among those with the lowest rates of hypertension awareness and control worldwide.[1]

Regarding the percentage of hypertensive people who have achieved optimal blood pressure values (Figure 12.2), an update on hypertension management prepared by Erdine for the European Society of Hypertension[9] reported that only a small minority of hypertensive patients achieve a satisfactory control of their blood pressure levels. Among the various European countries, only 12–36% of subjects (respectively in Poland and in Spain) are under effective control.

In other countries of the World, things are not going better.

It is therefore evident how easy and common it could be to encounter people who discover for the first time that they have hypertension when they arrive in the mountains, due to the physiopathological phenomena (already extensively described) associated with climbing to moderate or high altitudes.

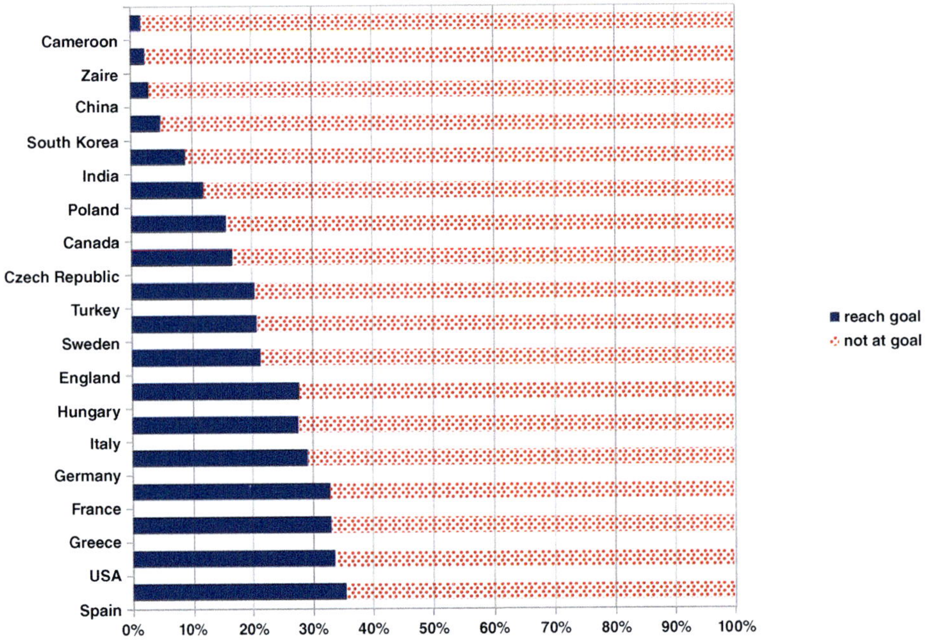

FIGURE 12.2 Percentage of patients achieving the blood pressure goal (<140/90) in various Countries of the World. Adapted from [9].

Tourists with Hypertension on the Alps

Around 40 million tourists visit the Alps every year;[10] a 2022 statistic reports that in Italian mountain resorts alone (of various altitudes), more than 10 million arrivals are recorded every year.[11] It could be deduced that – if the prevalence of hypertension were that detected on the occasion of the aforementioned World Hypertension Day – we would be faced with approximately 5–8 million people with hypertension (known or unknown) who reach mountain resorts of the Alps every year.

Even competitive athletes are not exempt from hypertension; a study conducted in the years 2010–2015[12] reports that approximately 3% of athletes had hypertension, both primary and secondary.

Hypertension and High Altitude

As we have previously noted (see Chapter 7), acute exposure to hypoxia (such as the hypobaric hypoxia characteristic of mountain altitudes) produces systemic vasodilation, which is both endothelium-dependent and endothelium-independent.[13] This vasodilation can lead to a reduction in blood pressure values in the first hours of climbing to altitude. After a few hours, however, this vasodilation is counterbalanced by an increase in sympathetic tone related to altitude (hypoxia stimulates peripheral chemoreceptors located in the carotid bodies), which consequently leads to a generalised increase in arteriolar vasoconstriction and an increase in heart rate, both at rest and during effort.

The net result is an increase in blood pressure, which is significant in the high mountains and is proportional to the altitude reached; the increase in blood pressure results to be also more pronounced in older people.[14]

The increase in blood pressure is more evident during the night: physiologically, a significant reduction in blood pressure values should occur at night, a phenomenon that does not occur when the person sleeps at high altitude. This situation persists for at least the first week (and up to 2 weeks) at high altitude and is also evident in healthy people, as in the climbers studied in 2022 by Salvi et al.[15] during an ascent in the Himalayas; in these climbers, systolic blood pressure showed a progressive, statistically significant but still rather modest increase, with the progressive rise from sea level up to 5,050 m AMSL; the maximum blood pressure values were reached after approximately 8 days of staying at altitude.

As regards hypertensive patients, they are particularly sensitive to increased altitudes due to an already present greater sensitivity of peripheral and central chemoreceptors to hypoxia and to an alteration of calcium homeostasis.[13] It must also be remembered that in hypertensive subjects there is an endothelial dysfunction linked to hypertension, which can significantly alter and reduce the vasodilatory response and instead facilitate the vasoconstrictive response to hypoxia.

The effects of exposure to altitude in hypertensive subjects were confirmed both by the study on Chinese high-altitude railway workers,[16] and by the HIGHCARE-Andes Lowlanders Study:[17] in both studies (see Chapter 7), with the ascent to altitude, the hypertensive subjects presented a further increase in blood pressure, greater than that of the normotensive subjects, especially during the night period.

We also need to remember that – in addition to the described phenomena related to hypobaric hypoxia – the reduction in environmental temperature leads to an increase in blood pressure, both systolic and diastolic, inversely proportional to the level of environmental temperature.[18]

Hypertension and Low-moderate Altitude

We have just reported that the increase in blood pressure and heart rate is proportional to the altitude reached. In fact, we have already seen how observations carried out in Austria on patients suffering from metabolic syndrome taken to an altitude of approximately 1,700 m did not show increases in blood pressure (but notice that all patients were under optimal medical treatment); on the contrary, a slight reduction was recorded starting from the second day in the mountains.[19] Furthermore, another observation conducted on a thousand people living in the Appalachian Mountains in the United States, a predominantly hilly or low-mountainous area, highlighted how the blood pressure values of these people were not substantially different from those found in people living in other non-mountainous areas.[20]

Now, what recommendations can we give to a hypertensive adult who wishes to go to the high mountains?[13]

Recommendations to Persons with Hypertension

First of all, since blood pressure values increase proportionally to the altitude reached, hypertensive patients should avoid very high altitudes, even if it seems that hypertensives with well-controlled blood pressure values can reach altitudes of up to 4,000 m AMSL without particular problems, provided that they take regularly all their therapy (Evidence: 1C).[17, 21] People suffering from severe hypertension or hypertension that is poorly controlled by therapy should avoid climbing to altitude (Evidence: 1C), because they could experience hypertensive crises and the possibility of organ damage.[16, 22]

It is extremely important that patients continue to take their current antihypertensive medications regularly and that they regularly check their blood pressure during their stay at altitude (Evidence: 2aB).

Well in advance of the planned mountain climbing period, they should discuss with their general practitioner or cardiologist the possible indications for Ambulatory Blood Pressure Monitoring (commonly called 'blood pressure Holter'), in order to evaluate the actual quality of blood pressure control, especially during the night hours.

Always with the GP or cardiologist, it will be necessary to evaluate the possible opportunity to introduce therapeutic changes. For example, if the patients were taking the non-selective β-blocker drug carvedilol, its possible replacement with the selective nebivolol should be considered (Evidence: 2aB). Both drugs have significant effects on blood pressure control, but the first (carvedilol) seems to reduce the peripheral arterial O_2 saturation of haemoglobin (a not useful effect at altitude) and the exercise capacity at high altitude (Evidence: 1B), while the second (nebivolol) does not have these negative effects (Evidence: 2aB) and seems also to achieve a better control of the nocturnal variation of blood pressure and allow better maintenance of exercise tolerance.[21]

As regards the use of angiotensin receptor blockers (sartans), long-acting ones, such as telmisartan, have been shown to be able to control the increase in blood pressure induced by climbing to altitude, both during the day and during the night: therefore, the patient (his/her GP) should evaluate the possibility of replacing ACE inhibitors or shorter-acting sartans with telmisartan. However, this positive effect of telmisartan was only verified up to an altitude of 3,400 m AMSL and it seems that it is lost at higher altitudes, since at higher altitudes the mechanisms that support hypertension appear to be very complex (not only linked to the activation of the RAA system).

Patients must also be instructed on any dosage adjustments or introduction of other medications, if they notice an increase in blood pressure during ascent to high altitude. For example, in patients who already use telmisartan, a possible increase in blood pressure related to altitude seems to be well controlled by the association with a dihydropyridine calcium channel blocker (nifedipine).[17] The patients will need to be informed about dosages and warned about side effects.

Acetazolamide, used for the prevention of mountain sickness (in particular high-altitude cerebral oedema; Evidence: 1A), was found to be able to contribute to the control of blood pressure at high altitude, as well as to reduce the appearance of sleep apnoea of central origin. The administration of this drug seems also to reduce the risk of sub-endocardial ischaemia at high altitude (Evidence: 2aC).[13, 17, 23]

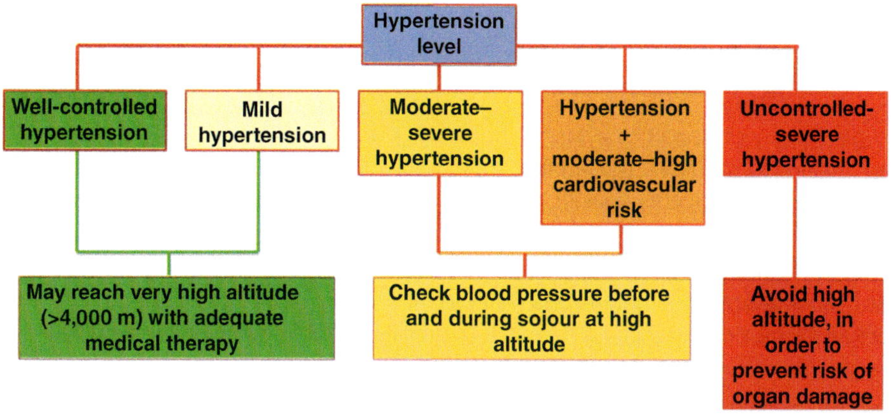

FIGURE 12.3 Clinical recommendations for patients with high blood pressure planning to go to high altitude. Adapted from [13].

In people with labile hypertension at low altitudes, the administration of O_2 during night hours when they sleep at high altitudes may be indicated, as it seems to help keep blood pressure values under control, especially in older people.[24]

In the event of a significant rise in blood pressure that is poorly responsive to pharmacological treatment, rapid evacuation to lower altitudes and to healthcare facilities with the possibility of monitoring and providing adequate treatment is recommended.

An **expert group from various medical societies**[13] has summarised the recommendations, which are reported in the flow chart (Figure 12.3).

In conclusion, however, we must report that no major complications (retinopathy, intracranial haemorrhage, myocardial infarction, stroke) have been reported in hypertensive patients exposed to moderate altitude (a study on 105 American veterans, exposed to an altitude of approximately 2,500 m AMSL);[25] another study on higher altitudes (a total of 14,050 workers employed at altitudes up to 5,000 m above sea level) was conducted on a selected group of people from which those who presented with hypertension ≥160/95 already at the valley bottom were excluded.[22]

Warnings

A report has warned of an increased incidence of sudden death in hypertensive patients, especially during downhill skiing (with an odd ratio of 9, which is much greater than the odd ratio of 1.5 presented by hikers), due to the increase in sympathetic activity related to skiing with possible appearance of arrhythmias, increased cardiac work and increased platelet aggregability.[26, 27]

Regarding the incidence of mountain sickness in patients with arterial hypertension, no increase has been reported.[28, 29]

References

1 Reuter H, Jordan J. Status of hypertension in Europe. Curr Opin Cardiol 2019; 34(4):342–349. https://doi.org/10.1097/HCO.0000000000000642.

2 Wolf-Maier K, Cooper RS, Banegas JR, Giampaoli S, Hense HW, Joffres M, Kastarinen M, Poulter N, Primatesta P, Rodríguez-Artalejo F, Stegmayr B, Thamm M, Tuomilehto J, Vanuzzo D, Vescio F. Hypertension prevalence and blood pressure levels in 6 European countries, Canada, and the United States. JAMA 2003; 289(18):2363–2369. https://doi.org/10.1001/jama.289.18.2363.

3 NCD Risk Factor Collaboration (NCD-RisC). Worldwide trends in hypertension prevalence and progress in treatment and control from 1990 to 2019: a pooled analysis of 1201 population-representative studies with 104 million participants. Lancet 2021; 398(10304):957–980. https://doi.org/10.1016/S0140-6736(21)01330-1. Erratum in: Lancet 2022; 399(10324):520. https://www.thelancet.com/action/showPdf?pii=S0140-6736%2821%2901330-1.

4 Istituto di Ricerca della SIMG, Società Italiana di Medicina Generale e delle Cure Primarie. VIII Report Health Search, Anno 2013/2014. [Research Institute of SIMG, Italian Society of General Medicine and Primary Care. 8th Report, years 2013/2014]. Firenze, November 2014. https://healthsearch.it/documenti/Archivio/Report/VIIIReport_2013-2014/VIII%20Report%20HS.pdf.

5 Torlasco C, Faini A, Makil E, Bilo G, Pengo M, Beaney T, Xia X, Borghi C, Poulter NR, Tocci G, Galletti F, Desideri G, Veglio F, Ferri C, Parati G. Nation-wide hypertension screening in Italy: data from May measurements month 2017-Europe. Eur Heart J Suppl 2019; 21(Suppl D): D66–D70. https://doi.org/10.1093/eurheartj/suz058.

6 Di Lonardo A, Donfrancesco C, Palmieri L, Vanuzzo D, Giampaoli S. Time trends of high blood pressure prevalence, awareness and control in the Italian general population: surveys of the national institute of health. High Blood Press Cardiovasc Prev 2017; 24(2):193–200. https://doi.org/10.1007/s40292-017-0201-8.

7 Tocci G, Presta V. Time trend analysis of hypertension prevalence, awareness, treatment and control in Italy: novel insights from recent national surveys in the general population. High Blood Press Cardiovasc Prev 2017; 24(2):103–105. https://doi.org/10.1007/s40292-017-0204-5.

8 Hengel FE, Sommer C, Wenzel U. Arterielle Hypertonie – Eine Übersicht für den ärztlichen Alltag [Arterial hypertension – an overview for everyday medical practice]. Dtsch Med Wochenschr 2022; 147(7):414–428. https://doi.org/10.1055/a-1577-8663.

9 Erdine S. How well is hypertension controlled in Europe? (revised version). European Society of Hypertension Scientific Newsletter: update on Hypertension Management. 2007; 8:3. https://www.eshonline.org/esh-content/uploads/2014/12/03r_Newsletter-How-Well-is-Hypertension-Controlled-in-Europe.pdf.

10 Burtscher M, Ponchia A. The risk of cardiovascular events during leisure time activities at altitude. Prog Cardiovasc Dis 2010; 52(6):507–511. https://doi.org/10.1016/j.pcad.2010.02.008.

11 Marasco A, Maggiore G, Morvillo A, Becheri E (Eds). Rapporto sul Turismo Italiano, XXV edizione [Report on Italian Tourism, 25th edition], 2020-2022. Edizioni Consiglio Nazionale delle Ricerche, Rome, 2022. https://www.iriss.cnr.it/wp-content/uploads/2023/01/XXV-Edizione-2020-2022-del-Rapporto-sul-Turismo-Italiano.pdf.

12 Caselli S, Vaquer Sequì A, Lemme E, Quattrini F, Milan A, D'Ascenzi F, Spataro A, Pelliccia A. Prevalence and Management of Systemic Hypertension in Athletes. Am J Cardiol 2017; 119(10):1616–1622. https://doi.org/10.1016/j.amjcard.2017.02.011.

13 Parati G, Agostoni P, Basnyat B, Bilo G, Brugger H, Coca A, Festi L, Giardini G, Lironcurti A, Luks AM, Maggiorini M, Modesti PA, Swenson ER, Williams B, Bärtsch P, Torlasco C. Clinical recommendations for high altitude exposure of individuals with pre-existing cardiovascular conditions: a joint statement by the European Society of Cardiology, the Council on Hypertension of the European Society of Cardiology, the European Society of Hypertension, the International Society of Mountain Medicine, the Italian Society of Hypertension and the Italian Society of Mountain Medicine. Eur Heart J 2018; 39(17):1546–1554. https://doi.org/10.1093/eurheartj/ehx720.

14 Parati G, Bilo G, Faini A, Bilo B, Revera M, Giuliano A, Lombardi C, Caldara G, Gregorini F, Styczkiewicz K, Zambon A, Piperno A, Modesti PA, Agostoni P, Mancia G. Changes in 24 h ambulatory blood pressure and effects of angiotensin II receptor blockade during acute and prolonged high-altitude exposure: a randomized clinical trial. Eur Heart J 2014; 35(44):3113–3122. https://doi.org/10.1093/eurheartj/ehu275.

15 Salvi P, Grillo A, Gautier S, Montaguti L, Brunacci F, Severi F, Salvi L, Pretolani E, Parati G, Benetos A. Haemodynamic adaptive mechanisms at high altitude: comparison between European lowlanders and Nepalese highlanders. J Clin Med 2022; 11(13):3843. https://doi.org/10.3390/jcm11133843.

16 Wu TY, Ding SQ, Liu JL, Yu MT, Jia JH, Chai ZC, Dai RC, Zhang SL, Li BY, Pan L, Liang BZ, Zhao JZ, Qi de T, Sun YF, Kayser B. Who should not go high: chronic disease and work at altitude during construction of the Qinghai-Tibet railroad. High Alt Med Biol 2007; 8(2):88–107. https://doi.org/10.1089/ham.2007.1015.

17 Bilo G, Villafuerte FC, Faini A, Anza-Ramírez C, Revera M, Giuliano A, Caravita S, Gregorini F, Lombardi C, Salvioni E, Macarlupu JL, Ossoli D, Landaveri L, Lang M, Agostoni P, Sosa JM, Mancia G, Parati G. Ambulatory blood pressure in untreated and treated hypertensive patients at high altitude: the high altitude cardiovascular research-Andes study. Hypertension 2015; 65(6):1266–1272. https://www.ahajournals.org/doi/epub/10.1161/HYPERTENSIONAHA.114.05003.

18 Fan P, Xue X, Hu J, Qiao Q, Yin T, Yang X, Chen X, Hou Y, Chen R. Ambient temperature and ambulatory blood pressure: an hourly-level, longitudinal panel study. Sci Total Environ 2023; 864:160854. https://doi.org/10.1016/j.scitotenv.2022.160854.

19 Schobersberger W, Schmid P, Lechleitner M, von Duvillard SP, Hörtnagl H, Gunga HC, Klingler A, Fries D, Kirsch K, Spiesberger R, Pokan R, Hofmann P, Hoppichler F, Riedmann G, Baumgartner H, Humpeler E. Austrian Moderate Altitude Study 2000 (AMAS 2000). The effects of moderate altitude (1,700 m) on cardiovascular and metabolic variables in patients with metabolic syndrome. Eur J Appl Physiol 2003; 88(6):506–514. https://doi.org/10.1007/s00421-002-0736-8.

20 Shandera-Ochsner AL, Han DY, Rose D, Aroor SR, Schmitt F, Bellamy LM, Dobbs MR. Comparing the trends of elevated blood pressure in Appalachian and non-Appalachian regions. J Clin Hypertens (Greenwich) 2014; 16(10):713–715. https://doi.org/10.1111/jch.12397.

21 Bilo G, Caldara G, Styczkiewicz K, Revera M, Lombardi C, Giglio A, Zambon A, Corrao G, Faini A, Valentini M, Mancia G, Parati G. Effects of selective and nonselective beta-blockade on 24-h ambulatory blood pressure under hypobaric hypoxia at altitude. J Hypertens 2011; 29(2):380-7. https://doi.org/10.1097/HJH.0b013e3283409014.

22 O'Brien E, Parati G, Stergiou G, Asmar R, Beilin L, Bilo G, Clement D, de la Sierra A, de Leeuw P, Dolan E, Fagard R, Graves J, Head GA, Imai Y, Kario K, Lurbe E, Mallion JM, Mancia G, Mengden T, Myers M, Ogedegbe G, Ohkubo T, Omboni S, Palatini P, Redon J, Ruilope LM, Shennan A, Staessen JA, vanMontfrans G, Verdecchia P, Waeber B, Wang J, Zanchetti A, Zhang Y; European Society of Hypertension Working Group on Blood Pressure Monitoring. European society of hypertension position paper on ambulatory blood pressure monitoring. J Hypertens 2013; 31(9):1731–1768. https://doi.org/10.1097/HJH.0b013e328363e964. Erratum in: J Hypertens 2013; 31(12):2467.

23 Parati G, Revera M, Giuliano A, Faini A, Bilo G, Gregorini F, Lisi E, Salerno S, Lombardi C, Ramos Becerra CG, Mancia G, Salvi P. Effects of acetazolamide on central blood pressure, peripheral blood pressure, and arterial distensibility at acute high altitude exposure. Eur Heart J 2013; 34(10): 759–766. https://doi.org/10.1093/eurheartj/ehs140.

24 Campbell AD, McIntosh SE, Nyberg A, Powell AP, Schoene RB, Hackett P. Risk stratification for athletes and adventurers in high-altitude environments: recommendations for preparticipation evaluation. Clin J Sport Med 2015; 25(5):404–411. https://doi.org/10.1097/JSM.0000000000000231. Erratum in: Clin J Sport Med 2015;25(6):553. https://doi.org/10.1097/01.jsm.0000473552.59434.45.

25 Roach RC, Houston CS, Honigman B, Nicholas RA, Yaron M, Grissom CK, Alexander JK, Hultgren HN. How well do older persons tolerate moderate altitude? West J Med 1995; 162(1):32–36. https://www.ncbi.nlm.nih.gov/pmc/articles/PMC1022590/pdf/westjmed00053-0034.pdf.

26 Burtscher M, Pachinger O, Mittleman MA, Ulmer H. Prior myocardial infarction is the major risk factor associated with sudden cardiac death during downhill skiing. Int J Sports Med 2000;21(8):613–615. https://doi.org/10.1055/s-2000-8481.

27 Niebauer J, Burtscher M. Sudden cardiac death risk in downhill skiers and mountain hikers and specific prevention strategies. Int J Environ Res Public Health 2021; 18(4):1621. https://doi.org/10.3390/ijerph18041621.

28 Rimoldi SF, Sartori C, Seiler C, Delacrétaz E, Mattle HP, Scherrer U, Allemann Y. High-altitude exposure in patients with cardiovascular disease: risk assessment and practical recommendations. Prog Cardiovasc Dis 2010; 52(6):512–524. https://doi.org/10.1016/j.pcad.2010.03.005.

29 Duke CB, Sallade TD, Starling J, Pant S, Sheets A, McElwee MK, Young DS, Taylor RA, Keyes LE. Hypertension and acute mountain sickness in Himalayan trekkers in Nepal: an observational cohort study. Wilderness Environ Med 2020; 31(2):157–164. https://doi.org/10.1016/j.wem.2020.01.004.

PART 4

Other Cardiovascular Aspects of the Exposure to High Altitude

CHAPTER 13

The Cardiovascular System of Pregnant Ladies at Altitude

Maternal Cardiovascular Modifications During Pregnancy: At Sea Level ... and at High Altitude

The **maternal cardiovascular adaptations to pregnancy** are well known since a rather long time. We can summarise the changes that occur during a pregnancy **at sea level**, as follows:[1–3]

- Cardiac output increases in early pregnancy, as a result of increased heart rate as well as of increased stroke volume (+10% in the first trimester, and +20% in the second and third trimesters). Cardiac output continues increasing until mid-pregnancy, when it is 30–50% greater than before pregnancy; afterwards, it remains stable or reduces slightly during the last weeks of pregnancy.
- Heart rate increases by 10–20 beats per minute, mainly during the third trimester.
- Blood pressure decreases in early pregnancy, reaching a minimum in mid-pregnancy (mean pressure reduced by 5–10 mmHg), then returning to pre-pregnancy levels at term.
- Peripheral vascular resistance is reduced throughout pregnancy by 40–70% as a result of the presence of the low-resistance circuit of the placenta, the increased vasculature of the uterus and a decrease of vascular resistance of skin and kidneys.
- Myocardial contractility seems to be increased during all trimesters of pregnancy and is accompanied by the development of a mild ventricular hypertrophy.
- A progressive increase of blood volume (by 30–50%, mainly due to increased plasma volume, with a resulting physiological haemodilution) leads to an increment of the preload that is accompanied by a slight enlargement of the left ventricle by 10–30%.

- Left atrial diameter increases already during early pregnancy, also due to the increased circulating volume.
- Pregnancy is also a state of hypercoagulability that is partially reversed by the haemodilution and the activation of the fibrinolytic system.

During labour, both cardiac output (+25%) and blood pressure increase.

After delivery, cardiac output shows a transient increase but begins to decrease within the first hour to reach baseline levels 2 weeks postpartum. Most cardiovascular parameters tend to return to the normal levels within 2 weeks postpartum; after 5 months, only a mild residual ventricular hypertrophy may persist.

The described adaptations aim to provide adequate supply of oxygenated blood to the utero-placental circulation to allow proper fetal development. At altitude, this physiological challenge is magnified, due to the reduced O_2 availability in hypobaric hypoxic conditions (Figure 13.1). Maternal physiological adaptations occur to try and counteract arterial hypoxaemia and to increase utero-placental blood flow.[4]

A recent study by Bailey et al. made evident that **pregnant ladies living at high altitude** (≥2,500 m AMSL) suffered alterations of the blood pressure course that was present both in normotensive and hypertensive subjects: their mean arterial pressures were higher during pregnancy in comparison to low-altitude women, due to lack of a mid-pregnancy blood pressure fall. They presented a 33% increased risk of hypertensive disorders of pregnancy (gestational hypertension, pre-eclampsia, eclampsia and HELLP[i] syndrome) in comparison with low-altitude women; their likelihood to suffer from eclampsia was 41% greater than in low-altitude women.[5]

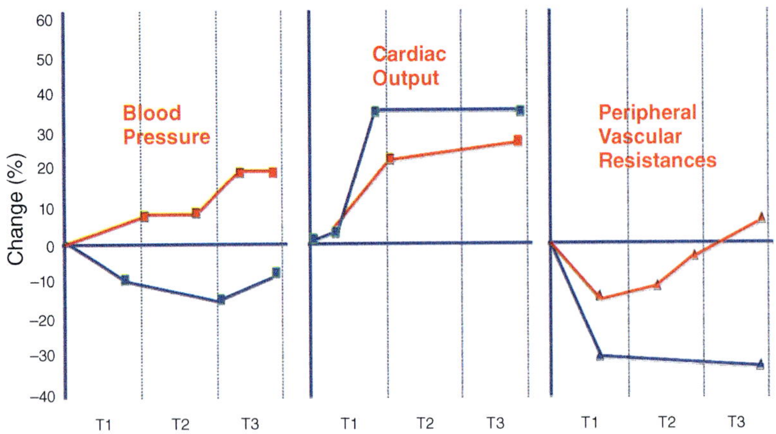

FIGURE 13.1 Some of the haemodynamic changes that occur during pregnancy are depicted; blue lines: women living at sea level; red lines: women living at high altitude. The percentages are approximate and for exemplification purposes only, according to data derived from literature.

[i]HELLP Syndrome = Haemolysis, Elevated Liver enzymes and Low Platelets (HELLP) Syndrome

Birth weights were lower (with twice as many births that were small for the gestational age) at high in comparison to low altitude; these newborns were 9% more likely to be admitted to a neonatal intensive care unit. No significant differences have been recorded in the gestational age or the frequency of preterm births.

Differently to what happens in pregnancies at sea level, it has been observed that at high altitude (La Paz-El Alto, Bolivia, 3,850 m AMSL), pregnancies later affected by pre-eclampsia and/or fetal growth restriction showed impaired maternal central haemodynamics (elevated systemic vascular resistances, reduced stroke volume) and increased uterine vascular resistance as early as at 10–16 gestational weeks.[6]

It should also be remembered that resting uterine artery blood flow has been found to be lower in residents at 3,100 m than in those at 1,600 m, and that flow is likely to decrease further during exercise, in proportion to its intensity and duration.[7, 8]

The above-mentioned studies confirm what was already described in 1999 by Palmer et al.:[9] they observed how living at high altitude led to an incidence of pre-eclampsia that increased with increasing altitude (3% at 1,260 m and 16% at 3,100 m) with an odd ratio of 3.6. Mean blood pressure fell until week 20 in normotensive pregnancy at 1,260 m (as in sea-level pregnancies), while it rose linearly at the altitude of 3,100 m even in women who remained normotensive. However, in a meta-analysis made in 2021 by Grand et al.,[10] it was not confirmed that the incidence of pre-eclampsia is increased in pregnant ladies exposed to high altitude (≥2,500 m AMSL), while it was confirmed that maternal blood pressure was higher at term, accompanied with an increased risk of gestational hypertension.

Placental Hypoxia

The exact mechanism by which hypobaric hypoxia increases maternal risk for the development of pre-eclampsia is not clear. There is evidence that placental hypoxia is a factor causally involved in the development of pre-eclampsia, and it seems to impact on several physiological systems of adaptation to pregnancy:[11] reduced utero-placental blood flow, circulating factors of placental origin, placental oxidative stress and increased maternal vascular reactivity.

The data exposed above on blood pressure modifications during pregnancy at high altitude seem partially to contrast with the findings by Kametas et al.[12] on pregnant ladies accustomed to the high altitude of Cerro de Pasco, Peru (4,370 m AMSL): in these ladies, mean arterial pressure was lower by approximately 8% than in controls living at sea level.

Lower Maternal Cardiac Output

Pregnant women at high altitude had 31% lower maternal cardiac output, due to 15% lower stroke volume and 11% lower heart rate. Their left ventricular systolic function showed signs of impairment (reduced longitudinal and transverse shortening).

Their intravascular space failed to expand to the same extent as the sea level group: cardiac output increased by 17% and left atrial diameter by 12%, values that were more than half in comparison to those found in the sea-level pregnant ladies.

At high altitude, pregnancy is furthermore characterised by greater blood viscosity (+38%) compared to sea level, as a result of increased haematocrit (+25%) and plasma viscosity (+7%); also, fibrinogen concentration increases at altitude by 25% in comparison to a sea-level pregnancy.[13]

Lower Newborn Weight

As regards low birth weight at high altitude, recent reviews of existing literature highlighted a clinically relevant association between birth weight reduction and maternal residence altitude beginning from sea level; the reduction of birth weight has been quantified roughly at about 100 g for every 1,000 m of increase in the mother's residence altitude.[14, 15] There is evidence that in pregnant residents at 2,500–4,300 m AMSL, hypoxia induces modifications of the structure of the placenta, with increased villous capillary density and thinning of the villous membranes (that are believed to be a beneficial adaptation as they increase oxygen diffusion capacity);[16] nonetheless, other studies observed a decreased villous surface area and a larger intervillous space in placentas at high altitude (3,600 m AMSL),[17] thus deducing that hypoxia reduces placental nutrient transporter densities. This situation may act in additive or synergistic fashion to other factors to reduce birth weight at high altitude. High-altitude hypoxia induces reduction of the uterine artery blood flow and impaired myometrial artery vasodilator response; the negative effects seem to be greater for women who moved from lower altitudes to higher altitudes, in comparison to women born and living at >3,000 m AMSL.[18]

In populations chronically living at high altitude, some kind of genetic adaptations to hypoxia are anyway present and reduce the negative effects of hypoxia on neonatal birth weight and height.[19, 20]

Hypobaric hypoxia induces an increase of the haemoglobin levels in all persons living at high altitude: pregnancies of women living at high altitude who had haemoglobin levels >15.5 g/dL showed higher risks for stillbirths (odd ratio 1.3), preterm (odd ratio 1.5) and small for gestational age births (odd ratio 2.1), which added to the other significant adverse effect of living at high altitude.[21] To further complicate matters, it should also be remembered that a percentage of pregnant women present anaemia of varying degrees: below 1,000 m AMSL, less than 10% of pregnant women suffer from anaemia, but at altitudes above 3,000 m AMSL, mild or moderate anaemia (haemoglobin values adjusted for altitude, as indicated by the WHO)[22] affects more than 31% of women and up to 47.1% at altitudes above 4,000 m.[23]

Physical Activity in Lowland Pregnant Women Going to Altitude

If a *lowlander pregnant lady goes to altitude and practices physical activities*, what could then happen?

It is well known that pregnant women performing regular light-to-moderate intensity physical activity at sea level (i.e. submaximal exercise at sea level, like walking, stepping and treadmill exercise) present a series of benefits that include improved cardiovascular function and limited pregnancy-related physical (such as limited weight gain and decreased musculoskeletal discomfort and lower limb oedema), psychological (mood stability) and metabolic problems (positive effects on gestational diabetes mellitus and gestational hypertension) (Evidence: 1B). Fetal benefits are also present with decreased fat mass, improved stress tolerance and advanced neurobehavioural maturation. Physical activity during pregnancy seems also to be accompanied by shorter labour and decreased incidence of operative delivery for women with normal pregnancies.[24, 25]

But is this the case also for activities performed by pregnant women at altitude?

A first thing to remember is that at altitude, there is a combined reduction of maternal arterial Oxygen content and a reduction of uterine flow (that worsens with increasing altitude), and that during pregnancy, anaemia is quite common (a fact that could further diminish oxygen delivery to the fetus).[7]

No study has specifically explored the limits of combined exercise and altitude exposure in pregnancy. Anyway, a study made by Artal et al.[26] many years ago may provide some highlights. As expected, lowlander pregnant women in the third trimester showed a reduction of the maximal oxygen uptake and of the maximum workload that they were able to sustain when exercising at altitude (1,820 m) in comparison to sea level. Both cardiac output and stroke volume showed higher values at rest and a lower reserve (lower range of increment) at altitude. Anyway, fetal heart rate responses to maternal exercise did not differ between the sea level and altitude conditions, thus indicating that pregnant women had some limitations in maximal exercise but could engage in short bouts of moderate exercise at moderate altitudes without adverse consequences for themselves and their fetuses.

The American College of Obstetricians and Gynaecologists indicated in 2020 that pregnant women, who live at sea level, can safely exercise up to 1,829 m (6,000 ft), and pregnant women who live at higher altitudes may be able to safely exercise above that altitude.[27] The 2018 Canadian guidelines suggest that after appropriate acclimatisation, pregnant lowlanders could perform moderate-intensity exercise at altitudes of 1,800–2,500 m but should avoid exercising above 2,500 m.[28] The main message is that a travel to high altitude, especially after 20 weeks of pregnancy, should be approached with caution; the acclimatisation process has to be respected to avoid acute mountain sickness (without taking drugs), and at least a few days of acclimatisation are required before exercising.[29]

The cited studies were, however, conducted in sedentary or non-athlete pregnant ladies.

Competitive Pregnant Athletes and Physical Activity at Altitude

For *competitive and elite athletes* who would like to continue training at altitude throughout their pregnancies, it is yet unknown whether they would have similar or different cardiovascular responses to exercise at altitude.[30] A study on a very small number of elite pregnant athletes (six in all),[31] performing submaximal exercise test at sea level, demonstrated that when they reached 90% of their maximal heart rate fetal bradycardia appeared, together with high umbilical artery pulsatility, and 50% reduction in mean uterine artery volume blood flow;

strenuous physical activity at high altitude could probably lead to similar effects at a lower workload, and reaching 90% of maximal heart rate should be discouraged in pregnant athletes at all altitudes.

Other aspects that should be considered are the increased danger of traumatization of mother and fetus during activities in impervious areas, or in case of sports requiring maintenance of balance or sudden changes of movement. Physical activity associated with high stress, such as marathon running, hampers thermoregulation in such a way that blood flow of the uterus is affected. Excess physical stress leading to exhaustion and dehydration/hypovolaemia (and hypotension and/or hypoglycaemia) of the pregnant woman definitely implies an adverse effect on the fetus.[32]

References

1 Duvekot JJ, Peeters LL. Maternal cardiovascular hemodynamic adaptation to pregnancy. Obstet Gynecol Surv 1994; 49(12 Suppl):S1–S14. https://doi.org/10.1097/00006254-199412011-00001.

2 Artal R, O'Toole M. Guidelines of the American College of Obstetricians and Gynecologists for exercise during pregnancy and the postpartum period. Br J Sports Med 2003; 37(1):6–12; discussion 12. https://doi.org/10.1136/bjsm.37.1.6.

3 Ruys TPE, Johnson MR, Roos-Hesselink JW. Coronary artery disease and pregnancy. In: Gaze D (Ed). Coronary Artery Disease - Current Concepts in Epidemiology, Pathophysiology, Diagnostics and Treatment. London: IntechOpen; 2012. ISBN 978-953-51-0262-5. https://www.intechopen.com/books/2038.

4 Julian CG. High altitude during pregnancy. Clin Chest Med 2011; 32(1):21–31. https://doi.org/10.1016/j.ccm.2010.10.008.

5 Bailey B, Euser AG, Bol KA, Julian CG, Moore LG. High-altitude residence alters blood-pressure course and increases hypertensive disorders of pregnancy. J Matern Fetal Neonatal Med 2022; 35(7):1264–1271. https://doi.org/10.1080/14767058.2020.1745181.

6 Wiegel RE, Baker K, Calderon-Toledo C, Gomez R, Gutiérrez-Cortez S, Houck JA, Larrea A, Lazo-Vega L, Moore LG, Pisc J, Toledo-Jaldin L, Julian CG. Impaired maternal central hemodynamics precede the onset of vascular disorders of pregnancy at high altitude. Am J Physiol Heart Circ Physiol 2025; 328(1):H174–H185. https://doi.org/10.1152/ajpheart.00520.2024.

7 Entin PL, Coffin L. Physiological basis for recommendations regarding exercise during pregnancy at high altitude. High Alt Med Biol 2004; 5(3):321–334. https://doi.org/10.1089/ham.2004.5.321.

8 Lorca RA, Lane SL, Bales ES, Nsier H, Yi H, Donnelly MA, Euser AG, Julian CG, Moore LG. High altitude reduces NO-dependent myometrial artery vasodilator response during pregnancy. Hypertension 2019; 73(6):1319–1326. https://doi.org/10.1161/HYPERTENSIONAHA.119.12641.

9 Palmer SK, Moore LG, Young D, Cregger B, Berman JC, Zamudio S. Altered blood pressure course during normal pregnancy and increased preeclampsia at high altitude (3100 meters) in Colorado. Am J Obstet Gynecol 1999; 180(5):1161–1168. https://doi.org/10.1016/s0002-9378(99)70611-3.

10 Grant ID, Giussani DA, Aiken CE. Blood pressure and hypertensive disorders of pregnancy at high altitude: a systematic review and meta-analysis. Am J Obstet Gynecol MFM 2021; 3(5):100400. https://doi.org/10.1016/j.ajogmf.2021.100400.

11 Zamudio S. High-altitude hypoxia and preeclampsia. Front Biosci. 2007;12:2967–2977. https://doi.org/10.2741/2286. https://pmc.ncbi.nlm.nih.gov/articles/PMC6428070/pdf/nihms-31956.pdf.

12 Kametas NA, McAuliffe F, Krampl E, Chambers J, Nicolaides KH. Maternal cardiac function during pregnancy at high altitude. BJOG 2004; 111(10):1051–1058. https://doi.org/10.1111/j.1471-0528.2004.00246.x.

13 Kametas NA, Krampl E, McAuliffe F, Rampling MW, Nicolaides KH. Pregnancy at high altitude: a hyperviscosity state. Acta Obstet Gynecol Scand 2004;83(7):627–633. https://doi.org/10.1111/j.0001-6349.2004.00434.x.

14 Grant ID, Giussani DA, Aiken CE. Fetal growth and spontaneous preterm birth in high-altitude pregnancy: a systematic review, meta-analysis, and meta-regression. Int J Gynaecol Obstet 2022; 157(2):221–229. https://doi.org/10.1002/ijgo.13779.

15 Yang L, Helbich-Poschacher V, Cao C, Klebermass-Schrehof K, Waldhoer T. Maternal altitude and risk of low birthweight: A systematic review and meta-analyses. Placenta 2020; 101:124–131. https://doi.org/10.1016/j.placenta.2020.09.010.

16 Zamudio S. The placenta at high altitude. High Alt Med Biol 2003; 4(2):171–191. https://doi.org/10.1089/152702903322022785.

17 Mayhew TM, Bowles C, Yücel F. Hypobaric hypoxia and villous trophoblast: evidence that human pregnancy at high altitude (3600 m) perturbs epithelial turnover and coagulation-fibrinolysis in the intervillous space. Placenta 2002; 23 (2–3):154–162. https://doi.org/10.1053/plac.2001.0775.

18 Gonzales GF. Impacto de la altura en el embarazo y en el producto de la gestación [Impact of high altitude on pregnancy and newborn parameters]. Rev Peru Med Exp Salud Publica 2012; 29(2): 242–249. Spanish. https://doi.org/10.1590/s1726-46342012000200013.

19 Julian CG, Vargas E, Armaza JF, Wilson MJ, Niermeyer S, Moore LG. High-altitude ancestry protects against hypoxia-associated reductions in fetal growth. Arch Dis Child Fetal Neonatal Ed 2007; 92(5):F372–F377. https://doi.org/10.1136/adc.2006.109579.

20 Rothhammer F, Fuentes-Guajardo M, Chakraborty R, Lorenzo Bermejo J, Dittmar M. Neonatal variables, altitude of residence and Aymara ancestry in northern Chile. PLoS One 2015;10(4):e0121834. https://doi.org/10.1371/journal.pone.0121834.

21 Gonzales GF, Steenland K, Tapia V. Maternal hemoglobin level and fetal outcome at low and high altitudes. Am J Physiol Regul Integr Comp Physiol 2009; 297(5):R1477–R1485. https://doi.org/10.1152/ajpregu.00275.2009.

22 World Health Organization. Haemoglobin concentrations for the diagnosis of anaemia and assessment of severity. World Health Organization. 2011; document WHO/NMH/NHD/MNM/11.1. https://iris.who.int/handle/10665/85839.

23 Muñoz del Carpio Toia A, Alarcón Yaquetto DE, Álvarez Cervantes G, Sánchez Guillén JC, Cornejo Roselló I, Rojas Pauca S, Iparraguirre Meza M, Cóndor Privat MH, Diaz del Olmo Calvo F, Bernabé Ortiz JC, Zubieta Calleja G. Anemia in pregnant women residing at different geographical altitudes in Arequipa, Peru. Rev Cuban Invest Bioméd 2023;42:e2084. http://scielo.sld.cu/pdf/ibi/v42/1561-3011-ibi-42-e2084.pdf.

24 Melzer K, Schutz Y, Boulvain M, Kayser B. Physical activity and pregnancy: cardiovascular adaptations, recommendations and pregnancy outcomes. Sports Med 2010; 40(6):493–507. https://doi.org/10.2165/11532290-000000000-00000.

25 Nascimento SL, Surita FG, Cecatti JG. Physical exercise during pregnancy: a systematic review. Curr Opin Obstet Gynecol 2012; 24(6):387–394. https://doi.org/10.1097/GCO.0b013e328359f131.

26 Artal R, Fortunato V, Welton A, Constantino N, Khodiguian N, Villalobos L, Wiswell R. A comparison of cardiopulmonary adaptations to exercise in pregnancy at sea level and altitude. Am J Obstet Gynecol 1995; 172(4 Pt 1):1170–1178; discussion 1178-80. https://doi.org/10.1016/0002-9378(95)91475-7.

27 Physical Activity and Exercise During Pregnancy and the Postpartum Period: ACOG Committee Opinion Summary, Number 804. Obstet Gynecol 2020; 135(4):991–993. https://doi.org/10.1097/AOG.0000000000003773.

28 Mottola MF, Davenport MH, Ruchat SM, Davies GA, Poitras VJ, Gray CE, Jaramillo Garcia A, Barrowman N, Adamo KB, Duggan M, Barakat R, Chilibeck P, Fleming K, Forte M, Korolnek J, Nagpal T, Slater LG, Stirling D, Zehr L. 2019 Canadian guideline for physical activity throughout pregnancy. Br J Sports Med 2018; 52(21):1339–1346. https://doi.org/10.1136/bjsports-2018-100056.

29 Jean D, Moore LG. Travel to high altitude during pregnancy: frequently asked questions and recommendations for clinicians. High Alt Med Biol 2012; 13(2):73–81. https://doi.org/10.1089/ham.2012.

30 McManis BG. Integrative review of exercise at altitude during pregnancy. Int J Environ Res Public Health 2021; 18(17):9272. https://doi.org/10.3390/ijerph18179272.

31 Salvesen KÅ, Hem E, Sundgot-Borgen J. Fetal wellbeing may be compromised during strenuous exercise among pregnant elite athletes. Br J Sports Med 2012; 46(4):279–283. https://doi.org/10.1136/bjsm.2010.080259.

32 Huch R. Reisen, Sport und Schwangerschaft [Travel, sports and pregnancy]. Geburtshilfe Frauenheilkd. 1985; 45(3):140–146. German. https://doi.org/10.1055/s-2008-1036221.

CHAPTER 14

Newborns and Children at High Altitude

After birth, during the first moments of life outside of the uterus, the **newborn's cardiovascular system** begins a series of dramatic changes that usually are completed in the first few days (up to the thirtieth day) of life. The most distinct feature is the rapid passage from the fetal pattern of both ventricles working in parallel to the newborn pattern of ventricles working in serial manner, under physiological conditions.

Besides the rapid closure of the umbilical veins that had brought oxygen and nutrients from the placenta during intrauterine life, the transition from the fetal to the neonatal circulatory pattern is immediately triggered by the newborn's first breath. With the inflation of the lungs, the blood pressure drops rapidly inside the pulmonary system, as well as in the right atrium and ventricle.[1] The inspiration of air (with its O_2 concentration) ensues a further significant fall of the *pulmonary vascular resistances*; arterial oxygen saturation increases from 60 to 70% at 1 minute to above 90% within 10 minutes following delivery.[2] The rise of PO_2 seems to be the most important mechanism for the reduction of the pulmonary vascular resistances and the increase of the pulmonary blood flow, which passes from about 35 ml/kg/min during intrauterine life to 160–200 ml/kg/min within a few minutes after birth.[3] A subsequent progressive regression of the medial muscle layer of the pulmonary arterioles allows further gradual and delayed reduction of the pulmonary vascular resistance and pulmonary artery pressure within 6–8 weeks after birth.

During intrauterine life, the *foramen ovale* had allowed the oxygenated blood coming from the placenta to pass from the right atrium to the left atrium and then to the systemic circulation (Figure 14.1); immediately after birth,[4] with the important drop of the pressure in the right circulation and the concomitant increase in systemic resistances (loss of the low-resistance placental circulation after the clamping of umbilical cord and release of catecholamines, renin, angiotensin and vasopressin during labour contractions) and increase in left atrial filling (increased pulmonary venous return), the flow of blood tends to reverse transiently through the foramen ovale, moving from the left to the right atrium. At this moment, the membrane of the foramen ovale is pushed to approach the foramen and then to adhere to its rims, causing its closure and abolishing right-to-left atrial flow. Within 1 year, the tissue

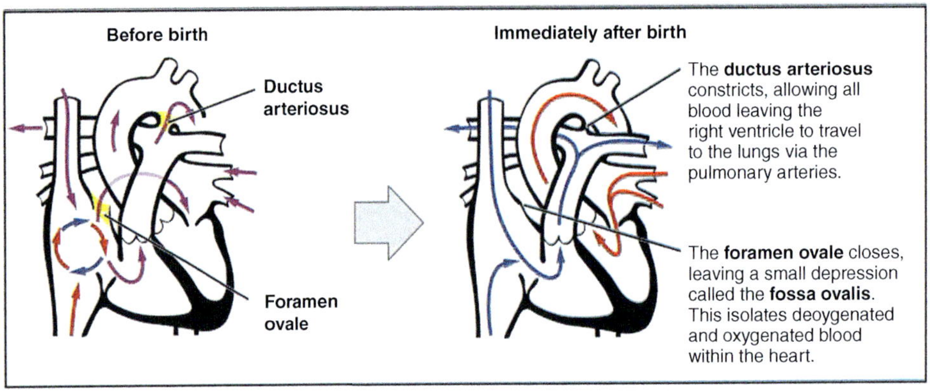

FIGURE 14.1 The newborn's circulatory system reconfigures immediately after birth: foramen ovale and ductus arteriosus close allowing separation between deoxygenated and oxygenated blood flows [5]. Oregon State University / https://open.oregonstate.education/anatomy2e/chapter/adjustments-infant-birth-postnatal/ / CC BY-SA 4.0 / last accessed Dec. 26, 2025.

flaps usually (in a great majority of infants) fuse over the shunt, turning the foramen ovale into the fossa ovalis.

During intrauterine life, the greatest part of the flow ejected by the right ventricle was shunted through the *ductus arteriosus* towards the descending aorta and towards the placenta. Immediately after birth, the pattern of flow through the ductus arteriosus is significantly altered, as lung compliance improves, pulmonary vascular resistance decreases and systemic vascular resistance increases; with the increase of the oxygen concentration of the blood passing through the ductus, it begins constricting (definitely beginning for PO_2 over 40–50 mmHg and being intensely constricted for PO_2 of 120–150 mmHg)[3] and then closes, becoming the ligamentum arteriosum. With the closure of the ductus arteriosus, which typically occurs within 24–48 hours of birth, the pulmonary artery pressure declines further. The response of the ductus arteriosus to Oxygen is highly related to the gestational age of the fetus: with advancing gestational age, the responsiveness to Oxygen and the magnitude of constriction increase.

With the closure of both foramen ovale and ductus arteriosus, all the blood returning from the periphery to the right atrium and the right ventricle is thus pumped through the pulmonary vessels, is oxygenated and reaches the left atrium and the systemic circulation without mixing with non-oxygenated blood.

Immediately after birth, there is also a significant increase of the *left ventricular (LV) output*, correlated to:

- increased heart rate,
- increased LV volume linked to increased return from the pulmonary circulation,
- increased contractility linked to the circulating catecholamines and
- increased LV compliance linked to the decreased volume of the right ventricle.

Over the first 1–2 days after birth, the high LV output decreases in relation to the constriction of the ductus arteriosus and, therefore, to the reduced venous return to the left atrium.[2]

Changes of the Newborn's Cardiovascular System at High Altitude

What has been described above is what happens in newborns at sea level. But what could be the evolution of the *circulation in newborns at high altitude*, in a hypobaric hypoxic environment?

When an infant is born at high altitude, a significant reduction of SaO_2 is present in comparison to newborns at sea level; the reduction shows a statistically significant gradient with higher altitudes, especially at altitudes of 2,250 m AMSL or more.[6] For an infant who continues to live at high altitude, the low fraction of O_2 in the inspired air and the consequent reduction of SaO_2 influence significantly the maturation of the *pulmonary vessels*. Although there is a great interpersonal variation, a close relationship has been identified between altitude of residence and the effects on the pulmonary vessels, which show persistence of the medial muscle with associated high pulmonary vascular resistance (and – thus – elevated pulmonary artery pressure).

Chronic hypobaric hypoxia for 3 days in newborn experimental animals (51 kPa, i.e. 382 mmHg, corresponding to more than 5,000 m AMSL) was associated with abnormal structural remodelling of the pulmonary vasculature.[7]

Pulmonary Vasculature Maturation and Pulmonary Pressure

Due to the great amount of medial smooth muscle in infants (greater than that present in older children), even relatively mild degrees of chronic hypoxia are sufficient to alter the normal pattern of pulmonary vascular maturation.[3] Thus, in newborns at high altitude, the fall of pulmonary arterial pressure during the first 3 days of life is less marked than at sea level. If the individual continues living in a high-altitude hypoxic environment, the increased pulmonary vascular resistance persists throughout childhood and adult life (although it is slowly reversible if the individual moves to live at sea level, as exposed in Chapter 6). The risk for chronic hypoxaemia and increased pulmonary resistance in children living at high elevations is modified also by other factors, such as nutrition, intercurrent lower respiratory infections, exposure to pollutants and toxins, socioeconomic status and access to medical care.[8]

It must be taken into account that there are also genetically inherited factors that lend protection to newborns against hypoxaemia at high altitudes: in Tibet, Niermeyer et al. found lower O_2 saturation values in infants born to Chinese Han immigrant mothers compared to the indigenous Tibetan infants.[9] The two groups of newborns showed differences in the susceptibility to the development of pulmonary artery hypertension, with evidence of medial hypertrophy of small pulmonary arteries, muscularisation of pulmonary arterioles and severe right ventricular hypertrophy and dilation in the Han infants at 4 months of age.

We must add also another observation about neonatal pulmonary hypertension and pulmonary vascular maturation. We have seen that pregnancies are affected by pre-eclampsia more frequently at high altitude: pre-eclampsia with fetal growth restriction is associated with increased fetal hypoxia that may impede normal development of the pulmonary circulation and may lead to adverse neonatal pulmonary vascular outcomes. Thus, birth to a pre-eclampsia woman at high altitude increases the risk of pulmonary hypertension in the neonate (but not later in infancy).[10] Other studies suggest that perinatal hypoxia could be associated with higher risk of excessive erythrocytosis[11] that could persist even in adult life, perhaps due to a disruption of the normal alveolarisation and microvascular development that lead to chronic impairment of gas exchange and/or pulmonary hypertension.[12]

Hypobaric Hypoxia and Ductus Arteriosus

In people born and continuing to live at high altitude, the patency of the *ductus arteriosus* (PDA) persists with a far greater incidence than in people born and living at sea level. From the studies of Peñaloza,[13] the incidence of PDA is about 30 times greater in people living at high altitude (4,500–5,000 m AMSL) than in people living at sea level.

In premature infants, PO_2 levels of 70–80 mmHg are not adequate to produce ductus constriction.[3]

In young patients with PDA living at high altitude (1,500–4,200 m AMSL), a larger ductal diameter was observed more frequently, being on average 4 mm, which is almost double compared to newborns living in the plains; anatomic type A (conical) and higher mean pulmonary artery pressure (on average 25 vs. 18 mmHg) were also present.[14]

In newborns in which ductus arteriosus remains patent, a significant left-to-right shunt would occur due to the progressive reduction of pulmonary vascular resistance. In these infants, pulmonary oedema develops about 6–10 weeks after birth (or earlier in case of premature babies).

Prevalence of Congenital Heart Diseases at Altitude

At this point, it is necessary to remember that there are some studies that report how congenital heart diseases (consisting mainly of atrial septal defect and patent ductus arteriosus) are generally 10–20 times more frequent among newborns[15, 16] and inhabitants of high altitudes than among those who reside at lower altitudes, although it cannot be excluded that this prevalence is also influenced by different living conditions and limited accessibility to health services (Figure 14.2).[17, 18] A second study recently carried out in Ecuador[19] highlighted a direct and very significant correlation between high altitudes and the prevalence of congenital heart diseases: at average altitudes of 2,619 m AMSL, 63 cases of congenital heart disease were observed per 10,000 live births; at average altitudes of 2,909 m, the cases of congenital heart disease were 72 per 10,000 live births; at average altitudes of 3,176 m, the cases of congenital heart disease increased to 86.6 per 10,000 live births.

Small ventricular septal defects close spontaneously, while larger defects persist – at sea level – in a percentage of adults of approximately 3 cases per 10,000 people.[20] In children (about 11 years of age) who live at high altitudes (about 4,000 m AMSL in Tibet) and, therefore,

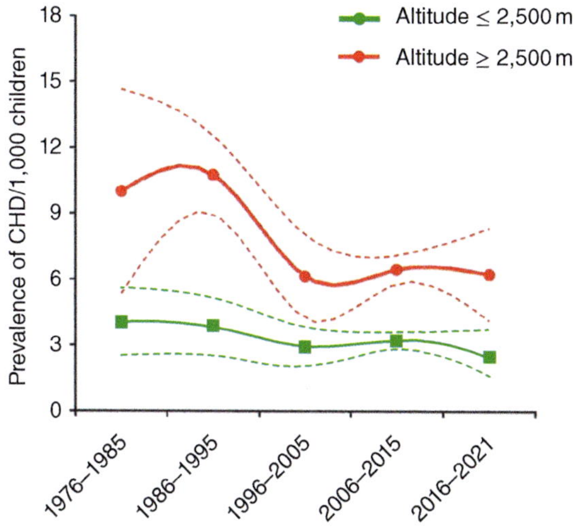

FIGURE 14.2 Prevalence of congenital heart diseases in China, in the years from 1976 to 2021. Red line: the prevalence in populations living at altitudes greater than 2,500 m above sea level; green line: prevalence in populations living at lower altitudes.[16] / Tech Science Press / CC BY 4.0.

in situations of chronic hypobaric hypoxia, it has been found that a ventricular septal defect is present in about 47 cases every 10,000 children, that is, with a prevalence approximately 16 times greater than that observed in populations living at sea level.[21]

It must be said that population screening for the detection of congenital heart diseases in newborns is not easily performed at high altitudes: echocardiography is not easily available, and the usually recommended evaluation of pulse-oximetry in newborn babies 24–48 hours after birth to screen for cyanotic heart diseases may lead to a certain percentage of false positives already at the moderate altitude of 1,646 m AMSL (a 43 times greater false-positive rate of 1.5% at moderate altitude in comparison to the false-positive rate of 0.035% at sea level).[22] Prevalence of congenital heart diseases at altitude may, thus, be rather different from the reported one.

Infants Acutely Exposed to Hypobaric Hypoxia

The effects of *brief acute exposure of newborns to altitude*, such as during rapid mountain ascents or during commercial flights (with median cabin pressurisation corresponding to an altitude of 1,894 m ≈ PiO_2 115 mmHg),[23] have not yet been adequately studied. However, it is estimated that about 19–34% of children 3–36 months old may suffer from acute mountain sickness (AMS) during a travel from 1,610 to 3,488 m;[23] in slightly older children (10 months to 14 years old), signs and symptoms of high-altitude pulmonary oedema (HAPE) may appear, with a reported incidence of 0–1.5% during exposure to high altitudes.[24]

Because of increased vascular reactivity, immature control of breathing and increased frequency of respiratory illnesses, children may develop HAPE either when travelling from low altitude to high altitude for vacation (classic HAPE), when returning to high-altitude homes after a travel to low altitude (re-entry HAPE) or even with a respiratory illness at high altitude without any change in elevation (high-altitude resident pulmonary oedema, HARPE). In these cases, HAPE could be the first sign of an underlying heart disease; thus, an evaluation for structural heart disease and pulmonary hypertension should be performed in these cases.[25] While lowland children probably have no increased risk of HAPE compared to adults, children resident at high altitude are more likely than adults to develop re-entry HAPE: HAPE appears to occur in Leadville, Colorado (at an altitude of 3,100 m), with an incidence of 140/100,000 children aged 1–14 years, when these children return to high altitude after a 2–7 days visit to a low altitude.[26]

In older children (>8 years), it is assumed that altitude illnesses will present in much the same way as it does in adults; in children <3 years of age, symptoms may be non-specific, such as behavioural changes, increased fussiness and difficulty sleeping.

Slow ascent is recommended to reduce the risk of appearance of AMS and HAPE in children; while prophylactic administration of acetazolamide can be performed in children, its use could lead to side effects such as paresthesiae, skin rashes and possible dehydration, so the use of the drug should be discouraged. Treatment of HAPE in children is achieved primarily by descent and administration of oxygen.[24]

Infants Chronically Exposed to Hypobaric Hypoxia

Children born and residing at high altitudes demonstrate ability to use a greater fraction of the inspired O_2 (62% greater O_2 extraction) in comparison to lowlanders, a result that probably derives from functional and structural alterations stimulated by fetal hypoxia.[27]

It is known since long time that infants born and living at high altitudes (3,770–4,350 m) present an increased *mass of the right ventricle* (right ventricular hypertrophy) that is normally present at birth but persists into adulthood and is related to the higher work performed by the right ventricle due to the presence of chronic pulmonary hypertension.[28]

Clinical observations performed in children born and living at high altitude (at 3,700 m, in Tibet) have shown the already described increase in mean pulmonary artery pressure and in the dimensions of the right heart and of the anterior wall thickness; it has been highlighted also that systolic and diastolic *function of both ventricles* were significantly depressed, in comparison to lowlander children.[29]

Linked to the described right ventricular hypertrophy, in the conventional 12-lead electrocardiogram differences appear between lowland and high-altitude newborns a few weeks after birth[30]: at high altitudes, an accentuated right axis deviation persists during infancy and childhood (expression of a delay in the morphological and electrical evolution of the right ventricle). For the same reasons, after the first weeks or months of life, the T wave becomes positive in the right precordial leads and remains so throughout infancy and childhood (while it usually persists negative in lowland children until late infancy).

It has been found also that healthy newborns in the Venezuelan Andes at altitudes >3,000 m had a significantly longer corrected QT interval than children born at lower altitudes;[31] what could be the prognostic significance of this finding (higher risk for tachyarrhythmias, syncope and sudden death?) is not yet clear.

Sudden Infant Deaths at Altitude

High altitude hypoxia appears to be related to sudden unexpected infant death (with a reported odd ratio of 1.93–2.3 in newborns at altitudes >2,400 m AMSL compared to newborns at altitudes <1,800 m),[32, 33] although there is still controversy on this point. In a 1998 retrospective study performed in Austria,[34] the risk of sudden infant deaths increased gradually at higher altitudes in a dose-response fashion (odds ratio 1.12/100 m), probably linked to the complex of relative environmental hypoxia for the infant, effects of maternal hypoxia on fetal growth and lower temperatures, associated with the prone position of the infant. There are experimental studies that postulate that postnatal hypoxia may delay the maturation of the cardiac conduction system and increase the risk of cardiac arrhythmias.[35]

References

1 Holmes H, Saini BS, Moir OJ, Darby JRT, Morrison JL, Sun L, Seed M. Pulmonary vascular regulation in the fetal and transitional lung. Clin Perinatol 2024; 51(1):1–19. https://doi.org/10.1016/j.clp.2023.11.003.

2 Wu TW, Azhibekov T, Seri I. Transitional hemodynamics in preterm neonates: clinical relevance. Pediatr Neonatol 2016; 57(1):7–18. https://doi.org/10.1016/j.pedneo.2015.07.002.

3 Rudolph AM. Congenital Diseases of the Heart. Chicago: Year Book Medical Publ; 1974.

4 Gowda S, Ball MK, Lakshminrusimha S, Rios DR, McNamara PJ. Hemodynamic instability in the transitional period after birth. Semin Perinatol 2024; 48(8):151986. https://doi.org/10.1016/j.semperi.2024.151986.

5 Oregon State University. 28.5 Adjustments of the infant at birth and postnatal stages. Anatomy and Physiology.https://open.oregonstate.education/aandp/chapter/28-5-adjustments-of-the-infant-at-birth-and-postnatal-stages.

6 Mier-Martínez M, García-Benítez L, Santiago-Vázquez V, Tamariz-Cruz O. Arterial oxygen saturation in healthy Mexican full-term newborns at different altitudes above sea level. Bol Med Hosp Infant Mex 2023; 80(4):242–246. https://doi.org/10.24875/BMHIM.23000032.

7 Haworth SG. Development of the normal and hypertensive pulmonary vasculature. Exp Physiol 1995;80(5):843–853. https://doi.org/10.1113/expphysiol.1995.sp003892.

8 Niermeyer S, Andrade Mollinedo P, Huicho L. Child health and living at high altitude. Arch Dis Child 2009; 94(10):806–811. https://doi.org/10.1136/adc.2008.141838.

9 Niermeyer S, Yang P, Shanmina, Drolkar, Zhuang J, Moore LG. Arterial oxygen saturation in Tibetan and Han infants born in Lhasa, Tibet. N Engl J Med 1995; 333(19):1248–1252. https://doi.org/10.1056/NEJM199511093331903.

10 Heath-Freudenthal A, Toledo-Jaldin L, von Alvensleben I, Lazo-Vega L, Mizutani R, Stalker M, Yasini H, Mendizabal F, Dorado Madera J, Mundo W, Castro-Monrroy M, Houck JA, Moreno-Aramayo A, Miranda-Garrido V, Su EJ, Giussani DA, Abman SH, Moore LG, Julian CG. Vascular disorders of pregnancy increase susceptibility to neonatal pulmonary hypertension in high-altitude populations. Hypertension 2022; 79(6):1286–1296. https://doi.org/10.1161/HYPERTENSIONAHA.122.19078.

11 Asas-Jinde M, González-Andrade F. Newborns physiological differences in low- and high-altitude settings of Ecuador. J Dev Orig Health Dis 2022; 13(4):494–499. https://doi.org/10.1017/S2040174421000532.
12 Julian CG, Gonzales M, Rodriguez A, Bellido D, Salmon CS, Ladenburger A, Reardon L, Vargas E, Moore LG. Perinatal hypoxia increases susceptibility to high-altitude polycythemia and attendant pulmonary vascular dysfunction. Am J Physiol Heart Circ Physiol 2015; 309(4):H565–H573. https://doi.org/10.1152/ajpheart.00296.2015.
13 Peñaloza D, Arias-Stella J, Sime F, Recavarren S, Marticorena E. The heart and pulmonary circulation in children at high altitudes: physiological, anatomical, and clinical observations. Pediatrics 1964; 34:568–582.
14 Białkowski J, Głowacki J, Zabal C, Garcia-Montes A, Bermudez-Canete R, Flores-Arizmendi R, Sagado-Sandova A, Diaz de Leon H, Delagadillo RM, Kreutzer J. Patent ductus arteriosus at low and high altitudes: anatomical and haemodynamic features and their implications for transcatheter closure. Kardiol Pol 2011; 69(5):431–436. https://journals.viamedica.pl/polish_heart_journal/article/view/79309/61307.
15 Hasan A. Relationship of high altitude and congenital heart disease. Indian Heart J 2016; 68(1): 9–12. https://doi.org/10.1016/j.ihj.2015.12.015.
16 Li JJ, Liu Y, Xie SY, Zhao GD, Dai T, Chen H, Mu LF, Qi HY, Li J. Newborn screening for congenital heart disease using echocardiography and follow-up at high altitude in China. Int J Cardiol 2019; 274:106–112. https://doi.org/10.1016/j.ijcard.2018.08.102.
17 Zhang S, Zhang B, Wu J, Luo Jshi H, Qi J, Yang H. The prevalence of congenital heart disease among school-age children in China: a meta-analysis and systematic review. Congenit. Heart Dis. 2023; 18(2):127–150. https://doi.org/10.32604/chd.2023.025616.
18 van der Linde D, Konings EE, Slager MA, Witsenburg M, Helbing WA, Takkenberg JJ, Roos-Hesselink JW. Birth prevalence of congenital heart disease worldwide: a systematic review and meta-analysis. J Am Coll Cardiol 2011; 58(21):2241–2447. https://doi.org/10.1016/j.jacc.2011.08.025.
19 González-Andrade F. High altitude as a cause of congenital heart defects: a medical hypothesis rediscovered in Ecuador. High Alt Med Biol 2020; 21(2):126–134. https://doi.org/10.1089/ham.2019.0110.
20 Minette MS, Sahn DJ. Ventricular septal defects. Circulation 2006; 114(20):2190–2197. https://doi.org/10.1161/CIRCULATIONAHA.106.618124. Erratum in: Circulation 2007; 115(7):e205. https://doi.org/10.1161/CIRCULATIONAHA.107.181352.
21 Chun H, Yue Y, Wang Y, Dawa Z, Zhen P, La Q, Zong Y, Qu Y, Mu D. High prevalence of congenital heart disease at high altitudes in Tibet. Eur J Prev Cardiol 2019; 26(7):756–759. https://doi.org/10.1177/2047487318812502.
22 Rao S, Goens MB, Myers OB, Sebesta EA. Pulse oximetry screening for detection of congenital heart defects at 1646 m in Albuquerque, New Mexico. Cardiol Young 2020; 30(12):1851–1855. https://doi.org/10.1017/S1047951120002899.
23 Samuels MP. The effects of flight and altitude. Arch Dis Child 2004; 89(5):448–455. https://doi.org/10.1136/adc.2003.031708.
24 Pollard AJ, Niermeyer S, Barry P, Bärtsch P, Berghold F, Bishop RA, Clarke C, Dhillon S, Dietz TE, Durmowicz A, Durrer B, Eldridge M, Hackett P, Jean D, Kriemler S, Litch JA, Murdoch D, Nickol A, Richalet JP, Roach R, Shlim DR, Wiget U, Yaron M, Zubieta-Castillo G Sr, Zubieta-Calleja GR Jr. Children at high altitude: an international consensus statement by an ad hoc committee of the

International Society for Mountain Medicine, March 12, 2001. High Alt Med Biol 2001; 2(3): 389–403. https://doi.org/10.1089/15270290152608561.

25 Liptzin DR, Abman SH, Giesenhagen A, Ivy DD. An approach to children with pulmonary oedema at high altitude. High Alt Med Biol 2018; 19(1):91–98. https://doi.org/10.1089/ham.2017.0096.

26 Scoggin CH, Hyers TM, Reeves JT, Grover RF. High-altitude pulmonary oedema in the children and young adults of Leadville, Colorado. N Engl J Med 1977; 297(23):1269–1272. https://doi.org/10.1056/NEJM197712082972309

27 Mortola JP, Frappell PB, Frappell DE, Villena-Cabrera N, Villena-Cabrera M, Peña F. Ventilation and gaseous metabolism in infants born at high altitude, and their responses to hyperoxia. Am Rev Respir Dis 1992; 146(5 Pt 1):1206–1209. https://doi.org/10.1164/ajrccm/146.5_Pt_1.1206.

28 Recavarren S, Arias-Stella J. Right ventricular hypertrophy in people born and living at high altitudes. Br Heart J 1964; 26(6):806–812. https://doi.org/10.1136/hrt.26.6.806.

29 Qi H, Xu S, Ma R, Jiang L, Li S, Mai S, Chen H, Ge M, Wang M, Liu H, Sun K, Zhang Y, Chen S, Cai Y, Li J. [Comparison of echocardiographic parameters in healthy Chinese children born and living at high altitude or at sea-level]. Zhonghua Xin Xue Guan Bing Za Zhi 2015; 43(9):774–881. Chinese. https://doi.org/10.3760/cma.j.issn.0253-3758.2015.09.006.

30 Peñaloza D, Gamboa R, Dreyer J, Echevarria M, Marticorena E. The influence of high altitudes on the electrical activity of the heart. I. Electrocardiographic and vectorcardiographic observations in the newborn, infants, and children. Am Heart J. 1960; 59:111–128. https://doi.org/10.1016/0002-8703(60)90390-2.

31 Fuenmayor AJ, Stock FU, Fuenmayor AC, Fuenmayor P AM. QT interval and final portion of T wave: measurements and dispersion in infants born at high altitude. Int J Cardiol 2002; 82(2): 123–126. https://doi.org/10.1016/s0167-5273(01)00616-7.

32 Katz D, Shore S, Bandle B, Niermeyer S, Bol KA, Khanna A. Sudden infant death syndrome and residential altitude. Pediatrics 2015; 135(6):e1442–e1449.https://doi.org/10.1542/peds.2014-2697.

33 Johnston R, Yan X, Anderson TM, Mitchell EA. Altitude and risk of sudden unexpected infant death in the United States. Sci Rep 2021; 11(1):2161. https://doi.org/10.1038/s41598-021-81613-w.

34 Kohlendorfer U, Kiechl S, Sperl W. Living at high altitude and risk of sudden infant death syndrome. Arch Dis Child 1998; 79(6):506–509. https://doi.org/10.1136/adc.79.6.506.

35 Neary MT, Breckenridge RA. Hypoxia at the heart of sudden infant death syndrome? Pediatr Res 2013; 74(4):375–379. https://doi.org/10.1038/pr.2013.122.

CHAPTER 15

Elderly Persons at Altitude

In 160 BC, the Latin playwright Publius Terentius Afro wrote the comedy 'Phormio',[1] titled from the name of one of the main characters, Phormio, a cunning 'schemer' who had managed to settle a couple of difficult marital situations with very unscrupulous manoeuvres and a series of intrigues (Figure 15.1). A story that surpasses any modern 'gossip'. In the first scene of the 4th act, Chremes, returning from a journey, which he had prolonged for secret romantic encounters with his lover, meets his brother Demipho, who asks him the reasons for the delayed return: the answer is 'I was held back by a disease'. 'What illness did you have?' To the question, Chremes answers evasively: 'Do you even have to ask? Old age is already an illness in itself'.

At the time of the play's performance, life expectancy at birth was 27 years, and the average lifespan was estimated to be around 40 years; it was rare to exceed 49 years of age, although the existence of cases of centenarians is known, like – according to what Pliny the Elder reported – Terentia, Cicero's first wife, who lived to be 103 years old.[2] It is also estimated, on the basis of sepulchral inscriptions and papyri, that in the imperial age Romans over 40 constituted 25% of the population, while over a third were young people under the age of 15; those over 60 do not seem to reach 6% of the population.[3]

The situation is radically different nowadays.

In 2022, in Italy, life expectancy at birth was estimated to be 82.6 years (80.5 years for males and 84.8 years for females).[4] In Europe, life expectancy at birth in 2022 was on average 80.6 years, increased by 0.5 years from the previous year: an expectancy of 77.9 years for males and 83.3 years for females.[5] In the United States, life expectancy in the same year was estimated to be much shorter: 77.5 years (74.8 for males and 80.2 for females).[6]

In the Italian population, the percentage of people over 60 years of age constitutes 30.5% of the population.[7] At least 42% of this elderly population is sedentary; however, this data – conversely – indicates that 58% perform some type of physical activity.[8]

In Europe, older adults represent 21.6% of the total population.[9] At least 36% of adult European residents (18–64 years old) can be classified as physically inactive, with Portugal having the highest prevalence (63.7%); in contrast, Sweden and Germany have the lowest rate of physically inactive adults (19% and 21%, respectively).[10]

In the United States, the 2020 Census reports that approximately 15% of population is 65 years of age or more.[11] The Global Observatory for Physical Activity[12] reports that approximately 32% of the US population is inactive (with a higher prevalence among women: 38% vs. 25% among men), and 10.1% of deaths are attributable to physical inactivity (worldwide, this percentage is 9%).

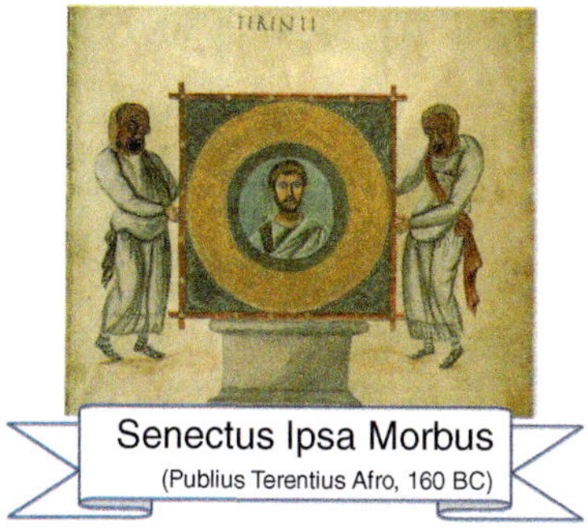

FIGURE 15.1 Portrait of Publius Terentius Afro from Codex Vaticanus Latinus 3868 f.2r (https://digi.vatlib.it/view/MSS_Vat.lat.3868) and the famous aphorism 'Old age is already an illness in itself'. https://commons.wikimedia.org/wiki/File:Vaticana,_Vat._lat._3868_(2r).jpg / Public domain / last accessed Dec. 27, 2025

For a mountainous Country like Nepal, the percentage of population aged over 60 is quite low (10%);[13] the percentage of physically inactive population is also low, estimated to be only 7% of the total population (males 8% and females 7%) with a percentage of deaths attributable to inactivity of approximately 3.6%. No data on the physically inactive population are available for another mountainous Country like Bolivia, where approximately 6% of the population is aged 65 or over[14] (with older people reaching 15–20% of the total population in some rural areas).

Thus, a large part of population in developed Countries results to be elderly and a large percentage is also physically inactive, much less so in developing Countries.

But can even elderly and often inactive people go to the mountains and perform some kind of physical activity there?

Advanced Age Persons and Ascent to Altitude

As for other pathological situations, even for 'advanced age disease', there is little scientific data about the potential cardiovascular problems these people may encounter when travelling to high altitude.

The few existing studies focus mainly on the risks linked to falls and traumas due to the imperviousness of the routes[15, 16] and on the need for adequate physical preparation and motivation before tackling mountain routes.[17]

In 2001, Burtscher et al.[18] studied the cardiopulmonary responses of a group of 20 healthy elderly persons (aged 55–77 years) during a 1-week hiking programme at low (600 m) and high (2,000 m) altitude. At high altitude, the study subjects demonstrated a rapid ventilatory adaptation at rest, but during exercise tests, SaO_2 was reduced compared to baseline, and blood lactate concentrations were increased; recovery from exercise was delayed. Overall, the Authors concluded that a 1-week hiking programme can be well tolerated by healthy older adults at both low and high altitude and suggested that heart rate and SaO_2 measurements should be used to estimate acclimatisation status and to monitor exercise intensity and duration in older adults at high altitude.

From a study on not particularly elderly people (i.e. 59 ± 5 years; we have no data on older people) who climbed Kilimanjaro,[19] it turned out that the hearts of elderly adults adapt to the altitude, up to at an altitude of 4,800 m AMSL, in a similar way to how the hearts of young persons do, although a greater increase in pulmonary artery pressure values has been observed in older adults (up to approximately 35 mmHg on average), as well as a greater increase of left ventricle end-diastolic pressures compared to younger people. It is also known that professional mountain guides of the Austrian army aged >50 years have a lower prevalence of overweight, arterial hypertension and diabetes mellitus compared to a control population of their peers; mountain activities carried out professionally at moderate and high altitudes allow them to maintain high physical fitness and reduced cardiovascular risk factors even beyond the age of 50.[20]

Two Popes and a President.

Pope Benedict XVI (Joseph Aloisius Ratzinger) in 2010 decided to give up his holidays in the mountains, also on the advice of doctors, due to his advanced age (83 years) and his arterial hypertension. In previous years, he had frequented some mountain resorts, whose altitudes, however, did not exceed 900 m above sea level.

On the other hand, at the age of 88, on 16 July 1984, the then President of the Italian Republic, Sandro Pertini, went to the *'Ai Caduti dell'Adamello'* refuge, at an altitude of 3,040 m above sea level, where he met Pope John Paul II (Karol Józef Wojtyła), then 64 years old, who had also taken a short skiing excursion.[21]

It should be noted that Sandro Pertini, in addition to his advanced age, had (probably) suffered from pulmonary tuberculosis[22] at the age of 34 – during his detention in the fascist prison on the island of Santo Stefano – and had also always been a heavy pipe smoker!

It is true that Pertini had reached that altitude by helicopter, but he remained there for a few hours, even walking on the snow on the Pope's arm from the landing area (Lobbia Alta pass, 3,015 m above sea level) to the refuge (Figure 15.2).

After a few hundred metres walk, Pertini (who was an old socialist) and the Pope sat down for lunch, like old friends, to talk freely and to enjoy the 'strangolapreti' (literally 'strangle the priests', a typical Trentino dish of green spinach gnocchi)!

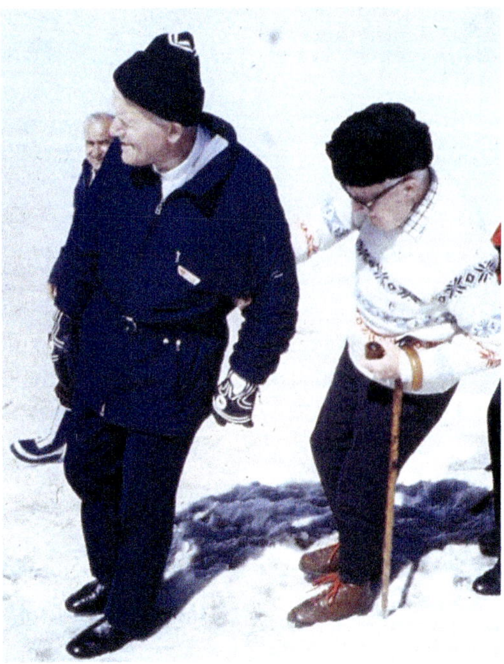

FIGURE 15.2 16 July 1984: President Sandro Pertini (aged 88) on the arm of Pope John Paul II (aged 64), walking towards the 'Ai Caduti dell'Adamello' refuge (3,040 m). Presidency of the Italian Republic / https://archivio.quirinale.it/aspr/fotografico/PHOTO-002-006331/presidente/alessandro-pertini/il-presidente-della-repubblica-sandro-pertini-e-papa-giovanni-paolo-ii-insieme-sulle-cime-adamello#n / last accessed Dec. 27, 2025

Another study that provides interesting data for our purposes is the one conducted by Puthon et al. in 2017; they submitted a group of healthy people aged between 60 and 70 years to a stress test under normoxic and hypoxic conditions (FiO_2 12%, i.e. corresponding to a simulated altitude of 4,800 m).[23] The study highlighted that these people had cardio-respiratory response and tissue oxygenation similar to those of young control subjects during moderate intensity effort; during hypoxic test, their desaturation and reduction of exercise tolerance were also comparable to those of younger people. From these data, we can, therefore, deduce that even people aged 60–70 years should be able to tackle climbs up to 4,800 m without problems, provided they are in good health.

But how many people of senile age are 'in good health'? We can draw indirect deductions from some studies conducted on people aged ≥40 years, so-called 'veteran athletes', subjected to cardiological evaluations with the aim of identifying those at high coronary risk.[24] These people regularly played endurance sports, although it is not reported how many of them practised mountain sports. However, it is important to note that in this group of people cardiovascular risk factors were present in 40.7% of cases and that an exercise test was abnormal in 12.4% of these athletes, both for ECG criteria (5.7%) and for the appearance of stress-induced ventricular arrhythmias (6.7%); on computerised tomography coronary angiogram, 25.7% of these athletes showed high cardiovascular risk due to the presence of calcified coronary plaques or stenoses.

Another recent study[25] observed that among Master athletes (note: age >35 years!; therefore, also young!), there were 2.8 cases of major cardiac events per 1,000 people per year; increasing age was correlated with an increased cardiovascular risk, and the classic tests (exercise test, echocardiogram) were not always adequate to recognise an underlying coronary disease in this group of people. The Authors came to the conclusion that it could be appropriate to suggest to have at least an ECG (and Holter Recording) and perhaps a coronary CT scan performed in athletes with abnormal ECG; they suggest also that a coronary CT scan should be performed in all Master athletes with a 10-year Framingham cardiovascular risk score[26] ≥10% and in those with suspected angina or dyspnoea. (The risks appear to be lower in female athletes: other observations show that veteran female athletes, aged 54 ± 8.5 years, have fewer coronary plaques and are less exposed to the risk of arrhythmias than male athletes of the same age.)[27]

We can thus imagine that similar (or even worse) data could be found in adult-senile people who frequent the mountains. At the same time, it is clear that it is not easily practicable to submit all adults and seniors to thorough testing before they venture into the mountains. We, therefore, return to the general recommendations already formulated more than 30 years ago by Hartsock et al.:[28]

'Requisites:

- *cardiovascular and musculoskeletal fitness, attainable through training;*
- *skills, acquired through schools or guide services;*
- *motivational psychology (usually reflecting positive qualities and attitudes toward life and the environment).'*

By acquiring these physical and psychological characteristics, recreational mountain activities (the Authors were referring specifically to climbing) could be enjoyed up to the seventh decade of life. Even for mountain trekking, it is of fundamental importance that elderly people follow adequate and regular physical training, aimed at the activity they intend to carry out, performed under medical supervision and monitored by experts in the sport.[29]

Multifactorial Pre-exposure Assessment in Aged Mountaineers

Anyway, before allowing a person of the 'third (or fourth) Age' to undertake physical activity in medium-high mountains, at least some multifactorial assessments must be carried out:[30]

1. type of disease by which the candidate is known to be (or is probably) affected;
2. his/her low altitude fitness: this can be evaluated through a Stress Test performed at low altitude (even if we have seen above how it has intrinsic limits) or – better – a Stress Test with FiO_2 12%;
3. altitude to reach (>2,000 m?);
4. speed of ascent (an ascent <300–400 m/day is recommended, to allow adequate acclimatisation; Evidence: 1C);
5. geographical location where the activity will take place;
6. type, duration and intensity of the planned activities;
7. availability of medical assistance and possibility of rescue in the event of the appearance of negative events.

Finally, regarding Points 5 and 7, it is helpful for tourists and the healthcare workers accompanying them to know what happens to people who crowd the high-altitude trails and go trekking every year. Among the 800,000 people who travel to Nepal every year, for example, 15% are over 60 years old; 30% are overweight and 4% are obese; 5% are smokers, and 2% report heart disease; 41% are being treated with one or more drugs, mainly for hypertension, hypercholesterolaemia, migraine and dysthyroidism.[31] Obtaining such drugs is potentially complicated in Nepal (as well as in other high-altitude locations); any complications or exacerbations of the aforementioned diseases that were to occur at high altitudes would create major logistical problems in those areas, where medical care is limited and evacuation presents enormous difficulties. People with the characteristics described should, therefore, be discouraged from travelling to those areas.

References

1 Publius Terentius Afer (Terence), Phormio. St. John Parry E, Ed. https://www.perseus.tufts.edu/hopper/text?doc=Perseus%3Atext%3A1999.02.0091. Full text of Phormio at: Phormio of Terence, translated into English prose by Morgan MH. J Wilson and Son, Cambridge, 1894. Available at: https://archive.org/details/phormiotranslate00tereuoft/page/n19/mode/2up.

2 Gaius Plinius Secundus. Naturalis Historia. Book 7, section 158. English translation by H.Rackham (1952). https://www.attalus.org/pliny/hn7c.html.

3 Frier BW. Demography. In: Alan K. Bowman AK, Garnsey P, Rathbone D (Eds). The Cambridge Ancient History. Part Va – Economy and Society. Cambridge University Press; 2000. https://www.academia.edu/105459729/The_Demography_of_the_Early_Roman_Empire.

4 ISTAT. Indicatori demografici, Anno 2022 [Italian Institute of Statistics. Demographic indicators, Year 2022]. https://www.quotidianosanita.it/allegati/allegato1680858531.pdf.

5 Eurostat. EU life expectancy at birth 80.6 years in 2022. https://ec.europa.eu/eurostat/web/products-eurostat-news/w/ddn-20240314-1#:~:text=In%202022%2C%20the%20life%20expectancy,by%200.5%20years%20from%202021.

6 CDC, National Center for Health Statistics. Life expectancy increases, However suicides up in 2022. https://www.cdc.gov/nchs/pressroom/nchs_press_releases/2023/20231129.htm#:~:text=Findings%20from%20Provisional%20Life%20Expectancy,(from%2076.4%20to%2077.5).

7 Tuttitalia. Popolazione per età, sesso e stato civile 2022 [Population by age, sex and marital status 2022]. https://www.tuttitalia.it/statistiche/popolazione-eta-sesso-stato-civile-2022.

8 Quotidiano sanità. Stili di vita e prevenzione [Lifestyles and prevention]. December 16, 2021. https://www.quotidianosanita.it/studi-e-analisi/articolo.php?articolo_id=100960.

9 Eurostat, Statistics Explained. Population structure and ageing. February 2025. https://ec.europa.eu/eurostat/statistics-explained/index.php.

10 Nikitara K, Odani S, Demenagas N, Rachiotis G, Symvoulakis E, Vardavas C. Prevalence and correlates of physical inactivity in adults across 28 European countries. Eur J Public Health 2021; 31(4):840–845. https://doi.org/10.1093/eurpub/ckab067.

11 United States Census Bureau. Exploring age groups in the 2020 census. https://www.census.gov/library/visualizations/interactive/exploring-age-groups-in-the-2020-census.html.

12 Global Observator for Physical Activity. Country cards. 2020. https://new.globalphysicalactivityobservatory.com/countrycards.

13 Chalise HN. Aging Trend and Pattern in Nepal. J Tikapur Mult Campus 2024; 7:142–156. https://www.researchgate.net/publication/378623257_Aging_Trend_and_Pattern_in_Nepal.

14 World Bank Group. Population ages 65 and above (% of total population); from: World Population Prospects, United Nations. 2025. https://data.worldbank.org/indicator/SP.POP.65UP.TO.ZS.

15 Amarowicz J, Kumorek A, Boczon K. Age and sex are strongly correlated to the rate and type of mountain injuries requiring search and rescue missions. Wilderness Environ Med 2019; 30(4): 378–385. https://doi.org/10.1016/j.wem.2019.06.016.

16 Lutter C, Schöffl V. Climbing in older athletes. In: Schöffl V, Schöffl I, Lutter C, Hochholzer T (Eds). Climbing Medicine. Springer, Cham; 2022. https://doi.org/10.1007/978-3-030-72184-8_15.

17 Wood C. Too Old for Long-Distance Walking? Not with these tips from former gold medallist, retired teacher and author. REI Co-op, August 20, 2018. https://www.rei.com/blog/hike/too-old-for-long-distance-walking.

18 Burtscher M, Bachmann O, Hatzl T, Hotter B, Likar R, Philadelphy M, Nachbauer W. Cardiopulmonary and metabolic responses in healthy elderly humans during a 1-week hiking programme at high altitude. Eur J Appl Physiol 2001; 84(5):379–386. https://doi.org/10.1007/s004210100393.

19 Stewart GM, Wheatley-Guy CM, Morris NR, Coffman KE, Stepanek J, Carlson AR, Issa A, Schmidt MA, Johnson BD. Myocardial adaptability in young and older-aged sea-level habitants sojourning at Mt Kilimanjaro: are cardiac compensatory limits reached in older trekkers? Eur J Appl Physiol 2020; 120(4):799–809. https://doi.org/10.1007/s00421-020-04319-3.

20 Puehringer R, Berger M, Said M, Burtscher M. Age-dependent health status and cardiorespiratory fitness in austrian military mountain guides. High Alt Med Biol 2020; 21(4):346–351. https://doi.org/10.1089/ham.2020.0092.

21 Punta Giovanni Paolo II (dalla legenda alla realtà. Storia di una croce) [Adamello. Crest of the Cross - Punta Giovanni Paolo II (from legend to reality. Story of a cross)]. Editrice Rendena, Tione, 1998. http://www.giornidistoria.net/adamello-1984-un-incontro-che-doveva-restare-segreto.

22 Letter from Palmiro Togliatti to Filippo Turati, October 30, 1930. http://www.pertini.it/cesp/doc_27.htm.

23 Puthon L, Bouzat P, Robach P, Favre-Juvin A, Doutreleau S, Verges S. Effect of ageing on hypoxic exercise cardiorespiratory, muscle and cerebral oxygenation responses in healthy humans. Exp Physiol 2017; 102(4):436–447. https://doi.org/10.1113/EP085949.

24 Dores H, de Araújo Gonçalves P, Monge J, Costa R, Tátá L, Malhotra A, Sharma S, Cardim N, Neuparth N. Subclinical coronary artery disease in veteran athletes: is a new preparticipation methodology required? Br J Sports Med 2020; 54(6):349–353. https://doi.org/10.1136/bjsports-2018-099840.

25 Morrison BN, Isserow S, Taunton J, Oxborough D, Moulson N, Warburton DER, McKinney J. Masters athlete screening study (MASS): incidence of cardiovascular disease and major adverse cardiac events and efficacy of screening over five years. Eur J Prev Cardiol 2023; 30(9):887–899. https://doi.org/10.1093/eurjpc/zwad090.

26 Wilson PWF. Framingham risk score for hard coronary heart disease. Estimates 10-year risk of heart attack. MD+Calc. https://www.mdcalc.com/calc/38/framingham-risk-score-hard-coronary-heart-disease.

27 Castelletti S, Gati S. The female athlete's heart: overview and management of cardiovascular diseases. Eur Cardiol 2021;16:e47. https://doi.org/10.15420/ecr.2021.29.

28 Hartsock LA, Feagin JA Jr, Ogilvie BC. Climbing and the older athlete. Clin Sports Med. 1991; 10(2):257–267.

29 Burtscher M. Endurance performance of the elderly mountaineer: requirements, limitations, testing, and training. Wien Klin Wochenschr 2004; 116 (21–22):703–714. https://doi.org/10.1007/s00508-004-0258-y.

30 Rimoldi SF, Sartori C, Seiler C, Delacrétaz E, Mattle HP, Scherrer U, Allemann Y. High-altitude exposure in patients with cardiovascular disease: risk assessment and practical recommendations. Prog Cardiovasc Dis 2010; 52(6):512–524. https://doi.org/10.1016/j.pcad.2010.03.005.

31 Keyes LE, Mather L, Duke C, Regmi N, Phelan B, Pant S, Starling J, McElwee M, Cole D, McConnell T, Paudel P, Sallade TD, Sheets A, Twillman D, Young DS, Basnyat B. Older age, chronic medical conditions and polypharmacy in Himalayan trekkers in Nepal: an epidemiologic survey and case series. J Travel Med 2016; 23(6):taw052. https://doi.org/10.1093/jtm/taw052.

CHAPTER 16

Ascent to High Altitudes and Risk of Arrhythmias

Some of the various factors that we have observed so far to be linked to ascent to altitude can trigger the appearance of arrhythmias or favour the worsening of pre-existing arrhythmias (Figure 16.1). We are referring in particular to the sympathetic activation with increased release of catecholamines, which appears following the hypobaric hypoxic stimulus, as well as to the changes in the ability of myocardial cells to control the transmembrane transport of potassium. Catecholamines directly increase cardiac excitability; added to these are the effects due to increased heart rate, possible myocardial ischaemia, pressure and volume overload of the right ventricle, hypokalaemia induced by respiratory alkalosis and the possible appearance of diarrhoea and vomiting. All these factors increase myocardial excitability and, therefore, predispose to the appearance of arrhythmias (sometimes malignant, with the possibility of sudden death, as we have already seen in Chapter 9), especially in patients with poorly controlled cardiovascular risk factors.

Besides this, during night, high-altitude hypoxia can associate with periodic breathing and exaggerate its effects, producing pronounced sinus arrhythmia and sinus bradycardia, in a way similar to what occurs at sea level in individuals with obstructive sleep apnoea.

In clinical practice, there are very few studies that have evaluated the incidence of arrhythmias in relation to ascent to altitude. Furthermore, patients with pre-existing high-grade arrhythmias have never been studied at high altitude, so that the available information is still scarce.

Already in 1990, it was observed that normal subjects exposed to simulated high altitude (Operation Everest II) showed cyclic variations in heart rate during sleep in relation to the appearance of periodic breathing, as well as **bradyarrhythmia's** down to 20 bpm with escape junctional rhythm as well as without escape rhythm, blocked P waves, sinus arrest, atrioventricular dissociation and idioventricular rhythm.[1] The occurrence of nocturnal episodes of pronounced sinus arrhythmia (with RR intervals up to 3.3 seconds, recorded with Holter method) had already been reported in 1979 in a 34-year-old mountaineer on Annapurna (Nepal), at 5,560 m above sea level.[2]

In a 2000 study,[3] it was observed with Holter recordings that going from an altitude of 200 m to one of 1,350 m above sea level resulted in a doubling of **supraventricular and**

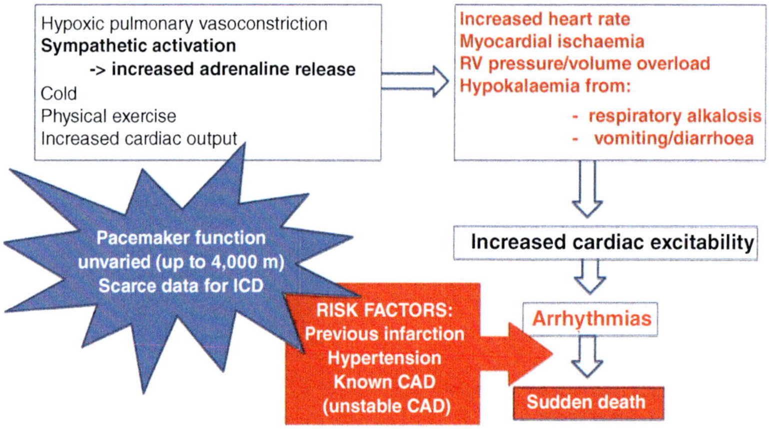

FIGURE 16.1 Mechanisms predisposing to major arrhythmias at high altitudes.

ventricular arrhythmias, but without a significant increase of sustained arrhythmias; the same Authors then observed how there was a progressive increase in arrhythmias proportionally with the increase in altitude (altitudes studied: 898, 1,764 and 2,632 m AMSL).[4, 5]

Based on these observations, it can be assumed that patients with pre-existing cardiac diseases and/or arrhythmias may have an increased incidence of arrhythmias at high altitude.

However, there is at least one study that would lead to opposite conclusions: Woods et al.[6] reported that the risk of dangerous arrhythmias seems to be low at high altitudes (over 5,000 m AMSL); these observations, however, were carried out in a very small number of young people (nine English soldiers) trained to perform physical exercise. Even Gibelli et al.,[7] through the study of T-Wave Alternans, came to the conclusion that there seems to be a low risk of dangerous arrhythmias, even when the subjects were submitted to physical exercise; anyway, this observation was again made in young and trained adults exposed to hypobaric hypoxia (an expedition to 8,150 m AMSL in Pakistan).

Instead, in another study (REVEAL High Altitude)[8] also conducted on young (military) subjects, in 9 out of 16 cases (=56%), arrhythmias appeared, which would suggest a pro-arrhythmic effect of exposure to high altitude: in 8 out of 15 subjects, **sinus pauses** and episodes of **atrioventricular block**, which increased in frequency with the altitude reached and the duration of the stay at altitude; in 1 subject, appearance of a nocturnal episode of high-frequency **atrial fibrillation** at 133 beats/min, which began after drinking cold water and lasted for 282 minutes; and in 1 other subject, an episode of **paroxysmal supraventricular tachycardia** at 207 bpm, occurring at 5,200 m AMSL after physical effort and lasted 31 seconds. It is likely that right atrial distention due to increased pressures in the pulmonary circulation induced by hypobaric hypoxia is responsible for the triggering of atrial arrhythmias in these subjects; these events could be resolved with descent or supplemental oxygen.

There is also another observation on a 65-year-old man, not acclimatised to high altitudes and without pre-existing heart disease, in whom **ventricular bigeminy** appeared during the climb to 5,895 m AMSL; the arrhythmia disappeared with the descent to lower altitudes.[9] A repeat study on the same subject at age 75 demonstrated the presence of an increased number of ventricular premature beats, with occurrence of runs of left **ventricular tachycardia** during ascent from 4,710 to 5,100 m, when arterial oxygen saturation reached 70%; the Author suggested that aging increases sympathetic response and/or sensitivity to hypoxia during exercise and even during sleep.[10]

Several other studies have reported the occurrence of ventricular arrhythmias during high-altitude ascents: they are mainly isolated ventricular ectopic beats, originating from the left ventricle. However, short runs of ventricular bigeminy have also been reported, while a study on members of a British military expedition to the Himalayas in 2008 identified a wide range of arrhythmic activity, including life-threatening ventricular arrhythmias (one episode of polymorphic ventricular tachycardia 'torsades de pointes' in a healthy, well-acclimatised mountaineer).

Anticoagulation in Mountain Environment

As regards patients with **permanent atrial fibrillation**, a relatively frequent situation in older subjects (around 5 people per 1,000 inhabitants are affected worldwide),[11] it is useful to remember that this arrhythmia can lead to a reduction in cardiac output even by 30% due to the loss of the atrial contribution to ventricular filling and the irregularity of the beat-to-beat interval;[12] this can, therefore, be a limiting factor when these patients intend to perform physical activity. Furthermore, even in patients with a well-controlled mean heart rate, hypoxia and the related sympathetic activation can induce an increase in heart rate. It should not be forgotten that these patients are subjected to chronic anti-coagulant treatment (which must be continued in the mountains, and – even more so – its effectiveness must be monitored; not an easy task); the relative dehydration associated with altitude and changes in diet can lead to significant changes in the level of anticoagulation. Physical activity in the mountains can cause trauma, which – in anti-coagulated patients – can be of greater relevance and more demanding than in other people.

In people with sinus rhythm but with situations predisposing to the appearance of atrial fibrillation, such as, for example, in cases with atrial enlargement due to hypertensive heart disease or in patients with valvular heart disease, the increase in sympathetic tone and the increase in systemic and pulmonary arterial pressure can act as a 'trigger' for the appearance of this arrhythmia. Even the fact that periodic breathing and sleep apnoea may appear (as happens at high altitudes) is a well-known factor that can induce the appearance of atrial fibrillation.[13]

Regarding the appearance of major and sustained arrhythmias, which can lead to **ventricular fibrillation** and **sudden death**, we have already discussed it in Chapter 9, to which reference should be made.

Patients with PMs or ICDs

Little is also known about patients with **Pacemakers** (PMs). The exposure of 13 patients to a simulated altitude of 4,000 m (reached in progressive steps of 500 m, with 5-minute breaks) did not determine any variation in the PM stimulation thresholds in the short term (30 minutes).[14] Patients with PM should be observed by a cardiologist before climbing to altitude, to evaluate any opportunity to increase the PM discharge frequency (increase the heart rate in view of the possible increase in the body's metabolic demands) or to change the settings of PM to DDD mode.

As regards the behaviour of **Implantable Cardioverter Defibrillators** (ICDs), even in this case, the data are extremely modest. A Swiss study on patients living at altitude (over 2,000 m AMSL) highlighted how the occurrence of defibrillator discharges was very low, such that it does not even discourage to carry out recreational activities of modest intensity.[15] Even during airline flights, in which the cabin is pressurised to values corresponding to altitudes no higher than 2,400 m (mostly around 1,800 m), no particular complications have been reported.[16]

If an ICD Shock Occurs at Altitude ...

The assessment of the suitability of a patient with an ICD to climb to altitude should, therefore, be based on the evaluation of his/her underlying pathology, while the presence of the ICD should not in itself constitute a contraindication.[17] However, it is necessary to remember that the possible increase of arrhythmias linked to climbing to altitude – as it happens in any case for activities requiring significant physical effort – could lead to a greater probability of intervention of the ICD, with the appearance of 'discomfort' for the patient, inability of the ICD to put an end to the arrhythmia (due to possible concomitant metabolic alterations, linked to exertion at altitude)[18] and possible trauma to the patient (fall) during defibrillator discharge.

Please also note that it has been reported[19] that both PMs and ICDs are built for altitudes (pressures) up to 4,000 m only; therefore, for higher altitudes, it is recommended to contact the manufacturer in advance.

In conclusion, the question of whether high altitude favours a dangerous increase in arrhythmic risk is still an unclear question, so much so that the International Union of Mountaineering Associations suggests caution in patients with known cardiac pathologies and awaits further studies on the topic.[19] The Clinical Recommendations[20] issued by some European Societies in 2018 suggest that patients prone to serious arrhythmias should not be exposed to altitudes above 3,000–3,500 m (particularly in case of ventricular arrhythmias) (Evidence 2C).

Pre-exposure Evaluation of Patients with Cardiac Arrhythmias

Before climbing to altitude, patients with ventricular arrhythmias related to ischaemic heart disease should undergo an exercise test to highlight whether physical effort could lead to an increase in frequency or severity of arrhythmias.

For patients with supraventricular arrhythmias (episodes of paroxysmal tachycardia, high-frequency atrial flutter), it could be useful to analyse the opportunity to perform ablation of the anatomical substrate of the arrhythmia, particularly if they are considering long sojourns at high altitude in remote areas.[20]

Patients with atrial fibrillation should be instructed on how to monitor the trend of their heart rate at altitude (nowadays, 'smart watches' could be useful for this purpose) and how to possibly modify the therapy in the event of significant increases of the heart rate (>90 beats/minute).

Patients with uncontrolled ventricular arrhythmias should be absolutely discouraged to expose to high altitudes. Those with a recent ICD implantation (<6 months) or recurrent ICD interventions (discharge or overpacing) for ventricular arrhythmias should not travel to remote geographic areas nor ascend to high altitude.[20]

Patients with arrhythmias should refrain from using alcohol or caffeine while hiking at altitude, as these substances can contribute to dehydration and may also interfere with the medications being used.

They must remember to carry all medications with them and continue to take them regularly, without interruptions; it seems also important to recommend to avoid remote locations, where medical facilities are scarce (Evidence: 2C).

References

1. Malconian M, Hultgren H, Nitta M, Anholm J, Houston C, Fails H. The sleep electrocardiogram at extreme altitudes (Operation Everest II). Am J Cardiol 1990; 65(15):1014–1020. https://doi.org/10.1016/0002-9149(90)91006-r.
2. Cummings P, Lysgaard M. Cardiac arrhythmia at high altitude. West J Med 1981; 135(1):66–68. https://pmc.ncbi.nlm.nih.gov/articles/PMC1272927/pdf/westjmed00215-0075.pdf.
3. Kujaník S, Snincák M, Vokál' J, Podracký J, Koval' J. Periodicity of arrhythmias in healthy elderly men at the moderate altitude. Physiol Res 2000; 49(2):285–287. http://www.biomed.cas.cz/physiolres/pdf/49/49_285.pdf.
4. Kujaník S, Snincák M, Galajdová K, Racková K. Cardiovascular changes during sudden ascent in a cable cabin to the moderate altitude. Physiol Res 2000; 49(6):729–731. http://www.biomed.cas.cz/physiolres/pdf/49/49_729.pdf.
5. Kujanik S, Mikulecky M. Circadian and ultradian extrasystole rhythms in healthy individuals at elevated versus lowland altitudes. Int J Biometeorol 2010; 54(5):531-8. https://doi.org/10.1007/s00484-010-0302-8.
6. Woods DR, Allen S, Betts TR, Gardiner D, Montgomery H, Morgan JM, Roberts PR. High altitude arrhythmias. Cardiology 2008; 111(4):239–246. https://doi.org/10.1159/000127445.
7. Gibelli G, Fantoni C, Anzà C, Cattaneo P, Rossi A, Montenero AS, Baravelli M. Arrhythmic risk evaluation during exercise at high altitude in healthy subjects: role of microvolt T-wave alternans. Pacing Clin Electrophysiol 2008; 31(10):1277–1283. https://doi.org/10.1111/j.1540-8159.2008.01178.x.
8. Boos CJ, Holdsworth DA, Woods DR, O'Hara J, Brooks N, Macconnachie L, Bakker-Dyos J, Paisey J, Mellor A. Assessment of cardiac arrhythmias at extreme high altitude using an implantable cardiac monitor: REVEAL HA Study (REVEAL High Altitude). Circulation 2017; 135(8):812–814. https://doi.org/10.1161/CIRCULATIONAHA.116.026584.

9 Alexander JK. Age, altitude, and arrhythmia. Tex Heart Inst J 1995; 22(4):308–316. https://www.ncbi.nlm.nih.gov/pmc/articles/PMC325279/pdf/thij00035-0036.pdf.

10 Alexander JK. Cardiac arrhythmia at high altitude: the progressive effect of aging. Tex Heart Inst J 1999;26(4):258–263. https://pmc.ncbi.nlm.nih.gov/articles/PMC325660/pdf/thij00019-0024.pdf.

11 Lippi G, Sanchis-Gomar F, Cervellin G. Global epidemiology of atrial fibrillation: an increasing epidemic and public health challenge. Int J Stroke 2021; 16(2):217–221. https://doi.org/10.1177/1747493019897870. Erratum in: Corrigendum. Int J Stroke 2020; 15(9):NP11–NP12. https://doi.org/10.1177/1747493020905964.

12 Lyon A, van Mourik M, Cruts L, Heijman J, Bekkers SCAM, Schotten U, Crijns HJGM, Linz D, Lumens J. Both beat-to-beat changes in RR-interval and left ventricular filling time determine ventricular function during atrial fibrillation. Europace 2021; 23(23 Suppl 1):i21–i28. https://doi.org/10.1093/europace/euaa387.

13 Diamond JA, Ismail H. Obstructive sleep apnea and cardiovascular disease. Clin Geriatr Med 2021; 37(3):445–456. https://doi.org/10.1016/j.cger.2021.04.006.

14 Weilenmann D, Duru F, Schönbeck M, Schenk B, Zwicky P, Russi EW, Candinas R. Influence of acute exposure to high altitude and hypoxaemia on ventricular stimulation thresholds in pacemaker patients. Pacing Clin Electrophysiol 2000; 23(4 Pt 1):512–515. https://doi.org/10.1111/j.1540-8159.2000.tb00836.x.

15 Kobza R, Duru F, Erne P. Leisure-time activities of patients with ICDs: findings of a survey with respect to sports activity, high altitude stays, and driving patterns. Pacing Clin Electrophysiol 2008; 31(7):845–849. https://doi.org/10.1111/j.1540-8159.2008.01098.x.

16 Katkat F. Flight safety in patients with arrhythmia. Anatol J Cardiol 2021; 25 (Suppl 1):24–25. https://doi.org/10.5152/AnatolJCardiol.2021.S109.

17 Badran H, Kolb C. Correspondence (letter to the editor): visiting high altitudes is possible. Dtsch Arztebl Int 2012; 109(25):445; author reply 446. https://doi.org/10.3238/arztebl.2012.0445a.

18 Lampert R, Olshansky B. Sports participation in patients with implantable cardioverter-defibrillators. Herzschrittmacherther Elektrophysiol 2012; 23(2):87–93. https://doi.org/10.1007/s00399-012-0181-2.

19 Donegani E, Hillebrandt D, Windsor J, Gieseler U, Rodway G, Schöffl V, Küpper T. Pre-existing cardiovascular conditions and high altitude travel. Consensus statement of the Medical Commission of the Union Internationale des Associations d'Alpinisme (UIAA MedCom) Travel Medicine and Infectious Disease. Travel Med Infect Dis 2014;12(3):237–252. https://doi.org/10.1016/j.tmaid.2014.02.004.

20 Parati G, Agostoni P, Basnyat B, Bilo G, Brugger H, Coca A, Festi L, Giardini G, Lironcurti A, Luks AM, Maggiorini M, Modesti PA, Swenson ER, Williams B, Bärtsch P, Torlasco C. Clinical recommendations for high altitude exposure of individuals with pre-existing cardiovascular conditions: a joint statement by the European Society of Cardiology, the Council on Hypertension of the European Society of Cardiology, the European Society of Hypertension, the International Society of Mountain Medicine, the Italian Society of Hypertension and the Italian Society of Mountain Medicine. Eur Heart J 2018;39(17):1546–1554. https://doi.org/10.1093/eurheartj/ehx720.

CHAPTER 17

Diabetes Mellitus and the Heart at High Altitude

Diabetes mellitus is a chronic disease, caused by deficient insulin production (type 1 diabetes) or ineffective use of the insulin produced (type 2 diabetes). It has been estimated[1] that the number of people living with diabetes worldwide in 2022 was approximately 830 million people, of which approximately 9.2 million people affected by type 1 diabetes.[2] Diabetes prevalence has increased dramatically over the past 30 years (in 1990, diabetes was estimated to affect 200 million people), especially in low- and middle-income countries, where 81% of diabetes cases are living and where, moreover, diabetes treatment coverage is often inadequate.

Based on the data above, it is estimated that 14% of adults aged 18 years and older are living with diabetes, and we also know that globally more than half (59%) of adults aged 30 years and over may be unaware of their diabetes or not following adequate treatment.[1]

Diabetes Mellitus: A Major Risk Factor for Cardiovascular Diseases

In the general population (and in high-mountain dwellers as well, in spite of the lower prevalence of the disease among them; see Chapter 20), diabetes mellitus is one of the major cardiovascular risk factors, as high glucose levels induce endothelial dysfunction, characterised by multiple events: reduced nitric oxide bioavailability with impaired endothelium-dependent vasodilation, increased permeability and inflammatory adhesion molecule expression, accumulation of advanced glycation end-products in the vascular walls and enhanced release of pro-inflammatory molecules. The frequent association of hyperglycaemia with dyslipidaemia can facilitate retention of atherogenic lipoproteins in the arterial intima, with their subsequent oxidative and enzymatic modification and generation of toxic products.[3]

The micro- and macro-vascular complications related to diabetes lead to a series of clinical manifestations that worsen the quality of life of the individuals and lead to a 2–4 times increased cardiovascular risk (further rising with worsening glycaemic control) and a 75% excess mortality in diabetic adults.[4] In persons with diabetes mellitus, the prevalence of coronary heart disease has been calculated to be approximately 14–21%, with greater frequency in females (hazard ratio of 1.48 in males and 1.81 in females). The prevalence of heart failure in diabetic persons is around 19–26%, and it is approximately twofold in men and fivefold in women in comparison to non-diabetic persons. Other major complications present also a high prevalence in diabetic patients: peripheral artery disease (16–29%), stroke (8–12%), retinopathy (34%), cardiac autonomic neuropathy (31–73%) and nephropathy (29–61%).[4]

No specific data are available about prevalence of diabetes among persons who frequent the high mountains, but, based on its high prevalence in the general population, a high prevalence could also be expected among those who frequent high mountain areas.

At altitude, as already presented in previous chapters, hypoxia induces some degree of hyperventilation that results in a decrease in $PaCO_2$. The lung transfer capacity for CO_2 seems to be modestly reduced in diabetic patients, especially type 2, together with lower ventilatory responses to hypoxia and a mild restrictive lung function impairment.[5] Anyway, peripheral arterial O_2 saturation seems to be similar in non-smoking subjects with uncomplicated type 2 diabetes compared to healthy individuals, at altitudes up to 4,167 m above sea level.

Acute altitude exposure increases heart rate, due to increased sympathetic activation. The physiological modifications of heart rate could be impaired in diabetic patients with cardiac autonomic neuropathy, especially if resting tachycardia is already present at low altitudes; diabetic patients with cardiac autonomic neuropathy should be discouraged to go to high altitudes.

With altitude, blood pressure can slightly increase in all persons; also in subjects with uncomplicated type 2 diabetes, only small non-significant differences have been found in systolic (3.7 ± 11.3 mmHg) and diastolic (1.5 ± 7.0 mmHg) blood pressure during a 12 day expedition to Mt. Toubkal (Morocco) at an altitude of 3,200 m in comparison to the values recorded at sea level.[5] At moderate altitude, observations made in Austria highlighted a slight reduction of blood pressure in patients with metabolic syndrome during a 2–3-week sojourn at 1,700 m.[6–8]

Heart work is usually increased by the increased heart rate together with the possible increase of blood pressure, especially in the first days or weeks of ascent; if diabetes is complicated by coronary artery disease (known or unknown), ischaemic cardiac manifestations may occur, with the onset of exertional angina, or symptoms of heart failure, or even lead to sudden cardiac death. It has already been cited in Chapter 9 that a retrospective study performed on Austrian Alps reported that among the hikers who died suddenly a history of diabetes was 6–7.4 times more frequent than the controls.[9, 10]

Exercise performance (evaluated as VO_2 max) decreases with ascent to mountain altitudes, already beginning at an altitude of 580 m in all persons;[11] this means that a certain degree of effort implies greater energy expenditure than if performed at low altitudes. It is known that at altitude, persons with coronary artery disease or heart failure (including patients with complicated diabetes) may experience symptoms at lower than usual physical effort. As regards persons with uncomplicated diabetes, little is known about how they could behave at moderate or high altitudes; at least two studies indicate that in uncomplicated type 1 diabetes, heart rate, blood pressure and echocardiographic parameters did not differ between type 1 diabetic patients and non-diabetic persons, even at the very high altitudes of 4,000–5,800 m.[5, 12]

Diabetic Patients with Diabetic Nephropathy at Altitude

About diabetic nephropathy, it is not known whether it could worsen during travel to, or prolonged stay at, altitude. In experimental animals, reduced O_2 content in the inhaled air results directly in reduced intrarenal tissue PO_2, and it is known that tissue hypoxia may worsen kidney disease;[13] scarce data are available for diabetic nephropathy in humans at high altitude.

Generally, during acute exposure of healthy persons to high altitude, renal blood flow decreases accompanied by a decrease of glomerular filtration rate; conversely, during chronic exposure to high altitude, renal blood flow continues to be reduced, but an increased activity of the Renin–Angiotensin–Aldosterone system causes glomerular hyper-filtration so that the glomerular filtration rate remains relatively unchanged.[14, 15]

It is interesting to remember that type 2 diabetic patients have higher proteinuria and higher serum creatine levels at altitudes greater than 1,727 m.[5] Plasma volume decreases with stay at altitude, and this could be a complicating factor in diabetic patients with more or less impaired kidney function. Chronically living at high altitudes at ≥2,000 m above sea level resulted to be an independent factor of progression to advanced kidney disease in persons with type 2 diabetes mellitus and diabetic nephropathy, anyway with important genetic differences.[16]

At high altitude, the reduced PiO_2 induces hyperventilation that usually leads to some degree of respiratory alkalosis; in normal persons, this respiratory alkalosis is compensated by excretion of bicarbonate with the urines. In persons with kidney dysfunction, the high-altitude respiratory alkalosis may not be adequately compensated. In diabetic persons with normal kidney function, a common metabolic disorder is metabolic alkalosis;[17] it may be exacerbated if diabetic patients with some degree of kidney failure reach altitudes that also induce respiratory alkalosis.

In diabetic patients with kidney dysfunction, metabolic acidosis becomes more frequent in parallel to the worsening of the renal function;[17] the combination of metabolic acidosis with respiratory alkalosis may lead to variable consequences and dynamic changes.

Metabolic acidosis (when severe) reduces myocardial contractility, is accompanied by electrolyte imbalance that predisposes patients to cardiac arrhythmias, causes vascular constriction and may reduce peripheral vascular resistance, blood pressure, hepatic blood flow and tissue oxygen release. These changes contribute to increased mortality and morbidity.[18, 19]

Glycaemia and Insulinaemia at Altitude

During acute exposure of lowlanders to high-altitude hypoxia, the tissue hypoxia together with the important activation of the sympathetic nervous system and the release of epinephrine and cortisol induce a state of transient (even though prolonged) insulin resistance and relative hyperglycaemia even in euglycaemic subjects, with glucose and insulin levels higher than at sea level for the first 2–3 days at altitude, followed by progressive normalisation within 1 week.[20, 21]

After acute exposure to high altitude, insulin resistance returns to baseline values upon returning to sea level.[22]

During prolonged exposure to altitude, fasting glucose concentrations appear to decrease with acclimatisation, while insulin concentrations remain unchanged;[5] in the group of chronic high-altitude residents who do not achieve adequate tissue oxygenation through compensatory mechanisms, insulin resistance persists, thus progressively causing the well-known related clinical complications.[22]

Numerous persons with type 1 and type 2 diabetes have climbed till now Mt. Kilimanjaro (5,895 m), and a few individuals also have reached the summit of Mt. Everest (8,848 m). The first person with type 1 diabetes to summit Mt. Everest was Will Cross, in May 2006;[23] Taylor Adams was the first person with type 1 diabetes to summit the Seven Summits.[24]

Diabetic patients may experience at altitude loss of glycaemic control with increase of the levels of HbA_{1c}, due to a combination of hypoxia-induced sympatho-adrenergic activity and cold-induced reduction of insulin absorption from the site of subcutaneous injection. Thus, they may experience episodes of hyperglycaemia, as well as episodes of hypoglycaemia especially in occasion of physical activity in the first days of exposure to altitude.

It is important to remember that in subjects with type 1 diabetes, the performance of physical activity, such as that sustained during trekking, is accompanied, on the one hand, by reductions in insulin requirement at lower altitudes and, on the other, by a progressive increase in insulin requirement at higher altitudes (>3,700–5,000 m), despite the physical exercise performed, together with a significant increase in blood lactate concentration.[12, 23] The reduced systemic tissue oxygenation due to the exposure to high altitude (hypobaric hypoxia) induces insulin resistance and a metabolic switch towards glycolysis that persists as long as tissue oxygenation is impaired.[22]

Besides the increase of counter-regulatory hormones (increased sympathetic output and increased catecholamine levels), other factors may alter greatly the glycaemic balance: degree and duration of physical effort at altitude, dietary changes (associated with reduced food intake due to high-altitude-induced anorexia),[25] possible intercurrent illnesses and possible mountain sickness.

Regular control of glycaemia is thus required by diabetic patients climbing to high altitudes, before, during and after and intense or prolonged effort (Evidence: 1B). In this purpose, it must be taken into account that glucometers (especially those using the glucose oxidase enzyme methods, which are dependent on oxygen in the surrounding environment) are affected with changes in altitude: they underestimate glucose levels by approximately 1–2% for each 300 m of elevation (after correction for changes in temperature and humidity) and may lead to use dosages of insulin lower than needed.[26] Glucometers based on glucose dehydrogenase reaction may overestimate glycaemia by 3.5–8% at altitude of 2,000 m. Anyway, the Wilderness Medical Society concluded that the reported differences were small enough to be of questionable clinical significance.[27]

During exposure to cold environment, with presence of cutaneous vasoconstriction, it is important also to properly choose the site of blood sampling. The need to administrate insulin could be complicated by the extreme excursions of temperature existing at very high altitudes, with very cold temperatures especially during the hours when sun is not out (possible freezing of insulin vials) and higher temperatures (insulin degradation) associated also with intense sunlight during day hours.[28]

Prolonged Exercise and Glycaemic Control

Prolonged exercise, lasting more than 60 minutes, has been shown to increase peripheral insulin sensitivity for up to 48 hours post-exercise, with possible appearance of post-exercise late-onset (typically nocturnal) hypoglycaemia in insulin-dependent diabetic patients.[29] Long-duration aerobic exercise is likely to cause hypoglycaemia, although less frequently and with great interindividual variations, also in type 2 diabetic patients treated with insulin or insulin secretagogues.[30]

Possible hypoglycaemia is a major concern for persons with diabetes when they are exercising in the wilderness as well as at high altitudes. Among the many symptoms of hypoglycaemia that can mimic acute mountain sickness (AMS) (and vice versa), palpitations, fatigue and sweating may be confused with cardiac symptoms. During hypoglycaemia, heart rate and systolic blood pressure increase, as well as myocardial contractility, stroke volume and cardiac output. These phenomena thus imply a great (although transient) increase of cardiac workload that may have dangerous consequences in older people with diabetes and underlying known or unknown coronary heart disease.[31] The reduced arterial elasticity that is present in patients with type 2 diabetes and in long-duration type 1 diabetes implies modification of the reflected pressure wave and reduction of the blood flow to the coronaries during diastole; this phenomenon, associated with the increased cardiac workload, may promote myocardial ischaemia, whose incidence is difficult to establish but seems to be rather elevated in type 2 diabetic patients.

During hypoglycaemia, the sympatho-adrenal activation, the direct effect of insulin and a direct inhibition of cardiac ion channels lead also to appearance of hypokalaemia, which is evident in the electrocardiogram (ECG) by flattening of the T waves and prolongation of the QT interval. At the same time, during an episode of hypoglycaemia, the profuse secretion of catecholamines increases cardiac excitability. The cardiac electrophysiological changes may increase the risk of cardiac arrhythmias that range from severe sinus bradycardia (that may progress to asystole) to appearance of atrial fibrillation, or episodes of ventricular tachycardia, to the risk of sudden death.[31, 32]

Increased erythrocyte concentration and plasma viscosity have been also described during hypoglycaemia, as well as pro-thrombotic effects (platelet activation and increment in factor VIII and von Willebrand factor) and pro-inflammatory effects; it also compromises the endothelial function.[31] All these changes are aggravated by the effects of altitude and may promote intravascular coagulation and thrombosis and pose the diabetic patient at risk of acute vascular events, myocardial infarction and sudden death.[25]

What is the incidence of hypoglycaemia in diabetic persons exercising at high altitude? There are only very few data on this topic. A study performed in 2022 on a very small group of type 1 diabetes individuals under simulated high altitude (4,200 m) demonstrated a greater decline in blood glucose levels during and after 1 hour exercise performed under acute hypoxia in comparison to effort performed at sea level.[33] During an ascent to Mt. Kilimanjaro (5,895 m), a few episodes of hypoglycaemia occurred among 11 individuals with type 1 diabetes, mainly after the first 2 days of climbing;[34] during an ascent to Mt. Uhuru (5,895 m), no cases of severe hypoglycaemia have been recorded among 19 trekkers with type 1 diabetes.[28] A 42-year-old climber with type 1 diabetes reported in 2017 his experience trekking to the Everest base camp (5,184 m): during the 18 days of trekking, only 2.5% of glycaemia measurements have been found below 70 mg/dl (3.9 mmol/L), while 78.7% of the measurements were higher than 140 mg/dl (7.8 mmol/L).[35]

Short High-intensity Exercise and Glycaemic Control

Brief bursts of high-intensity exercise (80% of individual's VO_2 max) have been shown to cause hyperglycaemia, sustained for 2 hours post-exercise, in normal subjects; in people with insulin-dependent diabetes mellitus, post-exercise hyperglycaemia seems to be of greater magnitude and duration.[36] Reductions of insulin doses (voluntary or due to malfunction of insulin infusion sets) can also trigger hyperglycaemic episodes. Other factors that can cause hyperglycaemia are stress, intercurrent illness, AMS and its treatment with dexamethasone (a drug that diabetics should use with caution because of the risk of hyperglycaemia; Evidence: 2C).

Hyperglycaemia

Hyperglycaemia may predispose to dehydration and electrolyte (Potassium, Magnesium and Phosphorous) loss through osmotic diuresis; dehydration in a hyperglycaemic person can be favoured at high altitude by the known high-altitude dehydration and by the use of diuretics or other cardiovascular drugs. Furthermore, climbers may experience reduced intake of water due to poor availability and adipsia. Adequate hydration is recommended in these cases (Evidence: 1C).

In healthy volunteers, a 14-day trekking in the mountains of Nepal was accompanied by increase in nocturnal glucose levels at all altitudes reached (3,600 m, 4650 m and 5,120 m); the increase was independent of energy intake and has been explained as a stress-induced relative insulin deficiency greater than the exercise-induced increase in insulin sensitivity.[37] The rate of ascent is also a modifying factor of the kind and intensity of glucose modifications during ascent to high altitude.[38] A significant increase in the mean daily glucose concentration was also observed by Matejko et al. in 18 type 1 diabetes mellitus patients during an ascent to the summit of Mt. Damavand (5,670 m; Iran); some severe episodes of hyperglycaemia occurred on days 2 and 3 of trekking, despite a reduction in carbohydrate consumption and a higher insulin delivery.[39]

It is well known that chronically elevated blood glucose levels lead to cardiovascular complications. The cardiac effects of short duration hyperglycaemia are less well known; however, a number of studies agree that glucose fluctuations and hyperglycaemia are triggers of inflammatory responses. Such inflammatory responses induced by one transient, short-term episode of hyperglycaemia may last for several days,[40, 41] eventually leading to endothelial dysfunction and impaired vasodilation[42] with possible reduction of myocardial perfusion,[43] in both healthy persons and type 2 diabetic patients,[44] as well as to impaired cardiac contractility.[45] While there is consensus on the long-term effects of hyperglycaemic peaks on cardiovascular risk,[46] it is still unclear what the short-term impact of these abnormalities may be in individuals operating at high altitudes.

Diabetic Ketoacidosis

Hyperglycaemia becomes a serious problem when it is associated with or triggered by AMS, a situation that exacerbates a metabolic derangement with possible development of diabetic ketoacidosis, mostly in persons with type 1 diabetes, especially if they are taking steroids or acetazolamide for prevention or treatment of mountain sickness or in case of non-compliance to a regular insulin intake. Anorexia, dehydration and physical exercise are all situations that exacerbate the generation of ketones. In these cases, hypokalaemia is often present and possibly severe,[47, 48] with appearance of cardiac arrhythmias that can lead to cardiac arrest. Hyperkalaemia may also be present in cases of diabetic ketoacidosis; it is usually considered a predictor of mortality in type 1 diabetes. An old review of the causes of deaths occurred among trekkers in Nepal between 1984 and 1987 reported that 3 out of a total of 40 deaths (among 275,950 trekkers) had been attributed to apparent diabetic ketoacidosis above 4,000 m in altitude,[19] and that 4 other people were reported to have died from heart attacks. In cases of suspect or possible appearance of ketoacidosis, frequent glucose monitoring and ketone checks are recommended (Evidence: 1C), which could indicate how to adjust insulin dosage (Evidence: 1B).

Cardiovascular Drugs in Diabetic Patients at High Altitude

As regards the use at high altitude of cardiovascular drugs in diabetic patients, the use of 'optimal' medical therapy is obviously recommended to treat concurrent diseases such as hypertension or hypercholesterolaemia.

In subjects with diabetes and hypertension that are taking ACE inhibitors or angiotensin receptor blockers, it seems advisable to continue with this therapy, as these drugs have known nephroprotective effects and could counteract the increase in proteinuria that occurs at high altitude.[49, 50] Because of the possible modifications with the exposure to hypobaric hypoxia, blood pressure should be monitored regularly while at high altitude.

The use of nifedipine or of phosphodiesterase type 5 inhibitors for prevention of high-altitude pulmonary oedema seems to have no particular negative effects in diabetic persons at high altitude.[5]

As in all persons reaching high altitudes, diuretics should be used with caution due to the presence of the hypoxic diuretic response and the relative high-altitude hypovolaemia with intravascular depletion.

In persons with diabetes, the use of acetazolamide therapy for the prophylaxis of AMS and high-altitude cerebral oedema may increase the risk of ketoacidosis (at least in type 1 diabetes mellitus;[34] with special relevance in patients with compromised kidney function),[51] and thus, it is not recommended (Evidence: 2C).[52] It must be noted that – together with the use of acetazolamide – in some cases, the increased development of ketoacidosis in these patients could have been caused by the reduction of insulin doses combined with dehydration and continued exertion.

The use of Aspirin (ASA, acetylsalicylic acid) is recommended in doses of 75–162 mg/day in individuals with type 2 diabetes with atherogenic risk factors (or previous cardiovascular events), due to its effect in primary and secondary prevention,[53] although some studies raise questions about its efficacy;[54] other anti-platelet drugs are also often used for this purpose. Exposure to high altitude may increase the risk of thrombosis in diabetic subjects even on chronic Aspirin treatment, while the stress to which these persons are subjected may increase the risk of gastrointestinal bleeding; the risk–benefit ratio of Aspirin use during high-altitude travel should, therefore, be assessed beforehand by a diabetologist or cardiologist, based on the patients' risk profile. Furthermore, there is no randomised trial on this topic, because people with diabetes have usually been excluded from intervention studies.[55]

Beta-blockers are often used in diabetics, especially in those with hypertension or coronary artery disease, because of their anti-anginal, anti-ischaemic and anti-arrhythmic properties.[56] In individuals with diabetes planning to ascend to high altitudes, the use of beta-blockers must be carefully evaluated before exposure: these drugs can mask possible hypoglycaemic episodes during exertion; by reducing heart rate, they may reduce exercise tolerance; the use of non-selective agents without intrinsic sympathomimetic activity (like Atenolol) can be involved in appearance of bronchoconstriction. If continued treatment with beta-blockers is necessary, the use of selective drugs (bisoprolol, nebivolol) should be considered.

Any other medication for coronary artery disease should be continued as prescribed at sea level; however, in this case, diabetic patients with known coronary artery disease should be evaluated before attempting ascent to high altitudes (see Chapter 19).

As regards possible cardiac effects of non-insulin anti-diabetic drugs, we should remember that Metformin, a medication commonly prescribed to the great majority of type 2 diabetes patients, may cause diarrhoea in 15% of patients,[57] thus predisposing to dehydration and hypokalaemia. Together with other factors described above, it may predispose to arrhythmias during strenuous efforts at high altitude. The drug can also induce lactic acidosis that could be favoured by intense physical activity and could be precipitated by concurrent use of acetazolamide.[27] By blocking glucose reuptake in renal tubules, SGLT2 inhibitors (Canagliflozin, Dapagliflozin and Empagliflozin) have a diuretic-like effect that could theoretically worsen high-altitude dehydration; volume depletion seems anyway rather rare,[58] and no supporting clinical evidence of increased risks at altitude is yet available. However, the use of non-insulin diabetes medications is not considered a contraindication to wilderness athletic involvement, provided that attention should be paid to the individual risks of each specific class of medication (Evidence: 1C).[27]

For further information, we recommend consulting the guidelines issued by the Wilderness Medical Society,[27] which contain valuable information for trekkers with diabetes who intend to venture into mountain areas. Another precious document is that issued by UIAA Medical Commission, with recommendations for mountaineers, hillwalkers, trekkers, and rock and ice climbers with diabetes.[52]

Going High with diabetes mellitus.

Useful tips from the diary of a mountaineer with type 1 diabetes.

In 2016, Mr. Gary Malcolm, a 42-year-old man who had type 1 diabetes for 30 years, decided to undertake a trek to the Everest Base Camp, Nepal, with the support of an English Multidisciplinary Physical Activity and Diabetes Clinic. He described his experiences in a paper, published in 2017 in the British Medical Journal of Sport and Exercise in Medicine.[35]

Here are some of the 'pearls' found in his travel diary.

A first set of observations concerns the *quality of glycaemic control* during high-altitude trekking; these observations may be particularly useful, especially for **people with T1DM**:

1. As the travel implies walking at increased altitude, it becomes important to monitor blood sugar levels and predict the climbs or descents to be faced in order to '*eat enough food to ensure my blood sugar did not rise too much, or fall below 6 mmol/L. In Nepal it meant that I tended to give less fast acting insulin*'. During acclimatisation at 3,800 m and then at 4,400 m, Mr. Malcolm reduced the dosage of his '*evening slow acting insulin. The 14 units I usually took at 11 pm before bed in the UK was replaced by 10 units at 9 pm.*' Such modifications are reasonable, but they need to be adjusted based on glucose monitoring and possible changes in morning insulin dosage.
2. Mr. Malcolm '*decided to have the same breakfast everyday (white coffee plus one fried egg and two rounds of toast)*', which allowed him to keep his glucose levels stable throughout the morning.
3. Keep in mind that when travelling in remote areas, the interval between breakfast and lunch is often very different from one day to the next; Mr. Malcolm reported: '*I brought with me a range of sugary snacks—some dextrose energy tablets and other cereal based snacks to give a longer term carbohydrate.*'
4. Despite these precautions, Mr. Malcolm suffered '*minor hypoglycaemic attacks ... in the first week,*' likely due to the demanding and prolonged physical activity he performed. Later, during the last part of the journey while descending from Pheriche (4,400 m) to Lukla (2,800 m), with longer and faster but not too intense treks, Mr. Malcolm has noticed that blood sugar levels dropped significantly and rapidly ('*my blood sugar levels had fallen to below 3 mmol/L*'), necessitating adequate intake of fast-acting foods and cessation of physical activity. So, he suggested to '*try to keep blood sugar levels at around 9 mmol/L, which will give you some leeway whilst trekking.*' However, by doing so, the time when glucose levels were between 3.9 and 7.8 mmol/L decreased, while the time when glucose levels were >7.8 increased to nearly 79% of readings during the trek.
5. An interesting observation is that Mr. Malcolm noticed that in the very cold climate '*injecting the insulin gave a sharp cold feeling as it was dispensed under the skin.*'

(continued)

Going High with diabetes mellitus. *(continued)*

Some additional observations and suggestions might also offer *useful tips for people with other chronic diseases, as well as for people with T1DM*:

Type 1 diabetes mellitus	Useful tips for other diseases
Preparing for the adventure	
Undertake activities to become fitter; for instance, walk at least 15,000 steps every day and take part in weekend hikes of varying difficulties. Monitor body weight and try to lose excess weight. Monitor HbA_{1c} (with regular physical activity, it should reduce, as happened in Mr. Malcolm from 63 mmol/mol to 56 mmol/mol in 6 months).	In addition to improving effort tolerance during the planned trek, these first two suggestions help reduce cardiovascular risk in the short and long term in everyone.
Learn to drink enough water (at least 2 L a day, enriched with electrolytes).	In high mountains, avoiding high-altitude dehydration will be crucial (both for people with diabetes and for mountaineers in general).
Blood glucose meters do not work properly when exposed to very low temperatures; there is a need to find alternatives. Mr. Malcolm switched from Accu-Chek© (which the manufacturer reports to be tested for altitudes up to 3,094 m) to a real-time continuous glucose monitoring device (Dexcom G4©). In fact, when Mr. Malcom reached the altitude of 5,100 m at Gorak Shep, he observed that the glucose monitoring devices were not working, due to a very cold environment at such altitude: '*Overnight it was −20°C in our room and using my standard blood glucose meter was not possible, even when taking it from my sleeping bag and being covered in a woolly hat.*' While trekking, Mr. Malcolm used a real-time continuous glucose monitoring device, but it was essential to calibrate it twice a day, using the conventional blood sugar meter as a reference. Protect the instruments from cold to allow them to function properly, '*wrapping the machine in a hat/warm clothes/next to body, so it would work during the calibration process.*'	The use of other devices, such as those used for coagulation monitoring, can also be critical at high altitudes. Cold and vasoconstricted skin, as occurs after exposure to low temperatures, can make the sample collected by skin prick inadequate. Coagulation devices appear to function properly in a temperature range of +10–+36 °C, temperatures not always present during a high-altitude travel. A patient undergoing chronic anti-coagulant treatment with vitamin K antagonists is exposed to the risk of inadequate monitoring of coagulation levels in case of prolonged travel to high altitudes; therefore, this should be avoided.

Going High with diabetes mellitus. *(continued)*

Type 1 diabetes mellitus	Useful tips for other diseases
Plan to carry spare packs of sensors '*to reduce the chance of the transmitter latches being broken off in transit.*' A caution is to keep '*batteries and blood sugar readers in internal pockets and inside the sleeping bag (to prolong their life).*'	Even for other types of devices, it is important to carry spare packs of sensors and batteries, without forgetting to carry adequate quantities of the medications in use.
During ascent	
At low altitude (Kathmandu, Nepal, 1,400 m), Mr. Malcolm observed that the delay between injection of the fast-acting insulin and the reduction of glycaemia was consistently increased by 20 minutes. Therefore, the correct time of insulin administration relative to meals had to be adjusted accordingly. At higher altitude (Gorak Shep, 5,100 m), a further significant delay occurred between the time of insulin injection and the onset of its effects, reaching 3 hours, thus forcing him to inject the insulin dose much earlier than usual.	For other injectable cardiovascular drugs (e.g. low molecular weight heparins), there are no studies on the effect of cold skin temperature on the possible delay of absorption, nor on their pharmacokinetics. Transdermal absorption of drugs such as clonidine may be variable: on the one hand, it is likely increased during exercise due to cutaneous vasodilation, augmented lymphatic drainage and the pumping effects of contracting muscles; on the other hand, cold environment may reduce percutaneous drug absorption due to reduced skin perfusion. At high altitude (3,600 m for 16 hours and 6 months), an increase in plasma concentrations of furosemide has been described.[59]
As there is no access to refrigerator while trekking, consider to '*carry [the insulin for immediate use] in the day bag to avoid direct sunlight, limiting temperature changes.*' Do not carry all your insulin supplies in one bag, but distribute them among the other members of the group ('*ensure I did not have all my eggs in one basket—i.e. lose a bag and so have NO insulin*').	This is also an important tip also for all other type of medications the traveller will need, especially essential ones.
Reduce the chances of contracting an intestinal infection, which could greatly complicate glycaemic control (and compromise the entire trip); use an antibacterial hand sanitizer, drink only bottled water, take dietary precautions.	Dehydration is a risk for all high-altitude trekkers; it can worsen the high-altitude hypovolaemia, and lead to symptomatic hypotension. Vomiting and diarrhoea can alter the intestinal absorption of drugs.
At high altitude, there is always the possibility of suffering from mountain sickness, which could represent an additional complicating factor. Preventive treatments should be considered.	Participants in a high-altitude trekking should discuss with their doctor in advance the potential interference between medications they are taking usually and those needed to prevent or treat mountain sickness.

(continued)

Going High with diabetes mellitus. *(continued)*

Type 1 diabetes mellitus	Useful tips for other diseases
A conclusive remark made by Mr. Malcolm is: '*Lastly, inform other trekkers and the tour organisers that you have diabetes and what symptoms to look out for, and how to deal with them.*'	All persons with chronic diseases should inform other trekkers, or at least the group leader, about their condition; in remote areas, it is vital to be able to receive support and essential medical care from fellow trekkers.

References

1 World Health Organization. Health Topic: Diabetes. November 14, 2024. https://www.who.int/health-topics/diabetes.

2 International Diabetes Federation. Type 1 diabetes. https://idf.org/about-diabetes/types-of-diabetes/type-1-diabetes.

3 Chait A, Eckel RH, Vrablik M, Zambon A. Lipid-lowering in diabetes: an update. Atherosclerosis. 2024; 394:117313. https://doi.org/10.1016/j.atherosclerosis.2023.117313.

4 Dal Canto E, Ceriello A, Rydén L, Ferrini M, Hansen TB, Schnell O, Standl E, Beulens JW. Diabetes as a cardiovascular risk factor: an overview of global trends of macro and micro vascular complications. Eur J Prev Cardiol 2019; 26(2_suppl):25–32. https://doi.org/10.1177/2047487319878371.

5 de Mol P, de Vries ST, de Koning EJ, Gans RO, Bilo HJ, Tack CJ. Physical activity at altitude: challenges for people with diabetes: a review. Diabetes Care 2014; 37(8):2404–2413. https://doi.org/10.2337/dc13-2302.

6 Schobersberger W, Schmid P, Lechleitner M, von Duvillard SP, Hörtnagl H, Gunga HC, Klingler A, Fries D, Kirsch K, Spiesberger R, Pokan R, Hofmann P, Hoppichler F, Riedmann G, Baumgartner H, Humpeler E. Austrian moderate altitude study 2000 (AMAS 2000). The effects of moderate altitude (1,700 m) on cardiovascular and metabolic variables in patients with metabolic syndrome. Eur J Appl Physiol 2003; 88(6):506–514. https://doi.org/10.1007/s00421-002-0736-8.

7 Mair J, Hammerer-Lercher A, Mittermayr M, Klingler A, Humpeler E, Pachinger O, Schobersberger W. 3-week hiking holidays at moderate altitude do not impair cardiac function in individuals with metabolic syndrome. Int J Cardiol 2008; 123(2):186–188. https://doi.org/10.1016/j.ijcard.2006.11.127.

8 Gutwenger I, Hofer G, Gutwenger AK, Sandri M, Wiedermann CJ. Pilot study on the effects of a 2-week hiking vacation at moderate versus low altitude on plasma parameters of carbohydrate and lipid metabolism in patients with metabolic syndrome. BMC Res Notes 2015; 8:103. https://doi.org/10.1186/s13104-015-1066-3.

9 Burtscher M. Risk of cardiovascular events during mountain activities. Adv Exp Med Biol 2007; 618:1–11. https://doi.org/10.1007/978-0-387-75434-5_1.

10 Niebauer J, Burtscher M. Sudden cardiac death risk in downhill skiers and mountain hikers and specific prevention strategies. Int J Environ Res Public Health 2021; 18(4):1621. https://doi.org/10.3390/ijerph18041621.

11 Fulco CS, Rock PB, Cymerman A. Maximal and submaximal exercise performance at altitude. Aviat Space Environ Med 1998; 69(8):793–801.

12 Pavan P, Sarto P, Merlo L, Casara D, Ponchia A, Biasin R, Noventa D, Avogaro A. Metabolic and cardiovascular parameters in type 1 diabetes at extreme altitude. Med Sci Sports Exerc 2004; 36(8):1283–1289. https://doi.org/10.1249/01.mss.0000135782.93008.6c.

13 Hansell P, Welch WJ, Blantz RC, Palm F. Determinants of kidney oxygen consumption and their relationship to tissue oxygen tension in diabetes and hypertension. Clin Exp Pharmacol Physiol 2013; 40(2):123–137. https://doi.org/10.1111/1440-1681.12034.

14 Wang SY, Gao J, Zhao JH. Effects of high altitude on renal physiology and kidney diseases. Front Physiol 2022; 13:969456. https://doi.org/10.3389/fphys.2022.969456.

15 Aoun M, Chelala D. Where do you live and what do you do? Two questions that might impact your kidney health. Front Nephrol 2022; 2:1011964. https://doi.org/10.3389/fneph.2022.1011964.

16 Zhao L, Wang X, Wang T, Fan W, Ren H, Zhang R, Zou Y, Xu H, Zhang J, Wu Y, Liu F. Associations Between High-Altitude Residence and End-Stage Kidney Disease in Chinese Patients with Type 2 Diabetes. High Alt Med Biol 2020; 21(4):396–405. https://doi.org/10.1089/ham.2020.0076.

17 Sotirakopoulos N, Kalogiannidou I, Tersi M, Armentzioiou K, Sivridis D, Mavromatidis K. Acid-base and electrolyte disorders in patients with diabetes mellitus. Saudi J Kidney Dis Transpl 2012; 23(1):58–62. https://journals.lww.com/sjkd/fulltext/2012/23010/acid_base_and_electrolyte_disorders_in_patients.11.aspx#:~:text=Abstract,calcium%20channel%20blockers%20or%20not.

18 Kraut JA, Kurtz I. Use of base in the treatment of severe acidemic states. Am J Kidney Dis 2001; 38(4):703–727. https://doi.org/10.1053/ajkd.2001.27688.

19 Shlim DR, Gallie J. The causes of death among trekkers in Nepal. Int J Sports Med 1992; 13 (Suppl 1):S74–S76. https://doi.org/10.1055/s-2007-1024601.

20 Sawhney RC, Malhotra AS, Singh T. Glucoregulatory hormones in man at high altitude. Eur J Appl Physiol Occup Physiol 1991; 62(4):286–291. https://doi.org/10.1007/BF00571554.

21 Sawhney RC, Malhotra AS, Singh T, Rai RM, Sinha KC. Insulin secretion at high altitude in man. Int J Biometeorol 1986; 30(3):231–238. https://doi.org/10.1007/BF02189466.

22 Adeva-Andany MM, Adeva-Contreras L, Carneiro-Freire N, Ameneiros-Rodríguez E, Vila-Altesor M, Calvo-Castro I. The impact of high altitude (hypobaric hypoxia) on insulin resistance in humans. J Physiol Biochem 2025; 81(1):35–55. https://doi.org/10.1007/s13105-025-01069-8.

23 de Mol P, de Vries ST, de Koning EJ, Gans RO, Tack CJ, Bilo HJ. Increased insulin requirements during exercise at very high altitude in type 1 diabetes. Diabetes Care 2011; 34(3):591–595. https://doi.org/10.2337/dc10-2015.

24 Valsan B. Scaling Everest: Taylor-made success story of diabetes. November 14, 2022. https://www.happiesthealth.com/articles/diabetes/diabetes-shouldnt-stop-anyone-from-reaching-the-top-of-the-world.

25 Vats P, Singh VK, Singh SN, Singh SB. High altitude induced anorexia: effect of changes in leptin and oxidative stress levels. Nutr Neurosci 2007; 10(5–6):243–249. https://doi.org/10.1080/10284150701722299.

26 Jendle J, Adolfsson P. Impact of high altitudes on glucose control. J Diabetes Sci Technol 2011; 5(6):1621–1622. https://doi.org/10.1177/193229681100500642.

27 VanBaak KD, Nally LM, Finigan RT, Jurkiewicz CL, Burnier AM, Conrad BP, Khodaee M, Lipman GS. Wilderness medical society clinical practice guidelines for diabetes management. Wilderness Environ Med 2019; 30(4S):S121–S140. https://doi.org/10.1016/j.wem.2019.10.003.

28 Richards P, Hillebrandt D. The practical aspects of insulin at high altitude. High Alt Med Biol 2013; 14(3):197–204. https://doi.org/10.1089/ham.2013.1020.

29 MacDonald MJ. Postexercise late-onset hypoglycemia in insulin-dependent diabetic patients. Diabetes Care 1987; 10(5):584–588. https://doi.org/10.2337/diacare.10.5.584.

30 Colberg SR. Key points from the updated guidelines on exercise and diabetes. Front Endocrinol (Lausanne) 2017; 8:33. https://doi.org/10.3389/fendo.2017.00033.

31 Frier BM, Schernthaner G, Heller SR. Hypoglycemia and cardiovascular risks. Diabetes Care 2011; 34 (Suppl 2):S132–S137. https://doi.org/10.2337/dc11-s220.

32 Tak S, Jain A. Severe hypoglycemia and cardiovascular disease. Curr. Opin. Endocr. Metab. Res. 2022; 24:100357. https://doi.org/10.1016/j.coemr.2022.100357.

33 Dugan CW, Maloney SK, Abramoff KJ, Panag SS, Davis EA, Jones TW, Fournier PA. Effects of simulated high altitude on blood glucose levels during exercise in individuals with type 1 diabetes. J Clin Endocrinol Metab 2022; 107(5):1375–1382. https://doi.org/10.1210/clinem/dgab881.

34 Moore K, Vizzard N, Coleman C, McMahon J, Hayes R, Thompson CJ. Extreme altitude mountaineering and Type 1 diabetes; the Diabetes Federation of Ireland Kilimanjaro Expedition. Diabet Med 2001; 18(9):749–755. https://doi.org/10.1046/j.0742-3071.2001.00568.x.

35 Malcolm G, Rilstone S, Sivasubramaniyam S, Jairam C, Chew S, Oliver N, Hill NE. Managing diabetes at high altitude: personal experience with support from a Multidisciplinary Physical Activity and Diabetes Clinic. BMJ Open Sport Exerc Med 2017; 3(1):e000238. https://doi.org/10.1136/bmjsem-2017-000238.

36 Mitchell TH, Abraham G, Schiffrin A, Leiter LA, Marliss EB. Hyperglycemia after intense exercise in IDDM subjects during continuous subcutaneous insulin infusion. Diabetes Care 1988; 11(4): 311–317. https://doi.org/10.2337/diacare.11.4.311.

37 Hill NE, Deighton K, Matu J, Misra S, Oliver NS, Newman C, Mellor A, O'Hara J, Woods D. Continuous glucose monitoring at high altitude-effects on glucose homeostasis. Med Sci Sports Exerc 2018; 50(8):1679–1686. https://doi.org/10.1249/MSS.0000000000001624.

38 Koufakis T, Karras SN, Mustafa OG, Zebekakis P, Kotsa K. The effects of high altitude on glucose homeostasis, metabolic control, and other diabetes-related parameters: from animal studies to real life. High Alt Med Biol 2019; 20(1):1–11. https://doi.org/10.1089/ham.2018.0076.

39 Matejko B, Gawrecki A, Wróbel M, Hohendorff J, Benbenek-Klupa T, Zozulińska-Ziółkiewicz D, Malecki MT, Klupa T. Physiological characteristics of type 1 diabetes patients during high mountain trekking. J Diabetes Res 2020; 2020: 8068710. https://doi.org/10.1155/2020/8068710.

40 El-Osta A, Brasacchio D, Yao D, Pocai A, Jones PL, Roeder RG, Cooper ME, Brownlee M. Transient high glucose causes persistent epigenetic changes and altered gene expression during subsequent normoglycemia. J Exp Med 2008; 205(10):2409–2417. https://doi.org/10.1084/jem.20081188. Erratum in: J Exp Med 2008; 205(11):2683. https://pmc.ncbi.nlm.nih.gov/articles/PMC2556800/pdf/jem2052409.pdf.

41 Mortuza R, Chakrabarti S. Glucose-induced cell signaling in the pathogenesis of diabetic cardiomyopathy. Heart Fail Rev 2014; 19(1):75–86. https://doi.org/10.1007/s10741-013-9381-z.

42 Kawano H, Motoyama T, Hirashima O, Hirai N, Miyao Y, Sakamoto T, Kugiyama K, Ogawa H, Yasue H. Hyperglycemia rapidly suppresses flow-mediated endothelium-dependent vasodilation of brachial artery. J Am Coll Cardiol 1999; 34(1):146-54. https://doi.org/10.1016/s0735-1097(99)00168-0. https://www.jacc.org/doi/10.1016/S0735-1097(99)00168-0.

43 Scognamiglio R, Negut C, de Kreutzenberg SV, Tiengo A, Avogaro A. Effects of different insulin regimes on postprandial myocardial perfusion defects in type 2 diabetic patients. Diabetes Care 2006; 29(1):95–100.

44 Esposito K, Nappo F, Marfella R, Giugliano G, Giugliano F, Ciotola M, Quagliaro L, Ceriello A, Giugliano D. Inflammatory cytokine concentrations are acutely increased by hyperglycemia in humans: role of oxidative stress. Circulation 2002; 106(16):2067–2072. https://doi.org/10.1161/01.cir.0000034509.14906.ae.

45 Singh RM, Waqar T, Howarth FC, Adeghate E, Bidasee K, Singh J. Hyperglycemia-induced cardiac contractile dysfunction in the diabetic heart. Heart Fail Rev 2018; 23(1):37–54. https://doi.org/10.1007/s10741-017-9663-y.

46 Standl E, Schnell O, Ceriello A. Postprandial hyperglycemia and glycemic variability: should we care? Diabetes Care 2011; 34 (Suppl 2):S120–S127. https://doi.org/10.2337/dc11-s206.

47 Miller SC. Diabetic ketoacidosis and acute mountain sickness: case report and review of treatment options in type 1 diabetes mellitus. Wilderness Environ Med 2015; 26(2):185–188. https://doi.org/10.1016/j.wem.2014.09.033.

48 Pandit K, Khanal S, Adhikari S, Acharya SP. Acute mountain sickness induced diabetic ketoacidosis managed with hemodialysis: a case report. Ann Med Surg (Lond) 2020; 56:165–168. https://doi.org/10.1016/j.amsu.2020.06.012.

49 Luks AM, Johnson RJ, Swenson ER. Chronic kidney disease at high altitude. J Am Soc Nephrol 2008; 19(12):2262–2271. https://doi.org/10.1681/ASN.2007111199.

50 Joyce KE, Delamere J, Bradwell S, Myers SD, Ashdown K, Rue C, Lucas SJ, Thomas OD, Fountain A, Edsell M, Myers F, Malein W, Imray C, Clarke A, Lewis CT, Newman C, Johnson B, Cadigan P, Wright A, Bradwell A. Hypoxia is not the primary mechanism contributing to exercise-induced proteinuria. BMJ Open Sport Exerc Med 2020;6(1):e000662. https://doi.org/10.1136/bmjsem-2019-000662.

51 Swenson ER. Safety of carbonic anhydrase inhibitors. Expert Opin Drug Saf 2014; 13(4):459–472. https://doi.org/10.1517/14740338.2014.897328.

52 Hillebrandt D, Gurtoo A, Kupper T, Richards P, Schöffl V, Shah P, van der Spek R, Wallis N, Milledge J. UIAA medical commission recommendations for mountaineers, hillwalkers, trekkers, and rock and ice climbers with diabetes. High Alt Med Biol 2023; 24(2):110–126. https://doi.org/10.1089/ham.2018.0043.

53 Buse JB, Ginsberg HN, Bakris GL, Clark NG, Costa F, Eckel R, Fonseca V, Gerstein HC, Grundy S, Nesto RW, Pignone MP, Plutzky J, Porte D, Redberg R, Stitzel KF, Stone NJ; American Heart Association; American Diabetes Association. Primary prevention of cardiovascular diseases in people with diabetes mellitus: a scientific statement from the American Heart Association and the American Diabetes Association. Diabetes Care 2007; 30(1):162–172. https://doi.org/10.2337/dc07-9917.

54 Tufano A, Cimino E, Di Minno MN, Ieranò P, Marrone E, Strazzullo A, Di Minno G, Cerbone AM. Diabetes mellitus and cardiovascular prevention: the role and the limitations of currently available antiplatelet drugs. Int J Vasc Med 2011; 2011: 250518. https://doi.org/10.1155/2011/250518.

55 Nieto Estrada VH, Molano Franco D, Medina RD, Gonzalez Garay AG, Martí-Carvajal AJ, Arevalo-Rodriguez I. Interventions for preventing high altitude illness: part 1. Commonly-used classes of drugs. Cochrane Database Syst Rev 2017;6(6):CD009761. https://doi.org/10.1002/14651858.CD009761.pub2.

56 Rehan N, Nasir K. Beta blockers: an important therapeutic modality for hypertensive diabetics. J Ayub Med Coll Abbottabad 2002; 14(2):31–34.
57 Garber AJ, Duncan TG, Goodman AM, Mills DJ, Rohlf JL. Efficacy of metformin in type II diabetes: results of a double-blind, placebo-controlled, dose-response trial. Am J Med 1997; 103(6):491–497. https://doi.org/10.1016/s0002-9343(97)00254-4.
58 Scheen AJ. SGLT2 Inhibitors: benefit/risk balance. Curr Diab Rep 2016; 16(10):92. https://doi.org/10.1007/s11892-016-0789-4.
59 Peng HT, Cheung B. A review on pharmacokinetic modeling and the effects of environmental stressors on pharmacokinetics for operational medicine: operational Pharmacokinetics. Defence Research and Development Canada, Technical Report 2009-037, Toronto, 2009. https://apps.dtic.mil/sti/html/tr/ADA509469/index.html.

CHAPTER 18

Prevention of Diseases related to High Altitude in Patients with Other Forms of Heart Disease

Most of the risks that patients with various forms of heart disease may face can be deduced from what has been described so far. The potential problems of exposure to altitude are those linked to the worsening of the volume and pressure overload of the two ventricles, as already analysed.

Patients with Pulmonary Hypertension of Different Origins

Pulmonary hypertension means mean pulmonary artery pressure values (PAPm) >20 mmHg (associated with pulmonary vascular resistance $\geq$ 3 Wood Units).[1] Normal resting values of PAPm are approximately 14 $\pm$ 3.3 mmHg, with a limit value of 20 mmHg; these normal values appear to be independent of age, sex and race.

Large cohort studies have clearly shown that mortality and the risk of hospitalisations progressively increase for values of PAPm already of 21–24 mmHg; it results that the increased PAPm and the increase in the systolic pressure beyond 30 mmHg are directly linked to the increase in mortality, regardless of whatever the origin of this pulmonary hypertension may be.[2] In the study by Strange et al., the 1- and 5-year mortalities have been estimated to be, respectively, 6.8 and 20.3% for persons with right ventricle systolic pressure (RVSP) <40 mmHg; the 1-year mortality raised to 23.9% and the 5-year mortality raised to 55.6% in persons with

RVSP 40.0–49.9 mmHg; in persons with higher RVSP, the 5-year mortality was estimated to be 68.8% for RVSP 50.0–59.9 mmHg and 78% for RVSP ≥60 mmHg. People with severely elevated RVSP were almost 10 times more likely to die within 5 years as compared with people with normal pulmonary artery pressure; advancing age and male sex contributed to the increased mortality risk.

Among the various forms of pulmonary hypertension, or rather of diseases that cause pulmonary hypertension, the most common are left ventricular failure (which we have already considered in Chapter 11) and chronic lung diseases, together with chronic hypoxia and hypoventilation syndromes.[3] Other forms of pulmonary hypertension are those secondary to pulmonary arteriolar obstruction caused by pulmonary embolism and those secondary to different diseases (such as sickle cell anaemia and sarcoidosis).

But what particularly interests us is **primary pulmonary hypertension**, that is, a form of pulmonary hypertension characterized by a primary pathology (i.e. not secondary to other causes) of the distal pulmonary arterioles; in these, structural alterations of the walls appear, linked to exaggerated proliferation of the cells of the vascular wall and inflammation (Figure 18.1).[4] It is estimated that there are approximately 25 cases of people with pulmonary hypertension per million inhabitants and that five new cases appear every year per million inhabitants.[5] These people experience a progressive increase in pressures in the right circulation and a consequent attempt of the right ventricle to adapt to them (chronic or pulmonale); however, the right ventricle undergoes progressive failure (right ventricle insufficiency) and therefore congestive heart failure appears.[4]

People who already have pulmonary hypertension at sea level experience worsening of pulmonary pressure levels when exposed to mountain altitudes (Figure 18.2), especially at elevations above 1,500–2,000 m AMSL and when they undergo physical effort.[7]

Based on a study conducted in simulated flight conditions at 1,700–2,500 m altitude,[8] it appears that patients with pulmonary hypertension treated with vasodilators may not, however, experience an acute worsening of their condition in the short term. However, it must be

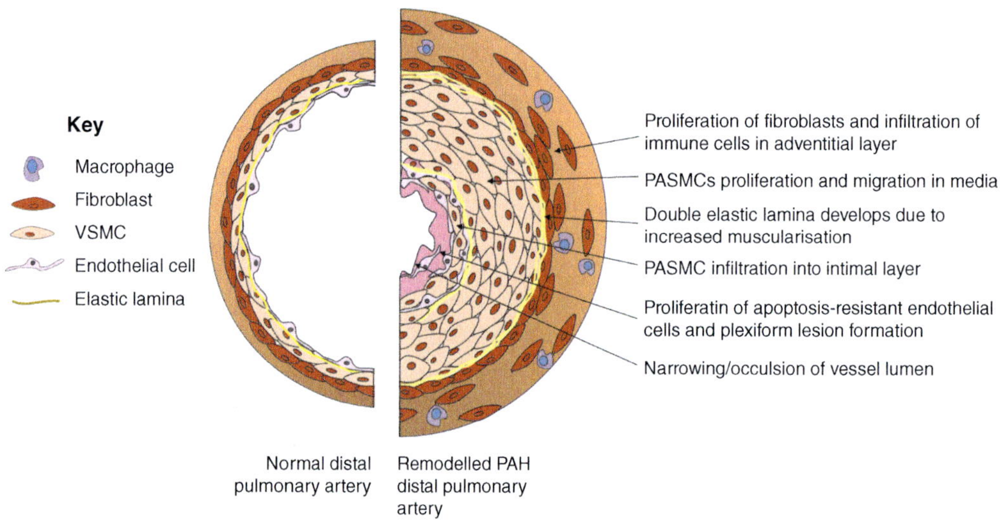

FIGURE 18.1 Vascular remodelling in pulmonary artery hypertension. [6] / Portland Press / CC BY 4.0.

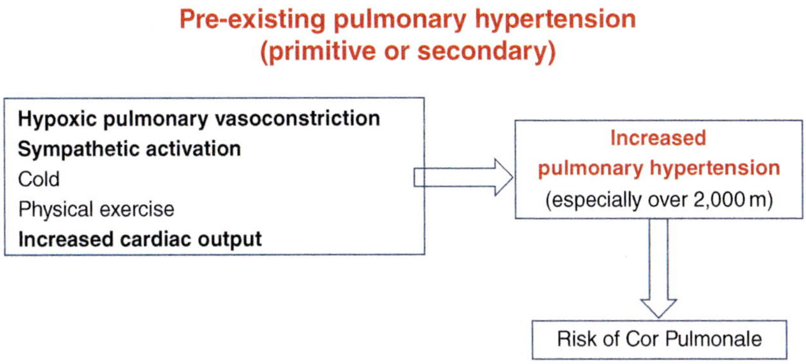

FIGURE 18.2 Effects of climbing to altitude in patients with pulmonary hypertension.

noted that, in this study, the patients were under special conditions, that is, they were observed at rest or were assessed during a light effort (equal to approximately 2 METs); they remained in such conditions for a short time, so that it is impossible to know how the situation would have evolved for longer exposure times. However, their already elevated systolic pressure in the pulmonary artery increased from 56 to 75 mmHg, which means an increase of 34% during the exposure to simulated altitude; in such conditions, also their feeling of fatigue (assessed according to the Borg scale) doubled at rest and tripled for light effort; in some of them PO_2 had dropped to less than 50 mmHg. We can therefore deduce that it is necessary to maintain the utmost caution towards this type of patient when exposed to light to moderate altitudes. The administration of supplementary oxygen may also be indicated.[9]

According to Rimoldi et al.,[10] going to altitude should be absolutely contraindicated for patients who present the following baseline conditions:

- Pulmonary hypertension with PAPm values >30 mmHg, or
- A gradient between the right ventricle and the right atrium >40 mmHg, and
- All those patients with pulmonary hypertension who are in NYHA functional class ≥ II, as well as,
- Those ones in unstable clinical conditions.

Patients with better clinical conditions should undergo an echocardiographic study with evaluation of right ventricular function and estimation of pulmonary pressure values; this study should be carried out in simulated altitude conditions, i.e. with mask administration of an air mixture with FiO_2 of 12% (that means simulated altitude of 4,500 m AMSL; the normal composition of atmospheric air has FiO_2 of 21%). Those who develop a right ventricle–right atrium gradient >40 mmHg in these conditions should be strongly discouraged from venturing into high mountains.

Persons with Trisomy 21

A special case is that of persons who are carriers of Trisomy 21.[11] In these subjects, an altered synthesis of nitric oxide (NO) by vascular endothelial cells and pulmonary alveolar epithelium has been detected, together with an inadequate availability of NO. This situation may constitute a defect capable of leading to an exaggerated response of the pulmonary arterioles to hypoxia and – consequently – to stress on the pulmonary capillaries, with leakage of liquids from the vessels and flooding of the pulmonary alveoli.[12]

These people are therefore at particular risk of developing exaggerated pulmonary hypertension and high-altitude pulmonary oedema (HAPE) even at relatively low altitudes. This risk also includes those who do not present cardiac dysfunction and also those who regularly practice physical activity on the plains.[11]

This observation is particularly important, given the growing number of young adults with Down syndrome participating in recreational and sporting activities in the mountains, including skiing and hiking. Before they start to engage in physical activity and prepare to climb the mountains, it is recommended that these people undergo a complete clinical cardiological evaluation, with echocardiographic evaluation of the estimated pressure values in the pulmonary circulation, under basic conditions and ideally also after having reached mountain altitudes (or after an echocardiogram in simulated altitude conditions, with inhalation of an air mixture with FiO_2 of 12%).

Patients with Intracardiac Shunts

The most common congenital heart defect is the persistence of a **patent foramen ovale (PFO)** (Figure 18.3). During intrauterine life, the foramen ovale allows the oxygenated blood coming from the placenta to pass from the right atrium to the left atrium and then to the systemic circulation; at the time of birth (or mostly within the first two years of life) the membrane of the foramen ovale closes this communication between the atria. In an estimated percentage of people reaching 25% (and perhaps 30%)[13] the closure of this foramen does not occur or occurs only partially, thus allowing the persistence of a communication between the right and left atrium: we therefore speak of persistence of patency of the foramen ovale, or PFO.[14] In approximately 6% of people, the atrial septal defect is of significant size (from a haemodynamic point of view).

During coughs, or during the pressure phase of the Valsalva manoeuvre (or even in some physiological states, such as pregnancy), the increased pressure in the right atrium allows the passage of a (more or less) small quantity of blood through the defect from the right atrium to the left atrium and then to the systemic circulation.

Now, we know that as we climb to altitude, pressures in the pulmonary circulation increase due to pulmonary vasoconstriction induced by hypoxia. This increase in pressure also occurs in the right ventricle and right atrium. Therefore, in people with PFO, it may happen that non-oxygenated blood passes from the right atrium to the left atrium and systemic circulation, causing some degree of peripheral desaturation. This desaturation, induced by venous blood passing from right to left, adds to the desaturation linked to altitude-induced hypoxaemia and can therefore contribute to a further worsening of the situation. The reduction in PO_2 due to the sum of the two phenomena can lead, especially in predisposed people, to a significant and acute increase in hypoxic pulmonary vasoconstriction and can trigger a vicious circle: altitude hypoxaemia → hypoxic pulmonary vasoconstriction → increase in pressure in the right circulation and therefore in the right atrium → shunt of non-oxygenated blood from the right atrium to the left atrium and systemic circulation through the PFO → worsening of hypoxaemia → further pulmonary vasoconstriction → further increase in pressure in the right circulation → increase in right-to-left shunt and so on.[10]

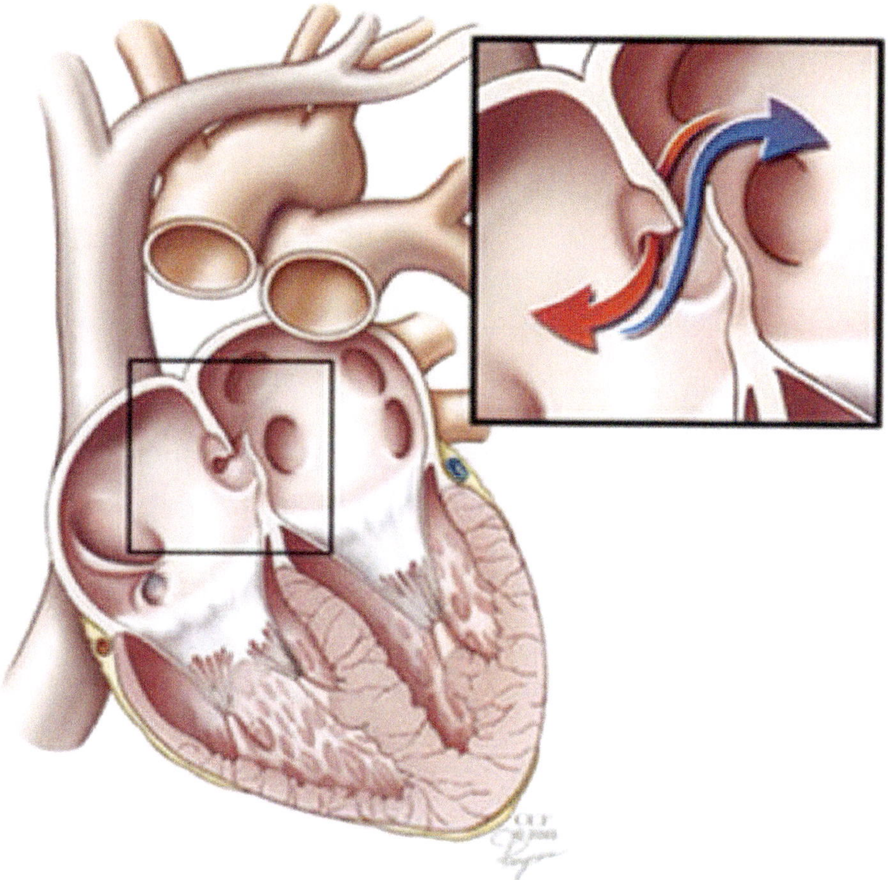

FIGURE 18.3 Patent foramen ovale; shunt of venous blood between the right to the left atrium. Creative commons license BY-NC-ND 3.0 (https://creativecommons.org/licenses/by-nc-nd/3.0/).

These patients with PFO appear to be more predisposed to HAPE(HAPE), as evidenced by the observation that among all those who suffer from HAPE, a PFO is found in a percentage 4–5 times higher than among those who have not had HAPE episodes.[15]

Left to Right Shunts

In 0.5–2 cases every thousand newborns, the persistence of a **patent ductus arteriosus (ductus Botalli)** is observed (i.e. a communication between the thoracic aorta and the pulmonary artery) (Figure 18.4)[16, 17], and in 2–7 cases per hundred newborns (or perhaps more)[18], a ventricular septal defect is present (Figure 18.5).

The ductus arteriosus generally closes spontaneously within the first three days of birth (or more rarely within the first weeks of life);[20] in a percentage of approximately 0.6% of infants,

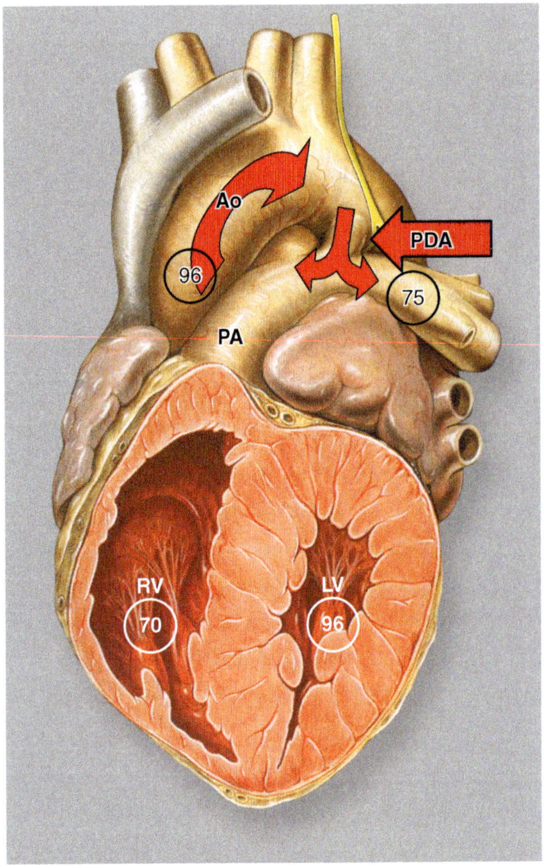

FIGURE 18.4 Patent ductus arteriosus (ductus Botalli, PDA); oxygen saturations (circled) in the various heart chambers are reported for a small PDA. Patrick J. Lynch / https://commons.wikimedia.org/wiki/File:Heart_patent_ductus_arteriosus.jpg / CC BY 2.5 / last accessed Dec. 27, 2025.

the ductus arteriosus remains patent until adulthood.[21] In populations living at 4,500–5,000 m above sea level, due to the chronic hypobaric hypoxia to which they are exposed, the persistence of the patent ductus arteriosus is approximately 30 times greater than in populations living at sea level.[19]

Of all the VSDs present at birth, a Danish study observed that 83.5% close spontaneously by one year of age, more frequently in the case of muscular septal defects and in smaller, single defects; thus, in 1-year-old children, the prevalence of VSDs has been estimated to be approximately 0.5%.[22] A study conducted in a middle-income country (Malaysia) demonstrated a lower percentage of cases with spontaneous closure of a VSD (55% of cases), while in another 25% a small defect remained present at age 2.3 years; episodes of congestive heart failure were present in one fourth of cases, and 3.6% presented persistent pulmonary hypertension.[23] An even smaller rate of spontaneous closure has been reported in a Korean study, in which spontaneous closure occurred only in 29.3% of the study cases after a median follow-up of 3 years.[24]

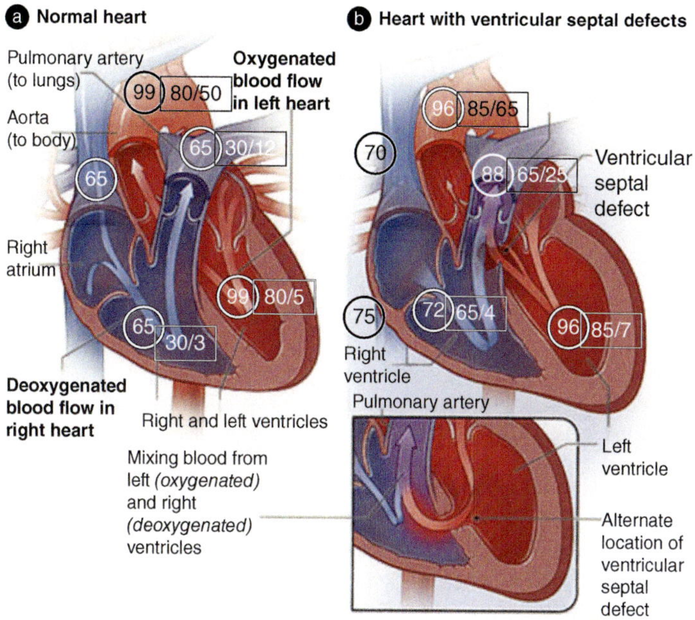

FIGURE 18.5 (a) shows the structure and blood flow in the interior of a normal heart; (b) shows two common locations for a ventricular septal defect. The defect allows oxygen-rich blood from the left ventricle to mix with oxygen-poor blood in the right ventricle; oxygen saturation (circled) and pressures (in squares) in the various heart chambers are reported for an infant with medium-sized VSD. Adapted from [19] / https://commons.wikimedia.org/wiki/File:VSD_image.jpg / Public domain / last accessed Dec. 27, 2025.

If we consider the high numbers of people who visit high mountains every year (estimated around 40 million only in the Alps),[25] it can be estimated that among all these tourists there could be thousands of persons with known or unknown atrial or ventricular septal defects of different magnitudes (mostly small) or other forms of heart defects with left-to-right shunt.

These congenital heart defects lead to an increase in flow and pressure regime in the pulmonary circulation, resulting in the progressive development of pulmonary hypertension (whose magnitude is correlated with the size of the defects). The consequences are those already reported for other causes of pulmonary hypertension.

Right to Left Shunts

Other diseases to consider in this chapter are **cyanotic congenital heart diseases** (i.e. all those malformations that involve the passage of blood from right to left); the best known is **Tetralogy of Fallot** (or 'Blue Disease' due to the colour of the mucous membranes of children affected by this pathology) (Figure 18.6). These are serious diseases, which require corrective surgery, and children or young adults with this disease are unlikely to be able to venture into the mountains. Patients with cyanotic heart disease are not recommended to live at high

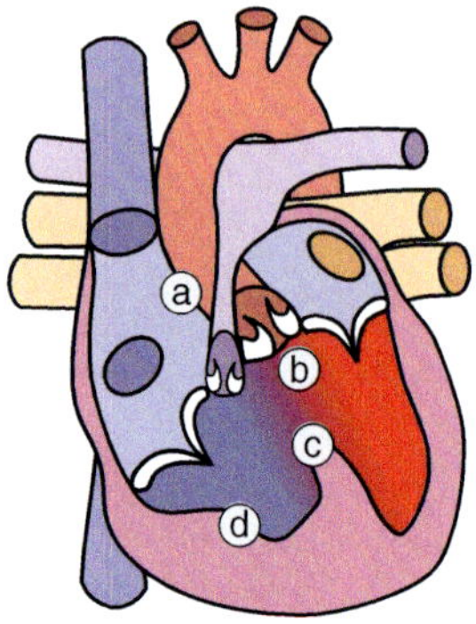

FIGURE 18.6 Heart presenting a Tetralogy of Fallot: (a) pulmonic stenosis; (b) overriding aorta; (c) ventricular septal defect (VSD); (d) right ventricular hypertrophy. Wapcaplet / https://commons.wikimedia.org/wiki/File:Heart_tetralogy_fallot.svg / CC BY-SA 2.5 / 2.0 / 1.0 / last accessed Dec. 27, 2025.

altitudes until the heart disease is surgically corrected. As far as we know so far, it seems that patients with surgically corrected congenital heart diseases do not present limitations in climbing to altitude, at least for short periods of exposure (such as travel time) and for altitudes up to 3,454 m AMSL,[26] provided that the cardiac pump function is preserved and there is no permanent pulmonary vascular damage.

The congenital heart diseases characterised by left-to-right shunts do not involve cyanosis (at least initially), except in the form called **Eisenmenger syndrome**. This is a complication of large uncorrected intracardiac left-to-right shunts or aorta-pulmonary artery shunts. Over time, the high flow and high pressures in the pulmonary circulation lead to the development of a progressive increase in pulmonary resistance, with severe pulmonary hypertension, and bidirectional shunt with a progressively increasing right-to-left shunt. In this situation, cyanosis and hypoxia can be expected to worsen significantly with exposure to mountain altitudes. However, there are no studies on sufficient numbers of patients to be able to evaluate the situation with certainty; there is a study [27] on 7 patients exposed to a simulated altitude of 2,468 m AMSL for a period of 1.5–7 hours and then exposed to real flight at altitudes of 1,767–1,829 m for 2.5 hours, in which SaO_2 decreased from approximately 86% to approximately 79% without the appearance of symptoms of dyspnoea or fatigue. The authors of this study hypothesised that in these patients with chronic hypoxaemia there is a mechanism similar to that which exists in inhabitants of high altitudes, in which the oxyhaemoglobin dissociation curve is modified, with facilitated release of oxygen to the tissues. Another study[28] retrospectively evaluated what had happened to 53 patients with Eisenmenger syndrome during a total of 1,157 airline flights: one patient presented a transient ischaemic attack during a flight and another needed to receive oxygen (but in an environment with the presence of cigarette smoking); other symptoms, such as headache, palpitations and oedema of the lower limbs, appeared with the same frequency as in control subjects. For this reason, the authors concluded that there are no reasons to prevent these patients from flying.

It is not possible to give a definitive answer as to whether these observations are also applicable to travelling to mountain heights; airplane flights are not the same as exposure to real mountain altitude.[10] However, it is suggested that – if these patients strongly desire to climb the mountains – a passive climb (i.e. transported) could be considered up to altitudes not exceeding 2,000–2,500 m AMSL and for a short duration. However, before doing this, patients should undergo an echocardiographic study of both the right and left ventricles while breathing in a mask at FiO_2 of 12%; the possible execution of an exercise test, and magnetic resonance imaging and Holter ECG should also be considered. Prevention and emergency treatment measures for possible complications related to hypoxaemia (oxygen therapy, pulmonary vasodilators) should also be made available.

In conclusion, the behaviour of SaO_2 in patients with congenital heart disease exposed to high altitudes does not appear to be easily predictable if only their baseline condition is considered; it is therefore suggested to carry out an exposure test to low concentrations of O_2 in these patients, preferably prolonged for three hours, in order to obtain more reliable data on their behaviour at altitude (be it a flight or – perhaps – a mountain climb).[29, 30]

The advice to be given to patients with congenital heart disease therefore depends on the type and severity of the pathology itself, and must be personalised in relation to the altitude they plan to reach.

Patients with Valvular Heart Diseases

Valvular heart disease is a major cause of cardiovascular morbidity and mortality worldwide. Of all deaths due to valvular heart disease, aortic valve disease accounts for 61% of cases, while mitral valve disease accounts for 15%.[31]

In an echocardiographic study, it was found that 2% of the population aged ≥65 years has manifest **calcific stenosis of the aortic valve**, and as many as 29% of this elderly population have age-related irregular sclerosis of the valve cusps, which is thought to be a mild form or precursor of frank stenosis.[32] In the elderly population, degenerative dilation of the aortic bulb is observed with a certain frequency, often linked (in addition to a series of other causes) to poorly controlled arterial hypertension; this dilation is often accompanied by **aortic valve insufficiency**.

These people can be almost asymptomatic until the relatively advanced stages of valve disease and can often be unaware of the pathology they carry. They may therefore wish to venture to even high mountain altitudes.

Mitral stenosis is nowadays much less frequent than in the past, at least in developed countries, thanks to the reduction in frequency of rheumatic heart disease since the 1970s. In patients who develop mitral stenosis, a symptom-free interval of 15–20 years is reported, and a further interval of 5–10 years for the symptoms to go from mild (NYHA class II) to severe (NYHA functional class III or IV).[33] Also **mitral valve insufficiency**, whatever its genesis (rheumatic disease, ischaemic heart disease, endocarditis, collagen disease), remains asymptomatic for a long time, until it reaches a significant extent of regurgitation; in contrast to mitral stenosis, the incidence of mitral insufficiency has progressively increased in the population in recent decades, linked to the progressive increase in the average lifespan of people.[34] **Mitral valve prolapse** is a form of mitral insufficiency that affects at least 1–2.5% (and up to 4% or perhaps more)[35] of the population; in most cases it does not involve significant haemodynamic alterations, at least for a long time. All these people can therefore, in this long period of time, climb to even high mountain altitudes.

So far, we do not have any studies that have evaluated systematically the effects of exposure to high altitude on these people with valvular heart disease, but we can deduce the main aspects from the pathophysiological elements previously exposed, especially regarding heart failure and pulmonary hypertension. We report here what Rimoldi wrote in his 2010 article:[10] *'The potential problems of high-altitude exposure in such patients are those related to the worsening of the pressure or volume overload associated with a particular valvular dysfunction'.* Figure 18.7 aims to summarise the main modifications induced by exposure to high altitude on valvular haemodynamics.

In aortic insufficiency and mitral insufficiency, exposure to high altitude can precipitate heart failure or the appearance of (cardiogenic) pulmonary oedema; in aortic stenosis, pressure overload and/or the volume reduction linked to dehydration can lead to a critical reduction in the anterograde output, with the appearance of episodes of syncope, heart failure, cardiogenic shock or pulmonary oedema. The patient with mitral stenosis may lose the compensatory state and slip into pulmonary oedema.

It follows that exposure to high altitudes of people with symptomatic or severe heart valve disease (NYHA class III or IV) is contraindicated.

However, as regards patients with milder forms of valvular disease, the same recommendations already set out for patients with heart failure apply: clinical and echocardiographic evaluation of the valvular disease and the state of compensation, and possible stress test (preferably during inspiration of FiO_2 12%).

Once they reach mountain altitude, people with valvular heart disease should check their body weight daily in order to detect any water retention early (a sudden increase in body weight can indicate the onset of heart failure). But they must also avoid dehydration linked to the possible loss of fluids in the high mountains and the reduced sense of thirst; hypovolaemia in a patient with valvular stenosis could lead to a critical reduction in cardiac output. Another recommendation for these patients (especially those with moderate or severe mitral or aortic insufficiency) is to frequently check their blood pressure, the trend of which can be very variable at altitude, especially during the first few days; patients should be instructed about the first measures to be adopted in order to control arterial hypertension according to their specific haemodynamic situation.

If the patients observe the appearance of arrhythmias (or arrhythmic palpitations), they must not underestimate the problem: any possible episode of new-onset atrial fibrillation (see below) requires adequate pharmacological treatments.

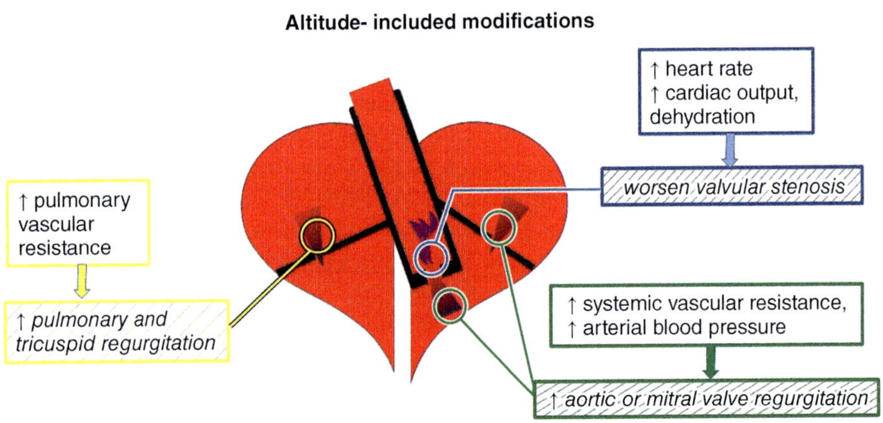

FIGURE 18.7 Main modifications induced by exposure to high altitude on valvular haemodynamics.

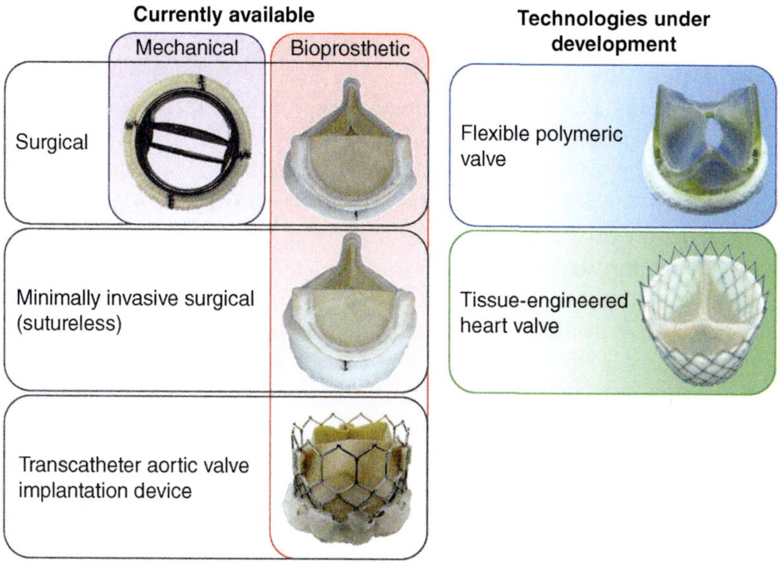

FIGURE 18.8 Available and under development prosthetic aortic valve technologies. From: Ref. [36]. Courtesy of the Authors; photographs adapted and modified from Figure 5 of Spühler et al. [37], Figure 1 of Capelli et al. [38], Figure 6 of Ghanbari et al. [39], and Figure 1 of Sanders et al. [40].

Patients with prosthetic valves (Figure 18.8) need to take continuous oral anti-coagulation, not only if the valve is mechanical but also biological, if in the mitral position, at doses adequate to maintain an INR between 2.5 and 3 (or 3.5) approximately, in order to avoid the possibility of thrombosis of the prosthesis or atrial thrombosis. Variations in the type of diet (frequent in environments other than the usual one), dehydration linked to altitude (due to increased release of atrial natriuretic peptide and decreased aldosterone synthesis), together with the possible onset of nausea and vomiting and high-altitude anorexia can lead to large fluctuations of INR. Reduced plasma volume, altered blood viscosity and the development of a pro-coagulatory state increase the risk of prosthetic valve thrombosis.[10] Patients should therefore be advised to always take the anti-coagulant drug regularly and should check whether a laboratory capable of performing a reliable INR test is available at the destination, or whether the patient is able to perform it independently using a self-monitoring kit and whether they are able to assess any dosage changes. In these patients, however, there is also the risk of haemorrhagic complications, given that activities at high altitude can expose them to possible trauma: such activities should therefore be strongly discouraged.

Heart Transplant Patients

The first human heart transplant was performed by Christiaan Barnard (1922–2001) on Louis Washkansky (1913–1967), on 3 December 1967, at the Groote Schuur hospital in Cape Town (South Africa); the patient survived 18 days. Adrian Kantrowitz, 3 days later, on December 6 1967, performed the second heart transplant at Maimonides Medical Center in Brooklyn, New York, on an 18-day-old male infant who, however, died 6½ hours after surgery.

In Europe, the first cardiac transplant was performed on 27 April 1968 by Christian Emile Cabrol (1925–2017) at Pitié-Salpêtrière Hospital in Paris, on the 66-year-old Clovis Roblain; unfortunately, the patient lived for only 53 hours. In the following years, the surgical techniques and the pharmacological treatments improved, so that the transplanted patients began progressively surviving many years. In 2022, the number of heart transplants performed in the European Region summed to 2,444, and in the region of Americas they totalled 4,996[41] (mainly performed in the USA, with 4,111 interventions).[42] It can be estimated that in the USA around 1 patient with heart transplant is currently living for every 10,000 population.[43]

In heart-transplanted patients, the response to stress (hypovolaemia, hypoxia, anaemia, exercise) is delayed, as it is based only on circulating catecholamines (due to cardiac denervation); so, the donor heart is slower to alter its heart rate during rest and exercise, and orthostatic hypotension is highly frequent. Coronary vasoregulation is also altered; pulmonary artery pressure may be elevated.

As regards the physical activity of people with heart transplants, it is known that many of these people are able to carry out significant physical and sporting activities. Regular physical activity is considered useful in heart transplant recipients and is generally recommended[44,45] as it contributes to improve the quality of life through the re-establishment and maintenance of physical 'fitness', it increases the individual's state of mental well-being (with positive influences on self-esteem) and reduces the impact of immunosuppressive drugs on the body's metabolic balance (in particular on lipid metabolism).[46] The World Transplant Games Federation has been staging for more than 40 years sporting events for transplant recipients, as well as promoting education of transplant recipients themselves and general public; besides many sessions of games all over the world, in 2024 the first Transplant Football World Cup has been organised.[47]

In spite of these activities, there is not enough information regarding the physical activity of these people in the mountains. What is known is that life at moderate altitudes appears to pose no additional danger; indeed, one study observed better survival in heart transplant recipients living at altitudes of 1,200 m AMSL or more, compared to those who live at lower altitudes or at sea level.[48]

As regards high altitudes, there is only one study,[49] which analysed the behaviour of two heart transplant women (aged 22 and 57, transplanted, respectively, 3 and 4 years earlier) who climbed Mount Kilimanjaro in 7 days, up to Uhuru peak at 5,895 m AMSL as part of an evaluation of the effects of high altitude on recipients of various types of transplants (Figure 18.9). No particular negative consequences were observed in these two ladies, who were not regular hikers. According to the authors of the study, the observations cannot, however, be considered of general value, due to the extremely small number of cases, who were very selected and trained for the purpose and were moreover accompanied by a medical team.

It is necessary to remember that heart transplant patients must also pay attention to environmental factors (e.g. exposure to cold), to dehydration and any trauma, and to possible infections favoured by the immunosuppressive therapy they are following; furthermore, they must be advised to ensure that they always take all prescribed medications on a regular basis.

In all of them, a cardiological examination with echocardiogram and a cardiopulmonary test (ideally at simulated altitude) are indicated before deciding to carry out activities in the mountains.

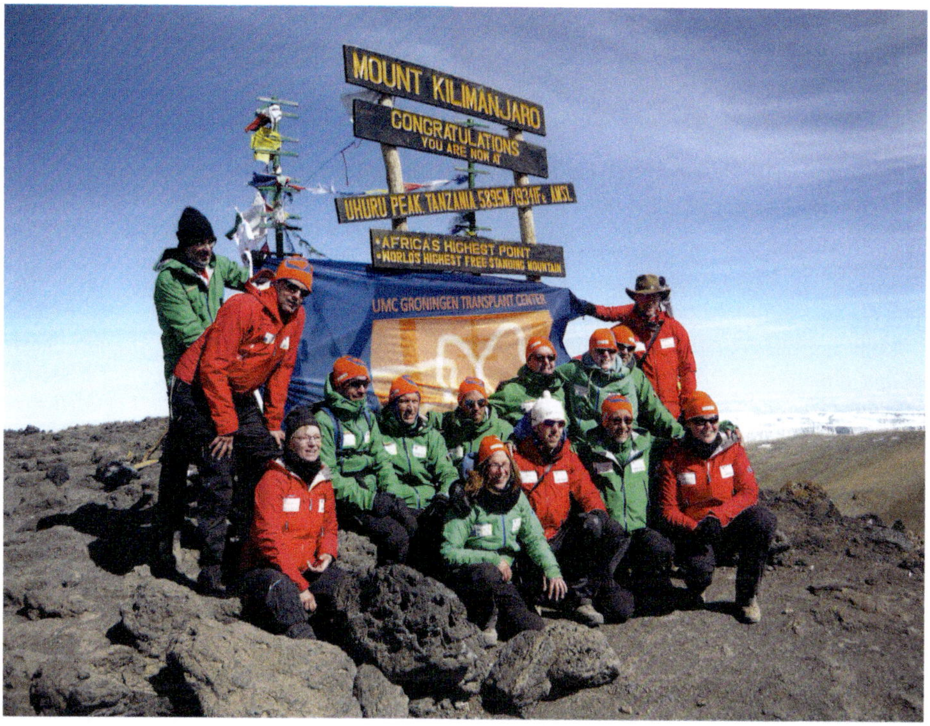
MOUNT KILIMANJARO
CONGRATULATIONS
YOU ARE NOW AT
UHURU PEAK, TANZANIA 5895M/19341Ft. AMSL
AFRICA'S HIGHEST POINT
WORLD'S HIGHEST FREE STANDING MOUNTAIN
UMC GRONINGEN TRANSPLANT CENTER

FIGURE 18.9 Two heart-transplanted ladies climbed Mount Kilimanjaro, up to 5,895 m a.s.l. in 2014. From: [49] / Van Adrichem / CC BY 4.0.

'A borrowed heart' at the top of Matterhorn, not to say of the other mountains.

She would never have expected what awaited her once she reached the top of Mt. Haleakala, Hawaii, 3,055 m high. Kelly Perkins and her fiancé Craig had climbed together other peaks since they had been dating. But that time was special. While atop the volcano, Craig positioned the camera so as to capture the entire scene, with *the sky [that] crackled red and orange as the sun began to rise above the sparkling water far below.* He pressed the timer and ran towards her; then, he took a small velvet-covered box from his pocket and presented her with the engagement ring. *'Will you marry me? He asked. My heart skipped a beat, then another, then another'.*

For their fifth wedding anniversary, in 1992 Kelly and Craig planned a trip to Europe. Zermatt and the Matterhorn were a key stop; anyway, that peak *'seemed much too daunting. For a peak bagger, the Matterhorn seemed the ultimate prize, but even I wasn't crazy enough to take on such a formidable challenge'.*

Soon after returning from this dreamt place, the first disturbances began: initially *a tiny flutter inside the chest* and the sensation of a fast heartbeat, especially at night; then a progressive reduction of effort tolerance with dyspnoea. Finally, it was detected that Kelly was suffering from episodes of sustained ventricular tachycardia. Further tests led to the diagnosis of a *serious situation*: a viral myocarditis. A complex drug therapy was necessary, together with the implantation of an ICD.

(continued)

'A borrowed heart' at the top of Matterhorn, not to say of the other mountains. *(continued)*

But, anyway, this was not the final solution. The clinical situation continued to progressively deteriorate (with *a downward health spiral*), until it became necessary to proceed with a heart transplant. After years of difficult emotional management, the transplant surgery took place in mid-November 1995.

After the first few months complicated by signs of initial rejection, a new therapy allowed the clinical picture to improve and stabilise.

Kelly noticed something extremely important and real in her new heart: the new heart was '*not automatically piloted by my nervous system. It is like a car engine without a starter. Fortunately, the body has its own, built-in backup – the adrenaline system. ... As I get active, ... triggering the 'fight or flight' response ... causes a release of adrenaline, thereby inducing an increase in heart rate to accommodate for my level of exertion. It's very efficient, but not as quick to respond, ... 2 to 10-minute delay*'.

And indeed, this is completely true. A transplanted heart is denervated and thus unable to respond to physical activity, emotions, or circadian rhythms with the normal autonomic control of its heart rate. It can only modify its end-diastolic volume in response to phenomena involving increased or decreased filling, or it can modestly vary its heart rate following systemic adrenergic discharge. On the other hand, the modification of peripheral adaptation mechanisms is extremely important; it is known that even in patients with total artificial hearts and in patients with left ventricle assist devices improved effort tolerance can be achieved through progressive physical training; the improvement results from a reduction of total peripheral resistances, a lower catecholamine level at rest and during effort, and improved oxygen extraction by working muscles.[50]

This is exactly what Kelly was able to achieve in the months and years following the transplant, once her clinical condition stabilised.

Four years after being diagnosed with severe heart failure and six months after heart transplant, Kelly and Craig returned to Lake Tahoe, on Sierra Nevada (1,900 m above sea level) for the first time, not without some apprehension. The hike went well and sparked planning for new adventures, such as hiking at Agnew Meadows pass (2,560 m), and planning to climb the challenging Half Dome at Yosemite (2,696 m) an undertaking that was successful ten months after the transplant. After a successful ascent to Mount Fuji, Japan (3,776 m; in July 1998), the ascent to Mount Kilimanjaro, Kenya (5,895 m; in October 2001) has, however, been accompanied by some complications, that could have proved dangerous if they had not been addressed quickly: nausea, vomiting, dehydration, hypotension and fainting. Thus, Kelly's experience can be considered '*a harsh reminder to everyone of my precarious condition*'.

However, at 42, this courageous lady decided to attempt what had been her dream for many years: climbing the Matterhorn, the mountain that 11 years before – while she was in full health – she had deemed *too daunting*. An intensive training programme was initiated and meticulous planning was organised to properly tackle that pyramid-shaped peak, which had claimed more than 500 lives among climbers who had attempted it. On August 25, 2003, Kelly Perkins became the first person with a transplanted heart to ascend the 4,478 m peak, with a total of 11.5 hours needed to ascend and descend. She is generally considered as a model for all heart transplant recipients as well as for all patients who are afflicted with serious illnesses.[51]

From: Perkins K. The climb of my life: scaling mountains with a borrowed heart. Rowman & Littlefield Pub Inc, Lanham, 2007.

References

1 Gelzinis TA. Pulmonary hypertension in 2021: part I-definition, classification, pathophysiology, and presentation. J Cardiothorac Vasc Anesth 2022; 36(6):1552–1564. https://doi.org/10.1053/j.jvca.2021.06.036.https://www.jcvaonline.com/action/showPdf?pii=S1053-0770%2821%2900572-3.

2 Strange G, Stewart S, Celermajer DS, Prior D, Scalia GM, Marwick TH, Gabbay E, Ilton M, Joseph M, Codde J, Playford D; NEDA Contributing Sites. Threshold of pulmonary hypertension associated with increased mortality. J Am Coll Cardiol 2019; 73(21):2660–2672. https://doi.org/10.1016/j.jacc.2019.03.482.https://www.sciencedirect.com/science/article/pii/S0735109719347187/pdf

3 Anderson JJ, Lau EM. Pulmonary hypertension definition, classification, and epidemiology in Asia. JACC Asia 2022; 2(5):538–546. https://doi.org/10.1016/j.jacasi.2022.04.008.https://www.ncbi.nlm.nih.gov/pmc/articles/PMC9823284/pdf/main.pdf.

4 Schermuly RT, Ghofrani HA, Wilkins MR, Grimminger F. Mechanisms of disease: pulmonary arterial hypertension. Nat Rev Cardiol 2011; 8(8):443–455. https://doi.org/10.1038/nrcardio.2011.87. https://www.ncbi.nlm.nih.gov/pmc/articles/PMC7097518/pdf/41569_2011_Article_BFnrcardio201187.pdf.

5 Maron BA, Abman SH, Elliott CG, Frantz RP, Hopper RK, Horn EM, Nicolls MR, Shlobin OA, Shah SJ, Kovacs G, Olschewski H, Rosenzweig EB. Pulmonary arterial hypertension: diagnosis, treatment, and novel advances. Am J Respir Crit Care Med 2021; 203(12):1472–1487. https://www.ncbi.nlm.nih.gov/pmc/articles/PMC8483220/pdf/rccm.202012-4317SO.pdf.

6 Morris HE, Neves KB, Montezano AC, MacLean MR, Touyz RM. Notch3 signalling and vascular remodelling in pulmonary arterial hypertension. Clin Sci (Lond) 2019;133(24):2481–2498.

7 Agostoni P, Cattadori G, Guazzi M, Bussotti M, Conca C, Lomanto M, Marenzi G, Guazzi MD. Effects of simulated altitude-induced hypoxia on exercise capacity in patients with chronic heart failure. Am J Med 2000; 109(6):450–455. https://doi.org/10.1016/s0002-9343(00)00532-5. https://www.researchgate.net/publication/12282708_Effects_of_simulated_altitude-induced_hypoxia_on_exercise_capacity_in_patients_with_chronic_heart_failure.

8 Seccombe LM, Chow V, Zhao W, Lau EM, Rogers PG, Ng AC, Veitch EM, Peters MJ, Kritharides L. Right heart function during simulated altitude in patients with pulmonary arterial hypertension. Open Heart 2017;4(1):e000532. https://doi.org/10.1136/openhrt-2016-000532. https://www.ncbi.nlm.nih.gov/pmc/articles/PMC5255554/pdf/openhrt-2016-000532.pdf.

9 Shrikrishna D, Coker RK; Air Travel Working Party of the British Thoracic Society Standards of Care Committee. Managing passengers with stable respiratory disease planning air travel: British Thoracic Society recommendations. Thorax 2011; 66(9):831–833. https://doi.org/10.1136/thoraxjnl-2011-200694.https://thorax.bmj.com/content/thoraxjnl/66/9/831.full.pdf.

10 Rimoldi SF, Sartori C, Seiler C, Delacrétaz E, Mattle HP, Scherrer U, Allemann Y. High-altitude exposure in patients with cardiovascular disease: risk assessment and practical recommendations. Prog Cardiovasc Dis 2010; 52(6):512–524. https://doi.org/10.1016/j.pcad.2010.03.005.

11 Richalet JP, Chenivesse C, Larmignat P, Meille L. High altitude pulmonary oedema, down syndrome, and obstructive sleep apneas. High Alt Med Biol 2008; 9(2):179–181. https://doi.org/10.1089/ham.2007.1062.

12 Sartori C, Allemann Y, Scherrer U. Pathogenesis of pulmonary oedema: learning from high-altitude pulmonary oedema. Respir Physiol Neurobiol 2007; 159(3):338–349. https://doi.org/10.1016/j.resp.2007.04.006.

13 Lovering AT, Elliott JE, Davis JT. Physiological impact of patent foramen ovale on pulmonary gas exchange, ventilatory acclimatization, and thermoregulation. J Appl Physiol 2016; 121(2):512–517. https://doi.org/10.1152/japplphysiol.00192.2015.https://journals.physiology.org/doi/epdf/10.1152/japplphysiol.00192.2015.

14 Homma S, Messé SR, Rundek T, Sun YP, Franke J, Davidson K, Sievert H, Sacco RL, Di Tullio MR. Patent foramen ovale. Nat Rev Dis Primers 2016; 2:15086. https://doi.org/10.1038/nrdp.2015.86.

15 Allemann Y, Hutter D, Lipp E, Sartori C, Duplain H, Egli M, Cook S, Scherrer U, Seiler C. Patent foramen ovale and high-altitude pulmonary oedema. JAMA 2006; 296(24):2954–2958. https://doi.org/10.1001/jama.296.24.2954.https://jamanetwork.com/journals/jama/fullarticle/204767.

16 Backes CH, Hill KD, Shelton EL, Slaughter JL, Lewis TR, Weisz DE, Mah ML, Bhombal S, Smith CV, McNamara PJ, Benitz WE, Garg V. Patent ductus arteriosus: a contemporary perspective for the pediatric and adult cardiac care provider. J Am Heart Assoc 2022; 11(17):e025784. https://doi.org/10.1161/JAHA.122.025784.https://www.ncbi.nlm.nih.gov/pmc/articles/PMC9496432/pdf/JAH3-11-e025784.pdf.

17 Ciuffreda M, Ferrero P. Pervietà del dotto arterioso. G Ital Cardiol (Rome) 2015; 16(4):232–239. Italian https://doi.org/10.1714/1848.20188.

18 Dickinson DF. Ventricular septal defect: (not) another epidemic? Cardiol Young 1998; 8(4):423–424. https://doi.org/10.1017/s1047951100007046.

19 Rudolph AM. Congenital Diseases of the Heart. Chicago: Year Book Medical Publisher, 1974.

20 Schneider DJ, Moore JW. Patent ductus arteriosus. Circulation 2006; 114(17):1873–1882. https://doi.org/10.1161/CIRCULATIONAHA.105.592063. https://www.ahajournals.org/doi/epub/10.1161/CIRCULATIONAHA.105.592063.

21 Mariager AF, Hammeken A, Malham M, Raja AA, Sellmer A, Skjellerup SL, Raja RA, Navne J, Sillesen AS, Vejlstrup N, Bundgaard H, Iversen KK, Garne E, Jeppesen DL. Age-related prevalence of open ductus arteriosus in full-term newborns. Neonatology 2023; 120(4):527–531. https://doi.org/10.1159/000529842. https://karger.com/neo/article-pdf/120/4/527/3988461/000529842.pdf.

22 Pihl C, Sillesen AS, Norsk JB, Vøgg ROB, Vedel C, Boyd HA, Vejlstrup N, Axelsson Raja A, Bundgaard H, Iversen KK. The prevalence and spontaneous closure of ventricular septal defects the first year of life. Neonatology. 2024; 121(6):742–751. https://doi.org/10.1159/000538810.

23 Bah MNM, Sapian MH, Anuar MHM, Alias EY. Survival and outcomes of isolated neonatal ventricular septal defects: A population-based study from a middle-income country. Ann Pediatr Cardiol. 2023; 16(5):322–330. https://doi.org/10.4103/apc.apc_130_23. https://pmc.ncbi.nlm.nih.gov/articles/PMC11098291/pdf/APC-16-322.pdf.

24 Kim AY, Tchah N, Lin CY, Park JM, Woo W, Kim CS, Jung SY, Choi JY, Jung JW. Predictive scoring system for spontaneous closure of infant ventricular septal defect: The P-VSD score. Pediatr Cardiol. 2025; 46(2):401–408. https://doi.org/10.1007/s00246-024-03434-8.

25 Burtscher M, Ponchia A. The risk of cardiovascular events during leisure time activities at altitude. Prog Cardiovasc Dis 2010; 52(6):507–511. https://doi.org/10.1016/j.pcad.2010.02.008.

26 Staempfli R, Schmid JP, Schenker S, Eser P, Trachsel LD, Deluigi C, Wustmann K, Thomet C, Greutmann M, Tobler D, Stambach D, Wilhelm M, Schwerzmann M. Cardiopulmonary adaptation to short-term high altitude exposure in adult Fontan patients. Heart. 2016; 102(16):1296–1301. https://doi.org/10.1136/heartjnl-2016-309682.

27 Harinck E, Hutter PA, Hoorntje TM, Simons M, Benatar AA, Fischer JC, de Bruijn D, Meijboom EJ. Air travel and adults with cyanotic congenital heart disease. Circulation 1996; 93(2):272–276. https://doi.org/10.1161/01.cir.93.2.272. https://www.ahajournals.org/doi/10.1161/01.cir.93.2.272?url_ver=Z39.88-2003&rfr_id=ori:rid:crossref.org&rfr_dat=cr_pub%20%200pubmed.

28 Broberg CS, Uebing A, Cuomo L, Thein SL, Papadopoulos MG, Gatzoulis MA. Adult patients with Eisenmenger syndrome report flying safely on commercial airlines. Heart 2007; 93(12):1599–603. https://doi.org/10.1136/hrt.2006.105239. https://www.ncbi.nlm.nih.gov/pmc/articles/PMC2095753/pdf/1599.pdf.

29 Naqvi N, Doughty VL, Starling L, Franklin RC, Ward S, Daubeney PEF, Balfour-Lynn IM. Hypoxic challenge testing (fitness to fly) in children with complex congenital heart disease. Heart 2018; 104(16):1333–1338. https://doi.org/10.1136/heartjnl-2017-312753.https://spiral.imperial.ac.uk/bitstream/10044/1/57916/2/FTF%20submitted%20version.docx.

30 Müller N, Herberg U, Breuer J, Kratz T, Härtel JA. Fitness to fly for children and adolescents after Fontan palliation. Front Cardiovasc Med. 2023; 10:1170275. https://doi.org/10.3389/fcvm.2023.1170275. https://www.ncbi.nlm.nih.gov/pmc/articles/PMC10326614/pdf/fcvm-10-1170275.pdf.

31 Aluru JS, Barsouk A, Saginala K, Rawla P, Barsouk A. Valvular heart disease epidemiology. Med Sci (Basel) 2022; 10(2):32. https://doi.org/10.3390/medsci10020032. https://www.ncbi.nlm.nih.gov/pmc/articles/PMC9228968/pdf/medsci-10-00032.pdf.

32 Otto CM, Lind BK, Kitzman DW, Gersh BJ, Siscovick DS. Association of aortic-valve sclerosis with cardiovascular mortality and morbidity in the elderly. N Engl J Med 1999; 341(3):142–147. https://doi.org/10.1056/NEJM199907153410302. https://www.nejm.org/doi/pdf/10.1056/NEJM199907153410302?articleTools=true.

33 Bonow RO, Carabello BA, Chatterjee K, de Leon AC Jr, Faxon DP, Freed MD, Gaasch WH, Lytle BW, Nishimura RA, O'Gara PT, O'Rourke RA, Otto CM, Shah PM, Shanewise JS; American College of Cardiology/American Heart Association Task Force on Practice Guidelines. 2008 focused update incorporated into the ACC/AHA 2006 guidelines for the management of patients with valvular heart disease: a report of the American College of Cardiology/American Heart Association Task Force on Practice Guidelines (Writing Committee to revise the 1998 guidelines for the management of patients with valvular heart disease). Endorsed by the Society of Cardiovascular Anesthesiologists, Society for Cardiovascular Angiography and Interventions, and Society of Thoracic Surgeons. J Am Coll Cardiol 2008;52(13):e1–142. https://doi.org/10.1016/j.jacc.2008.05.007. https://www.sciencedirect.com/science/article/pii/S0735109708018330?via%3Dihub#sec5.

34 Perone F, Peruzzi M, Conte E, Sciarra L, Frati G, Cavarretta E, Pingitore A. An overview of sport participation and exercise prescription in mitral valve disease. J Cardiovasc Dev Dis 2023; 10(7):304. https://doi.org/10.3390/jcdd10070304. https://www.ncbi.nlm.nih.gov/pmc/articles/PMC10380819/pdf/jcdd-10-00304.pdf.

35 Freed LA, Levy D, Levine RA, Larson MG, Evans JC, Fuller DL, Lehman B, Benjamin EJ. Prevalence and clinical outcome of mitral-valve prolapse. N Engl J Med 1999; 341(1):1–7. https://doi.org/10.1056/NEJM199907013410101.https://www.nejm.org/doi/pdf/10.1056/NEJM199907013410101?articleTools=true.

36 Marom G, Einav S. New Insights into Valve Hemodynamics. Rambam Maimonides Med J 2020; 11(2):e0014.

37 Spühler JH, Jansson J, Jansson N, Hoffman J. 3D fluid-structure interaction simulation of aortic valves using a unified continuum ALE FEM model. Front Physiol 2018; 9:363.

38 Capelli C, Corsini C, Biscarini D, Ruffini F, Migliavacca F, Kocher A, Laufer G, Taylor AM, Schievano S, Andreas M, Burriesci G, Rath C. Pledget-armed sutures affect the haemodynamic performance of biologic aortic valve substitutes: a preliminary experimental and computational study. Cardiovasc Eng Technol 2017; 8:17–29.

39 Ghanbari H, De Mel A, Seifalian AM. Cardiovascular application of polyhedral oligomeric silsesquioxane nanomaterials: a glimpse into prospective horizons. Int J Nanomedicine 2011; 6:775–786.

40 Sanders B, Loerakker S, Fioretta ES, Bax DJP, Driessen-Mol A, Hoerstrup SP, Baaijens FPT. Improved geometry of decellularized tissue engineered heart valves to prevent leaflet retraction. Ann Biomed Eng 2016; 44:1061–1067.

41 Statista. Estimated number of heart transplantations worldwide in 2022, by region. https://www.statista.com/statistics/1319797/global-estimation-of-heart-transplantations-by-region/#:~:text=In%202022%2C%20there%20were%20a,worldwide%20in%202022%2C%20by%20region.

42 Statista. Number of heart transplantations in the U.S. from 1975 to 2022. https://www.statista.com/statistics/671451/heart-transplants-number-us/#:~:text=In%202022%2C%20there%20were%20approximately,U.S.%20from%201975%20to%202022.

43 Health Resources and Services Administration, Scientific Registry of Transplant Recipients. OPTN/SRTR 2019 Annual Data Report: Heart. https://srtr.transplant.hrsa.gov/annual_reports/2019/Heart.aspx.

44 Janaudis-Ferreira T, Mathur S, Deliva R, Howes N, Patterson C, Räkel A, So S, Wickerson L, White M, Avitzur Y, Johnston O, Heywood N, Singh S, Holdsworth S. Exercise for solid organ transplant candidates and recipients: a joint position statement of the Canadian society of transplantation and CAN-RESTORE. Transplantation 2019; 103(9):e220–e238. https://doi.org/10.1097/TP.0000000000002806. https://journals.lww.com/transplantjournal/fulltext/2019/09000/exercise_for_solid_organ_transplant_candidates_and.5.aspx.

45 Schmidt T, Bjarnason-Wehrens B, Predel HG, Reiss N. Exercise after heart transplantation: typical alterations, diagnostics and interventions. Int J Sports Med 2021; 42(2):103–111. https://doi.org/10.1055/a-1194-4995. https://www.thieme-connect.com/products/ejournals/pdf/10.1055/a-1194-4995.pdf.

46 Ministero della Salute, Centro Nazionale Trapianti. Trapianto... e adesso sport, i risultati del primo studio sugli effetti dell'attività fisica, NOTIZIA. 11 Ott 2012. [Italian Ministry of Health, National Transplant Center. Transplant... and now sport, the results of the first study on the effects of physical activity, NEWS. 11 Oct 2012]. https://www.trapianti.salute.gov.it/trapianti/dettaglioComunicatiNotizieCnt.jsp?lingua=italiano&area=cnt&menu=media&sottomenu=news&id=320.

47 World Transplant Games Federation: https://wtgf.org.

48 Wozniak CJ, Baird BC, Stehlik J, Drakos SG, Bull DA, Patel AN, Selzman CH. Improved survival in heart transplant patients living at high altitude. J Thorac Cardiovasc Surg 2012; 143(3):735–741.e1. https://doi.org/10.1016/j.jtcvs.2011.11.012. https://www.jtcvs.org/article/S0022-5223(11)01286-4/fulltext.

49 van Adrichem EJ, Siebelink MJ, Rottier BL, Dilling JM, Kuiken G, van der Schans CP, Verschuuren EA. Tolerance of organ transplant recipients to physical activity during a high-altitude expedition: climbing Mount Kilimanjaro. PLoS One 2015; 10(11):e0142641. https://doi.org/10.1371/journal.pone.0142641. Erratum in: PLoS One 2015; 10(12):e0145566. https://www.ncbi.nlm.nih.gov/pmc/articles/PMC4659574/pdf/pone.0142641.pdf.

50 Bellotto F, Compostella L, Agostoni P, Torregrossa G, Setzu T, Gambino A, Russo N, Feltrin G, Tarzia V, Gerosa G. Peripheral adaptation mechanisms in physical training and cardiac rehabilitation: the case of a patient supported by a CardioWest total artificial heart. J Card Fail 2011; 17(8):670–675. https://doi.org/10.1016/j.cardfail.2011.04.006.

51 Kapp C. Heart transplant recipient climbs the Matterhorn. 42-year-old Kelly Perkins becomes the first person with a heart transplant to ascend the 4478-m peak. Lancet 2003; 362(9387):880–881. https://doi.org/10.1016/s0140-6736(03)14351-6.

CHAPTER 19

Pre-exposure Screening for High Altitudes

When evaluating people who intend to tackle the mountains and the risks they may face, it is first of all necessary to remembered that some multifactorial considerations are necessary, relating to:

Multifactorial Pre-exposure Assessment

- type of disease possibly presented by the individual being evaluated, its severity, the state of circulatory compensation, the symptoms present, the therapy in use, recent interventions the person has undergone and their results;
- the individual's physical fitness at low altitude and whether or not the candidates are accustomed to physical activity and the limitations they present;
- the altitude the subject intends to reach (will it be above 2,000 m?);
- the speed of ascent (which – as we have seen – should ideally be <300–400 m/day; Evidence: 1C);
- the geographical location where the ascent would take place;
- the kind and intensity of the activities planned once the altitude has been reached (challenging? light activities?);
- the availability of medical assistance on site and the possibility of rescue (and its labouriousness and possibly costs in terms of human and economic commitment) in the area of the excursion.

It is also essential to keep in mind that:

- The screening we will carry out is NOT intended to give the 'green light' for the mountain adventure; its purpose is to identify those factors or conditions that can put the individual at risk, either by increasing the risk of complications of his/her disease and by favouring the appearance of other altitude-related diseases.

- Sporting activities and – in general – physical activity carried out in the mountains are not equivalent to similar activities carried out on the plains or at low altitudes, both because the activities are performed in hypobaric hypoxia and because they take place in a generally 'hostile' environment (physical barriers, cold, bad weather, ...).
- There are no standardised guidelines, and the indications that can be found in the literature are mostly based on observation of a limited number of cases or on expert opinions, and no randomised studies are yet available.

The observations made will aim to provide suggestions and guidance to the patient, athlete, or high-altitude hiker, clarifying any risks that may arise and their potential severity in relation to his/her specific physical situation (in addition, obviously, to the general risks associated – as is known – with climbing to high altitudes).

Based on what can be identified during the interview with the individual (also taking into account the subject's wishes) and during the collection/analysis of his/her health data, it will be possible to carry out a targeted health education action, addressing the subject's doubts and providing information and suggestions on how to behave at altitude, both in situations of well-being and in the event of the appearance of pathological or potentially pathological manifestations.

Aims and Topics of the Evaluation

From a clinical point of view, the evaluation must be aimed at emphasizing the specific aspects related to ascent to altitude. In particular, it will be necessary to analyse how the ascent will be carried out (trekking, climbing, ascent by plane), how long the ascent will take, and how long the stay at altitude will last.

It will be important to check whether the individual has previously climbed to similar altitudes and what potential problems may have occurred on these occasions.

An attempt must be made to identify the presence of physical or clinical conditions that could put the individual's life at risk once he or she goes to high altitude or even simply performs physical activity (for example, consider the presence of ischaemic heart disease or major arrhythmias); in particular, as far as we are concerned, we will have to try to identify and evaluate any pulmonary or cardiovascular pathological conditions. Existing physical disabilities, or pre-existing conditions that may cause or aggravate a disability must also be carefully assessed; similarly, the possible presence of conditions or pathologies that may predispose to injury or illness must be assessed.

For an adequate classification, it will be essential to collect an accurate clinical history and possibly seek the opinion of specialists for the evaluation of specific diseases (present or suspected).

Relevant health topics should be discussed with the prospective mountaineer. The individual (and – with his consent – also the other participants in the climb to high altitude) must be informed of the existing chronic diseases, of the extent and type of physical effort that the individual may be able to sustain, of how he/she must behave with the drugs in use, which checks are to be carried out during the ascent and upon arrival at altitude (e.g. measurement of blood pressure and saturation, measurement of glycaemia) and how to modify medications if necessary (changes in dosage, or addition of other medications, and potential interferences or side effects).

It will also be useful to advise the patient to abstain from caffeine and alcohol, which can impair his/her physical condition or interfere with his/her judgement.

Categories of Risk

Based on what has been described by Campbell et al.[1] and by Luks et al. (Wilderness Medical Society),[2, 3] we can divide patients into three large categories relating to the extent of the risk they may incur by going to high altitude:

Low Risk:

- Are those individuals WITHOUT any history of mountain sickness, who – starting from ≈1,200 m – climb (and stop to sleep) at less than 2,800 m.
- Individuals who – starting from ≈1,200 m – take ≥2 days to reach 2,500–3,000 m, with subsequent increases in overnight altitude ≈500 m/day, with 1 extra day of acclimatisation every 1,000 m.

Moderate risk:

- Individuals WITH a history of mountain sickness, who – starting from ≈1,200 m – climb to 2,500–2,800 m in 1 day (and stop there to sleep).
- Individuals WITHOUT a history of mountain sickness, who - starting from ≈1,200 m – climb to more than 2,800 m in 1 day (and stop there to sleep).
- All those individuals who – starting from ≈1,200 m – climb >500 m/day to altitudes above 3,000 m (and stop there to sleep), maintaining; however, 1 extra day of acclimatisation every 1,000 m.

High risk:

- Individuals WITH a history of mountain sickness, who – starting from ≈1,200 m – climb to altitudes of 2,800 m or higher in 1 day (and stop there to sleep).
- All the individuals with a history of high-altitude pulmonary oedema or cerebral oedema.
- All those individuals who – starting from ≈1,200 m – climb to more than 3,500 m in 1 day (and stop there to sleep).
- All those individuals who – starting from ≈1,200 m – climb >500 m/day to altitudes higher than 3,000 m (and stop there to sleep), without an extra day of acclimatisation every 1,000 m.
- Very rapid ascents (e.g. climbing Kilimanjaro in less than 7 days).

Everything we have seen so far refers to the measures to be taken in the immediate vicinity of the high-altitude climb.

Special Support by Specific 'Health Coach'

But, in the case of people who often frequent the high mountains, and in the case of sports groups or tourist groups who intend to reach high altitudes on more than one occasion, for example, the more than 3 million members of the European Mountaineering Association,[4] or those who rely on specialised travel agencies to go trekking in exotic mountain areas,[i] it would be a good idea to organise special and continuous 'support', like that experienced in various areas of the world, to try to improve the cardiovascular health of particular groups of people.

We are referring to that activity, which has been defined as '**health coaching**';[5, 6] this activity, however, has so far been applied for the prevention of cardiovascular diseases in the general population, and never tested for the prevention of complications in frequenters of high mountains. However, the model is interesting and it could be worth studying its possibility of application in mountain contexts. In the original trial, the population group involved underwent an initial health assessment, with identification of existing diseases and cardiovascular risk factors; a prognostic assessment was formulated and recommendations regarding behavioural modifications were provided. These activities were similar to those described so far for those who intend to visit the high mountains. It is interesting to observe the intervention should not be limited to the initial diagnosis and recommendations, but that this first phase should constitute the start of an intervention repeated over time, which – as far as our purposes are concerned – we could adapt as follows:

- Provide periodic encouragement for behavioural modification; in our case, this would involve stimulating progressive physical training and completing assessments of the individual's health and fitness.
- Collaborate in solving any problems observed or that emerge during the intervention period; also create simulations regarding possible problems that could arise at altitude, studying with the participants the possible solutions to be undertaken.
- Evaluate participants' adherence to the recommendations provided and the results achieved.

In prevention studies conducted on the general population, personnel from various sources were used for this purpose: from dieticians and pharmacists to health volunteers. For the most part, therefore, personnel not directly involved in the healthcare sector were employed, who had the task of contacting the people entrusted to them and of reinforcing the recommendations that the participants had already received. Paramedics with specific training in mountain medicine issues should ideally be involved.

The following tables (Tables 19.1–19.10) summarise the **Recommendations** formulated by the Italian and the European Societies of Cardiology and of Hypertension and by the Italian

[i]Just to give an example, it appears that every year there are between 6 and 9 thousand Italians who travel to Nepal (Kathmandu is at 1,400 m above sea level) and many of them reach the laboratory-observatory of the Italian Pyramid, located at 5,050 m above sea level; on the other side of the world, it seems that every day a few dozen Italians go to visit Machu Picchu (2,430 m above sea level, province of Urabamba, Peru). Nepal Tourism Board (NTB) reported that a total of more than 1 million foreign tourists entered the country in 2023, coming from all over the world: https://www.nepaltrekkinginhimalaya.com/pages/total-number-of-tourists-arrival-in-each-months-of-2023. And a similar number of tourists (about 1.2 million) travel to Machu Picchu every year: https://www.machupicchutrek.net/how-many-tourists-visit-machu-picchu-annually.

and the International Societies of Mountain Medicine,[7] as well as the recommendations issued by various authors for patients with cardiovascular problems who intend to expose themselves to high altitudes.[1, 8–19] As reported by Parati et al.,[7] it must be taken into account that the strength of these recommendations is to be weighted in the light of the limited evidence available on non-acclimatised individuals with cardiovascular disease exposed to high altitudes. Due to the paucity of existing studies, some of the following recommendations are based on consensus or personal experience of experts and are not accompanied here by statements on the strength of evidence; however, the summarised recommendations are considered reasonable to ensure patient safety.[9]

For more details, we recommend to refer to the mentioned papers.

Summary of Recommendations and Pre-exposure Assessment in Various Cardiovascular Diseases

TABLE 19.1 **Coronary artery disease.**

Clinical Condition	Pre-exposure Assessment and Recommendations	R/E
Coronary Artery Disease		
All patients with known ischaemic heart disease	Consider to perform a pre-exposure activity (sport)-specific evaluation (including maximal exercise testing)	
	At high altitude, continue without interruption or changes any pre-existing medication (especially dual anti-platelet therapy, after DES)	1C
	Direct transportation to an altitude above 3,000 m should be avoided, when possible	
	Physical exertion should be avoided for the duration of a 3–5-day acclimatisation period	
	Above 2,000 m, sleeping altitude should be increased by not more than 300–350 m per night	
	If not regularly engaged in physical exertion at low altitude → should not engage in physical activity at high altitude	
After uncomplicated AMI/ CABG:	Patients should wait at least 6 months before exposure to high altitude	1C
Asymptomatic, revascularisation < 6 month	Consider symptom-limited exercise testing according to coronary status, as a prerequisite to travel	

TABLE 19.1 (continued)

Clinical Condition	Pre-exposure Assessment and Recommendations	R/E
After AMI/CABG: Asymptomatic, revascularisation > 6 month	Symptom-limited exercise testing If not conclusive → exercise testing with imaging modality	
After coronary stenting	Patients should wait at least 6–12 months before high-altitude exposure	2aC
Asymptomatic, reduced LVEF	Exercise testing If not conclusive → exercise testing with imaging modality Transthoracic echocardiography at rest	
Chronic CAD patients in CCS 1[20]	May safely ascend up to 4,200 m AMSL; avoid higher elevations If patient performs physical activity at sea level, he/she may practice light-to-moderate physical exertion at altitude (up to a target HR 70–80% of their low-altitude ischaemic endpoint)	2aC
Chronic CAD patients in CCS 2–3	May carefully ascend up to 2,500 m AMSL May practice only light physical exertion If angina is worsened on ascent → bed rest, oxygen, anti-anginal therapy, descent to lower altitudes	2aC
Chronic CAD patients in CCS 4	Exposure to altitude is contraindicated	1C
Unstable angina	Absolute contraindication to high-altitude exposure	
Exercise testing positive for signs or symptoms of ischaemia at low to moderate workload (<80 W or <5 METs)	Absolute contraindication to high-altitude exposure	
Individuals without known CAD, but very high-cardiovascular disease risk (e.g. SCORE >10%,[21] strong family history, or familial hypercholesterolaemia) who want to engage in high- or very high-intensity exercise	A symptom-limited exercise test is mandatory Consider a functional imaging test, coronary computed tomography angiography, or carotid or femoral artery ultrasound imaging	
Patients with triple antithrombotic therapy (double platelet antiaggregation and oral anti-coagulation)	Exposure to high altitude should be strongly discouraged	

TABLE 19.2 Heart failure.

Clinical Condition	Pre-exposure Assessment and Recommendations	R/E
Heart failure		
Reduced LVEF, any cause	Exercise testing (possibly with evaluation of peak VO_2)	
	Transthoracic echocardiography at rest	
	Carefully evaluate comorbidities (e.g. pulmonary hypertension, anaemia, sleep apnoea)	1C
	Carefully evaluate HF drugs (diuretics, Potassium supplementation, β_1 selective vs. non-selective beta-blockers)	1B
	Recommend slow ascent (300–500 m/day when above 2,000–2,500 m AMSL)	1C
	Give instructions for treatment adjustments if heart failure develops (advise to check body weight daily in order to identify any fluid retention early)	
Stable NYHA I-II patients	May safely reach altitudes up to 3,500 m (slow ascent)	2aC
	No more than light or moderate physical activity is recommended at altitude, particularly during the first days of exposure	2aC
Stable NYHA III patients	May safely reach altitudes up to 2,500–3,000 m, if needed, for a short period	2aC
	Only light physical activity allowed at altitude	2aC
People with symptomatic heart failure at their resident altitude Decompensated or unstable heart failure (NYHA IV), at present Decompensated heart failure in the past 3 months	Avoid high-altitude exposure	1C
Patients with heart transplant	Pre-exposure resting and stress transthoracic echocardiography for cardiac function and pulmonary artery pressure	
	Exposure to altitude contraindicated if pulmonary artery pressure >40 mmHg	
	Probably safe to travel up to moderate altitude (<3,000 m) in medically stable and physically fit patients; adequate acclimatisation needed	

TABLE 19.3 Arterial hypertension.

Clinical Condition	Pre-exposure Assessment and Recommendations	R/E
Arterial hypertension		
All hypertensive patients	Check blood pressure before and during sojourn at high altitude	
Well-controlled hypertension or mild hypertensive patients	May reach very high altitude (>4,000 m AMSL), with adequate medical therapy	1C
Labile hypertension at low altitudes	Administration of O_2 during night hours, when they sleep at high altitudes, may be indicated	
Not optimally controlled pressure at low altitude	Ambulatory blood pressure recording	
	Consider therapy modifications (especially regarding diuretics, β_1 selective vs. non-selective beta-blockers)	2aC
Moderate-severe hypertension and hypertensive patients with moderate-high cardiovascular risk	Instructions for self-monitoring of blood pressure before and during high-altitude sojourn	2aB
	Instruct about possible use of nifedipine (or α-adrenergic blockers) in case of hypertensive crisis	
	Prepare a plan about other treatment adjustments if uncontrolled hypertension or hypotension develops	
	Use of nocturnal oxygen at high altitude may be useful, especially in the elderly	
Poorly controlled arterial blood pressure (BP >160/100 mmHg at rest, or >220 systolic BP during exercise test) or severe hypertensive patients	Absolute contraindication to high-altitude exposure, in order to prevent risk of organ damage	1C

TABLE 19.4 **Pulmonary artery hypertension.**

Clinical Condition	Pre-exposure Assessment and Recommendations	R/E
Pulmonary artery hypertension		
Pulmonary hypertension, any cause	Echocardiographic assessment of RV function and of pulmonary artery pressure under simulated high altitude (FIO_2 12%)	
Marked pulmonary hypertension: • mean pulmonary artery pressure >30 mmHg, • RV-RA gradient >40 mmHg, or • if functional class > I, and/or • presence of markers of poor prognosis ∘ right heart failure, ∘ short distance at a 6-minute walk test or ∘ Peak O_2 consumption <12 $mL \cdot min^{-1} \cdot kg^{-1}$ at a cardiopulmonary exercise test, or ∘ increasing levels of NT-proBNP or Troponin T or I, or ∘ right atrial pressure >15 or Cardiac Index ≤2.0 $L \cdot min^{-1} \cdot m^{-2}$ on hemodynamic study[22]	Exposure contraindicated; patients should be strongly discouraged from a sojourn at even modest altitude	1C
Patients with moderate Pulmonary Hypertension (mean <30 mmHg or systolic value <50 mmHg)	May probably travel safely to altitudes <3,000 m, with prophylactic use of Nifedipine (30 mg twice daily) or Tadalafil (10 mg twice daily) for the duration of their sojourn	
	During stay at altitude, monitor O_2 saturation with portable oximeter → Supplemental oxygen should be available in the event of deterioration	1C
	Avoid travel into remote areas	
	Avoid rapid ascent to altitude and take enough time to acclimatise, even for low altitudes; limit physical activity	

TABLE 19.5 Valvular heart diseases.

Clinical Condition	Pre-exposure Assessment and Recommendations
Valvular heart diseases	
Symptomatic and/or severe valvular heart disease	High-altitude exposure contraindicated
Mild aortic stenosis/insufficiency or mild mitral regurgitation	Exercise testing, transthoracic echocardiography at rest before travelling; in case of doubts: expose to isobaric hypoxia under supervision of a physician prior to travel
	Instructions for self-monitoring of blood pressure and treatment adjustments if uncontrolled hypertension or hypotension develops
	Warn that new-onset arrhythmia, particularly AF, is a concern and would merit descent
	In anticoagulated patients: give instructions for self-monitoring of international normalised ratio (INR) and dose adaptation
Patients with prosthetic heart valves on anti-coagulant therapy	Consider an increased risk of haemorrhage → give instructions for self-monitoring of INR and doses adaptation
	Suggest to avoid activities with risk of severe traumatic injury; possible use of a helmet when climbing

TABLE 19.6 Congenital heart diseases.

Clinical Condition	Pre-exposure Assessment and Recommendations	R/E
Congenital heart diseases		
Acyanotic or cyanotic	Exposure contraindicated if functional class > I	
	Exercise testing and echocardiographic assessment of left and right ventricular function and pulmonary pressure under simulated high altitude (FIO_2 12%; if RV-RA gradient > 40 mmHg patients should be strongly discouraged)	
	Warn of the potential for developing HAPE; instruct to take nifedipine prophylactically to reduce their risk	
Cyanotic forms, with right-to-left shunt	Living at high altitude is not recommended	1C
Left-to-right shunt	Warn of the risk of pulmonary hypertension and recommended to stay at low altitude (<1,500 m)	1C

(continued)

TABLE 19.6 (continued)

Clinical Condition	Pre-exposure Assessment and Recommendations	R/E
Patients with simple congenital heart diseases, surgically treated	May safely ascend to high altitudes	1C
Patients with operated aortic coarctation	Consider evaluation of 24-hour ambulatory blood pressure monitoring	
Patent foramen ovale, asymptomatic (functional class I)	No evidence of contraindication to travel to high altitude	

TABLE 19.7 Thromboembolic events.

Clinical Condition	Pre-exposure Assessment and Recommendations
Thromboembolic events	
Event in the previous 3 months	Absolute contraindication to exposure to altitude

TABLE 19.8 Arrhythmias.

Clinical Condition	Pre-exposure Assessment and Recommendations	R/E
Arrhythmias		
Associated with CAD/CHF	Exercise testing	
Benign premature atrial contractions	Usually, no significant risk at high altitude	
Supraventricular tachycardia/atrial flutter	Consider catheter ablation before high-altitude exposure (particularly in those considering long high-altitude sojourns in remote areas)	
Paroxysmal or persistent atrial fibrillation	Exercise testing and Holter-ECG prior to exposure, to ascertain level of HR control Instruction for heart rate self-monitoring and therapy adjustments in case of insufficient rate control (>90 beats per minutes at rest) Instruct patient on possible use of rescue medication	
Poorly controlled or possibly dangerous arrhythmias (atrial or ventricular)	Absolute contraindication to high-altitude (3,000–3,500 m) exposure	2C
Pacemaker	PM function seems to be unchanged at altitudes up to 4,000 m Testing only if VVIR, DDDR or AAIR mode to adapt PM rates	1C

TABLE 19.8 (continued)

Clinical Condition	Pre-exposure Assessment and Recommendations	R/E
ICD implanted more than 6 months earlier	Possible safe sojourn at altitudes up to 2,000–2,500 m AMSL	1C
	Sport activities limited by underlying disease	
	Warn about possibility of increased arrhythmias and ICD shock (even inappropriate shocks) in case of exercise- or altitude-induced high HR	1A
ICD implantation in the previous 3–6 months	Exposure to high altitude contraindicated	
	Do not travel to remote geographic areas	
Episode of ICD intervention for ventricular arrhythmias in the previous 3–6 months	Exposure to high-altitude contraindicated	
	Do not travel to remote geographic areas	

Abbreviations: AAIR, atrium paced, atrium sensed, and pacemaker inhibited in response to sensed atrial beat and rate-adaptive. DDDR, atrial and ventricular pacing, atrial and ventricular sensing, dual response, and rate-adaptive. VVIR, ventricular pacing, ventricular sensing, inhibition response, and rate-adaptive.

TABLE 19.9 Cerebrovascular diseases.

Clinical Condition	Pre-exposure Assessment and Recommendations	R/E
Cerebrovascular diseases		
All conditions	Avoid trekking or climbing alone	1C
Ischaemic stroke or TIA < 90–(180) days before	Avoid travelling to higher altitudes (>2,000–2,500 m)	1C
	Avoid air travel	
Ischaemic stroke or TIA > 90–(180) days before, thorough workup of the stroke has been performed and risk factors are treated adequately	Avoid extreme altitude > 4,500 m	
Stenosis or occlusion of a major extra- or intracranial cerebral artery	Avoid travelling to altitude >2,000–2,500 m	
Hypertensive haemorrhage	Travel to high altitude only if blood pressure is controlled	
	Do not travel to high altitude before 90 d after the event	1C
Haemorrhage as a result of amyloid angiopathy	Avoid high altitude	
Known cerebral aneurysm, arteriovenous malformation, or cerebral cavernoma	Check blood pressure	
	Avoid extreme altitude >4,500 m	

TABLE 19.10 Diabetes mellitus.

Clinical Condition	Pre-exposure Assessment and Recommendations	R/E
Diabetes Mellitus		
All diabetic patients planning high-altitude travel	Undergo comprehensive risk assessment for cardiovascular disease with their primary care provider and/or endocrinologist/diabetologist	1B
	(including screening for diabetic retinopathy)	1C
All diabetic patients planning to travel to high altitude	Prepare and carry an adequate supply of drugs (2–3 x the anticipated need) and glucose monitoring devices (and spare supplies) for the duration of the travel	1C
	Obtain information about the availability of medical care in the travel area	
	Familiarise the patient with medication storage (low/high temperatures, exposure to sunlight)	1B
All diabetic patients during travel to high altitude	Recommend frequent glucose monitoring at altitude, before, during and after intense/prolonged effort, because of: • possible hypoglycaemia (exercise, appetite loss) • possible hyperglycaemia (high-altitude illnesses, rapid ascents, extreme altitudes)	1B
Athletes with diabetes	Undergo additional and more frequent evaluations with primary care provider or diabetologist/endocrinologist	1C
Suspected silent ischaemia (especially type 1 diabetes) or suggestive symptoms ECG abnormalities Known coronary artery disease	ECG screening	2C
	Exercise stress test: consider exercise stress test under simulated hypoxia. (Note: these tests are not recommended by the American Diabetes Association nor the American College of Sports Medicine, while the American Heart Association recognises a possible value).[15]	1B
	Echocardiogram (or stress echocardiogram) to detect segmental kinetic abnormalities	
Known autonomic nervous system dysfunction	Holter recording to evaluate heart rate variability.	
	Exercise stress test to evaluate heart rate response to physical effort	
	Try to discourage the patient from tackling high altitudes	
Diabetic patients with peripheral neuropathy or peripheral vascular disease	Increased risk of frostbite with exposure to cold environment; plan adequate protection	2C
Diabetic cardiomyopathy	Echocardiogram, with evaluation of LVEF and pulmonary pressure	

TABLE 19.10 (continued)

Clinical Condition	Pre-exposure Assessment and Recommendations	R/E
Physically inactive diabetic patient	Clinical examination, with identification of concomitant risk factors and assessment of 10 y cardiovascular disease risk	1B
	If risk factors are present: exercise stress test (better: cardiopulmonary exercise test; possibly performed with FiO_2 comparable to the expected altitudes)	
	Adequate training period, with monitoring of blood sugar levels and assessment of glycaemic response	2C
Unsatisfactory control of glycaemia, with hyperglycaemia	Increase insulin (or secretagogue medications) dosage; modifications must be planned in advance with care provider	1B
	Recommend frequent glucose monitoring and ketone check, and teach how to adjust insulin dosage	1C
	Recommend adequate hydration	1C
	Recommend the patients to stay close to their hiking companions, for help and possible need of emergent removal or evacuation to definitive care	2C
Previous episodes of hypoglycaemia	Consider reduction of insulin (or secretagogues) dosage, in view of the expected physical effort	1B
	Recommend frequent glucose monitoring (need for adequate supplies) and teach how to adjust insulin dosage	1C
	Recommend regular intake of (fast acting) carbohydrates	1B
	Inform and instruct fellow travellers and expedition leaders of your diabetes and its treatment, including emergency medical treatment (e.g. glucagon injection); recommend the patients to stay close to them	1C
Prevention of acute mountain sickness	Use of acetazolamide: caution!	2C
	Use of dexamethasone: caution! (risk of hyperglycaemia)	2C

References

1 Campbell AD, McIntosh SE, Nyberg A, Powell AP, Schoene RB, Hackett P. Risk stratification for athletes and adventurers in high-altitude environments: recommendations for preparticipation evaluation. Clin J Sport Med 2015; 25(5):404–411. https://doi.org/10.1097/JSM.0000000000000231. Erratum in: Clin J Sport Med 2015; 25(6):553.

2 Luks AM, Auerbach PS, Freer L, Grissom CK, Keyes LE, McIntosh SE, Rodway GW, Schoene RB, Zafren K, Hackett PH. Wilderness medical society clinical practice guidelines for the prevention and treatment of acute altitude illness: 2019 update. Wilderness Environ Med 2019; 30(4S):S3–S18. https://doi.org/10.1016/j.wem.2019.04.006.

3 Luks AM, Beidleman BA, Freer L, Grissom CK, Keyes LE, McIntosh SE, Rodway GW, Schoene RB, Zafren K, Hackett PH. Wilderness medical society clinical practice guidelines for the prevention, diagnosis, and treatment of acute altitude illness: 2024 update. Wilderness Environ Med 2023: S1080–6032(23)00167-9. https://doi.org/10.1016/j.wem.2023.05.013.
4 EUMA, European Mountaineering Association: https://www.european-mountaineers.eu.
5 Vale MJ, Jelinek MV, Best JD, Dart AM, Grigg LE, Hare DL, Ho BP, Newman RW, McNeil JJ; COACH Study Group. Coaching patients On Achieving Cardiovascular Health (COACH): a multicenter randomised trial in patients with coronary heart disease. Arch Intern Med 2003; 163(22):2775–2783. https://doi.org/10.1001/archinte.163.22.2775.
6 Sathe A, Flowers E, Mathur A, Garcia DM, Kotrys J, Gandhi R, Molina C, Mathur A. A culturally specific health coaching program targeting cardiovascular disease risk in South Asians: rationale, design, and baseline data. Ethn Dis 2013; 23(3):304–309.
7 Parati G, Agostoni P, Basnyat B, Bilo G, Brugger H, Coca A, Festi L, Giardini G, Lironcurti A, Luks AM, Maggiorini M, Modesti PA, Swenson ER, Williams B, Bärtsch P, Torlasco C. Clinical recommendations for high altitude exposure of individuals with pre-existing cardiovascular conditions: a joint statement by the European Society of Cardiology, the Council on Hypertension of the European Society of Cardiology, the European Society of Hypertension, the International Society of Mountain Medicine, the Italian Society of Hypertension and the Italian Society of Mountain Medicine. Eur Heart J 2018; 39(17):1546–1554. https://doi.org/10.1093/eurheartj/ehx720.
8 Kobza R, Duru F, Erne P. Leisure-time activities of patients with ICDs: findings of a survey with respect to sports activity, high altitude stays, and driving patterns. Pacing Clin Electrophysiol 2008; 31(7):845–849. https://doi.org/10.1111/j.1540-8159.2008.01098.x.
9 Rimoldi SF, Sartori C, Seiler C, Delacrétaz E, Mattle HP, Scherrer U, Allemann Y. High-altitude exposure in patients with cardiovascular disease: risk assessment and practical recommendations. Prog Cardiovasc Dis 2010; 52(6):512–524. https://doi.org/10.1016/j.pcad.2010.03.005.
10 Mieske K, Flaherty G, O'Brien T. Journeys to high altitude - risks and recommendations for travelers with preexisting medical conditions. J Travel Med 2010; 17(1):48–62. https://doi.org/10.1111/j.1708-8305.2009.00369.x.
11 Donegani E, Hillebrandt D, Windsor J, Gieseler U, Rodway G, Schöffl V, Küpper T. Pre-existing cardiovascular conditions and high altitude travel. Consensus statement of the Medical Commission of the Union Internationale des Associations d'Alpinisme (UIAA MedCom) Travel Medicine and Infectious Disease. Travel Med Infect Dis 2014; 12(3):237–252. https://doi.org/10.1016/j.tmaid.2014.02.004.
12 Niebauer J, Burtscher M. Sudden cardiac death risk in downhill skiers and mountain hikers and specific prevention strategies. Int J Environ Res Public Health 2021; 18(4):1621. https://doi.org/10.3390/ijerph18041621.
13 de Mol P, de Vries ST, de Koning EJ, Gans RO, Bilo HJ, Tack CJ. Physical activity at altitude: challenges for people with diabetes: a review. Diabetes Care 2014; 37(8):2404–2413. https://doi.org/10.2337/dc13-2302.
14 Mohajeri S, Perkins BA, Brubaker PL, Riddell MC. Diabetes, trekking and high altitude: recognizing and preparing for the risks. Diabet Med 2015; 32(11):1425–1437. https://doi.org/10.1111/dme.12795.
15 VanBaak KD, Nally LM, Finigan RT, Jurkiewicz CL, Burnier AM, Conrad BP, Khodaee M, Lipman GS. Wilderness medical society clinical practice guidelines for diabetes management. Wilderness Environ Med 2019; 30(4S):S121–S140. https://doi.org/10.1016/j.wem.2019.10.003.

16 Budts W, Pieles GE, Roos-Hesselink JW, Sanz de la Garza M, D'Ascenzi F, Giannakoulas G, Müller J, Oberhoffer R, Ehringer-Schetitska D, Herceg-Cavrak V, Gabriel H, Corrado D, van Buuren F, Niebauer J, Börjesson M, Caselli S, Fritsch P, Pelliccia A, Heidbuchel H, Sharma S, Stuart AG, Papadakis M. Recommendations for participation in competitive sport in adolescent and adult athletes with Congenital Heart Disease (CHD): position statement of the Sports Cardiology & Exercise Section of the European Association of Preventive Cardiology (EAPC), the European Society of Cardiology (ESC) Working Group on Adult Congenital Heart Disease and the Sports Cardiology, Physical Activity and Prevention Working Group of the Association for European Paediatric and Congenital Cardiology (AEPC). Eur Heart J 2020; 41(43):4191–4199. https://doi.org/10.1093/eurheartj/ehaa501.

17 Borjesson M, Urhausen A, Kouidi E, Dugmore D, Sharma S, Halle M, Heidbüchel H, Björnstad HH, Gielen S, Mezzani A, Corrado D, Pelliccia A, Vanhees L. Cardiovascular evaluation of middle-aged/senior individuals engaged in leisure-time sport activities: position stand from the sections of exercise physiology and sports cardiology of the European Association of Cardiovascular Prevention and Rehabilitation. Eur J Cardiovasc Prev Rehabil 2011; 18(3):446–458. https://doi.org/10.1097/HJR.0b013e32833bo969.

18 Corrado D, Pelliccia A, Bjørnstad HH, Vanhees L, Biffi A, Borjesson M, Panhuyzen-Goedkoop N, Deligiannis A, Solberg E, Dugmore D, Mellwig KP, Assanelli D, Delise P, van-Buuren F, Anastasakis A, Heidbuchel H, Hoffmann E, Fagard R, Priori SG, Basso C, Arbustini E, Blomstrom-Lundqvist C, McKenna WJ, Thiene G; Study Group of Sport Cardiology of the Working Group of Cardiac Rehabilitation and Exercise Physiology and the Working Group of Myocardial and Pericardial Diseases of the European Society of Cardiology. Cardiovascular pre-participation screening of young competitive athletes for prevention of sudden death: proposal for a common European protocol. Consensus Statement of the Study Group of Sport Cardiology of the Working Group of Cardiac Rehabilitation and Exercise Physiology and the Working Group of Myocardial and Pericardial Diseases of the European Society of Cardiology. Eur Heart J 2005; 26(5):516–524. https://doi.org/10.1093/eurheartj/ehi108.

19 Niebauer J, Börjesson M, Carre F, Caselli S, Palatini P, Quattrini F, Serratosa L, Adami PE, Biffi A, Pressler A, Schmied C, van Buuren F, Panhuyzen-Goedkoop N, Solberg E, Halle M, La Gerche A, Papadakis M, Sharma S, Pelliccia A. Recommendations for participation in competitive sports of athletes with arterial hypertension: a position statement from the sports cardiology section of the European Association of Preventive Cardiology (EAPC). Eur Heart J 2018; 39(40):3664–3671. https://doi.org/10.1093/eurheartj/ehy511.

20 Canadian Cardiovascular Society grading of angina pectoris: https://ccs.ca/wp-content/uploads/2020/12/Ang_Gui_1976.pdf.

21 SCORE, European High Risk Chart: https://www.escardio.org/static-file/Escardio/Subspecialty/EACPR/Documents/score-charts.pdf.

22 Task Force for Diagnosis and Treatment of Pulmonary Hypertension of European Society of Cardiology (ESC); European Respiratory Society (ERS); International Society of Heart and Lung Transplantation (ISHLT); Galiè N, Hoeper MM, Humbert M, Torbicki A, Vachiery JL, Barbera JA, Beghetti M, Corris P, Gaine S, Gibbs JS, Gomez-Sanchez MA, Jondeau G, Klepetko W, Opitz C, Peacock A, Rubin L, Zellweger M, Simonneau G. Guidelines for the diagnosis and treatment of pulmonary hypertension. Eur Respir J. 2009 Dec; 34(6):1219–1263. https://doi.org/10.1183/09031936.00139009. https://erj.ersjournals.com/content/34/6/1219.long.

CHAPTER 20

Prevention of Cardiovascular Diseases Through Activities at Altitude

The Venetian Marco Polo (who lived between 1254 and 1324) in his book 'Il Milione'[1] recounts his travels and his life at the court of the emperor of China (Figure 20.1); he also reports an interesting observation on the health effects of high-altitude climbing, in this case positive effects: ... *The air is so pure in those summits and the living there so healthy that the men who live in the city and in the plains and valleys, as soon as they feel attacked by the fever of some fate or other accidental infirmity, immediately ascend the mountain and they stay there two or three days and find themselves healthy due to the excellence of the air...* (Chapter 5). Certainly, the purity of the air and the cooler temperatures in the mountains can help to improve some disease situations (we will see later what the indications for cardiovascular health could be), but the statement is certainly not generalisable and above all, we cannot apply it so simply to the high-altitude climbing.

Already a few years ago, the question about the usefulness of climbing mountains (especially high mountains) had been posed in scientific terms by Gasser et al., who wanted to address the issue: *Climb to moderate altitudes and practice physical activity there: may it be useful in the prevention of cardiovascular diseases?*[2]. These authors studied four pairs of climbers who ascended up to 2,501 m AMSL on the Pfriendler peak, in the canton of Bern, CH, for a total of 7 different ascent difficulties (difficulties between grades 4b and 5c(+) on the French scale),[3] in the time of just under 6 hours. The climbers were equipped with a cardiac monitoring system, which made it possible to study the trend of their heart rate during sustained efforts. The increase in heart rate detected allowed them to deduce that the activity (substantially moderate for the subjects under study, but prohibitive for 'normal' people!) was able

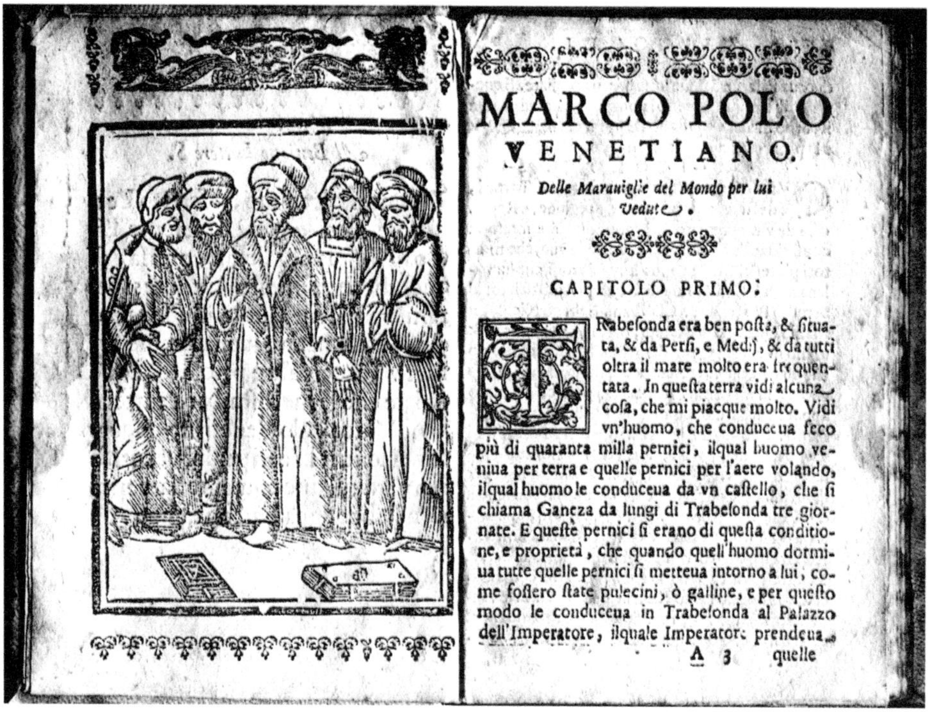
MARCO POLO
VENETIANO.
Delle Marauiglie del Mondo per lui vedute.
CAPITOLO PRIMO.
Trabeſonda era ben poſta, & ſituata, & da Perſi, e Medi, & da tutti oltra il mare molto era frequentata. In queſta terra vidi alcuna coſa, che mi piacque molto. Vidi vn'huomo, che conduceua ſeco più di quaranta milla pernici, ilqual huomo veniua per terra e quelle pernici per l'aere volando, ilqual huomo le conduceua da vn caſtello, che ſi chiama Ganeza da lungi di Trabeſonda tre giornate. E queſte pernici ſi erano di queſta conditione, e proprietà, che quando quell'huomo dormiua tutte quelle pernici ſi metteua intorno a lui, come foſſero ſtate pulecini, ò galline, e per queſto modo le conduceua in Trabeſonda al Palazzo dell'Imperatore, ilquale Imperatore prendeua
A 3 quelle

Courtesy of National Central Library of Rome

FIGURE 20.1 The initial pages of a copy of Marco Polo's 'Il Milione', in an ancient edition of the 17th century. (1627). With permission from Biblioteca Nazionale Centrale 'Vittorio Emanuele II', Rome; signature RA 526, identification code BVEE113078; available at: http://digitale.bnc.roma.sbn.it/tecadigitale/libroantico/BVEE113078/BVEE113078/8.

to stimulate lipid metabolism; from this, the authors underlined how carrying out physical activity at altitude could have a potential effect on the prevention of metabolic diseases.

We have long known that performing physical activity constitutes an effective form of prevention of cardiovascular diseases, both in sedentary but essentially healthy people and in those who have already had some form of cardiac disease: carrying out regular physical activity is considered as 'a cardiovascular therapy'.[4]

In fact, in a study conducted 25 years ago on a group of pensioners in Honolulu, Hawaii, it was observed that mortality was significantly reduced over the 12 years of observation in relation to the amount of daily walking they did, starting a from distance of approximately 1.5–3 km (1–2 miles) per day.[5] It can be commented that walking in Hawaii is presumably inviting and that the environment can clearly stimulate the desire to practice some form of physical activity, even in the laziest. However, it must be said that there is also at least another study, conducted a few years earlier, that reached similar conclusions to those of the Honolulu study: this study was conducted in the United States, in the city of Boston, and involved students (and former students) of that prestigious University.[6] Certainly Boston and its alumni work environments are not Hawaii; but also in this study the observations highlighted how mortality rates from all causes were significantly lower among those who were physically active, and how – among those who had reached the age of 80 – the fact of having carried out and continuing to carry out physical exercise added from one to more than two years of life in comparison to sedentary people.

Other studies[7] have confirmed that – at least in males – the level of physical performance (their effort tolerance) is directly linked to a clear reduction in the age-adjusted mortality risk, both in healthy subjects and in people with heart disease; this is true even when persons used to practice only slight or moderate physical exercise, and the reduction in the mortality rate can exceed 45%. Other studies[8] have confirmed that performing physical activity for at least two and a half hours a week leads to equally protective results against cardiovascular diseases even in women, and also in young women. Practising running even for just 7–10 minutes a day at low speed (less than 10 km/hour) leads to a 30–45% reduction in both cardiovascular and all-cause mortality, both in men and women, and also among smokers.[9–11]

Up to this point, we talked about physical activity essentially carried out on the plains.

Will physical activity carried out in the mountains have the same protective value? (Obviously taking into account all the limitations and attentions that we have seen in the previous chapters).

Some studies help us understand the situation.

In 2008, some Austrian scholars[12] accompanied a group of 18 adults (average age 55 years), suffering from metabolic syndrome (Figure 20.2), to a 3-week period of mountain excursions in Obertauern at 1,700 m AMSL; the participants were followed by doctors during these excursions, which were carried out 4 times a week, with physical effort corresponding to approximately 55–65% of their maximum heart rate, for a total of 29 hours of physical exercise. The analysis of various parameters (exercise tolerance, echocardiographic measurements of the systolic and diastolic function of the left ventricle and evaluation of pulmonary artery pressure,

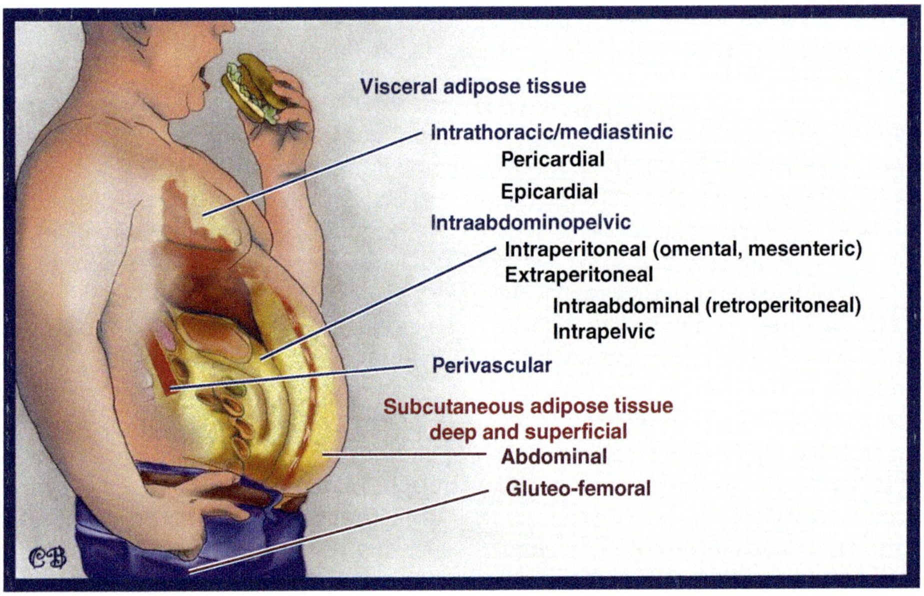

FIGURE 20.2 Classification of adipose tissue deposits in patients with metabolic syndrome; courtesy of © the author, Dr. Clara Bambace Alexandersson, from her PhD Doctoral Thesis 'Characterisation of epicardial adipose tissue and myocardial fat infiltration in humans', University of Verona, Italy, 2013.

and various blood chemistry measurements) did not highlight any negative cardiovascular effects, while resting blood pressure was significantly reduced.

Lower Prevalence of Metabolic Syndrome at Moderate-high Altitude

Similar effects were also confirmed by another study conducted in 2015, again on subjects suffering from metabolic syndrome and with a protocol quite similar to the previous study;[13] the authors of this study confirmed that physical activity performed during the 2 weeks of guided excursions at moderate altitudes (1,900 m AMSL) seems more effective in reducing various parameters of lipid metabolism (reduction of total and LDL cholesterol) in comparison to a similar period of training carried out on the plains or at low altitude. Thus, it seems reasonable to conclude that at least in patients with metabolic syndrome, no negative effects have been observed (on the contrary) when performing physical activity at moderate altitudes.

Other two studies performed in Spain and Ecuador by a group of Spanish Researchers confirmed that living at high altitude (2,758–2,787 m AMSL in Ecuador and 457–2,297 m AMSL in Spain) was associated with a lower prevalence of metabolic syndrome, hypercholesterolaemia and hyperglycaemia, compared to the control participants living at sea level.[14, 15] An epidemiological study conducted in Peru[16] highlighted that abdominal obesity was highly prevalent (affecting approximately 34% of the population studied), but it presented a significant inverse correlation with the altitude of residence above 3,000 m, although female gender and advanced age were also significant modifiers.

Body Weight Reduction at Moderate, High and Extreme Altitudes

However, doubts have also been raised as to whether it is the performance of regular physical activity in itself that allows an improvement of the metabolic picture, and not so much the fact of living at altitude rather than on the plains.[17]

In this regard, it should be noted that a systematic review and meta-analysis conducted in 2019[18] highlighted that in people exposed to moderate, high and extreme altitudes, a decrease in pooled mean body weight appeared in all subgroups, with larger changes occurring at higher altitudes. When participants were active, they experienced more pronounced decreases in body weight, but body weight reduction also occurred in passive individuals (Figure 20.3). The reduction was greater for more prolonged exposure (especially when the duration of the exposure exceeded 42 days). Another notable observation from this review is that body weight significantly decreased even when caloric intake was matched or increased relative to output, indicating hypoxia as a possible trigger for body composition changes in these persons.

Also, post-menopausal women can obtain positive results: arterial stiffness is reduced when they perform physical activity in a hypobaric hypoxic environment, at a simulated altitude of

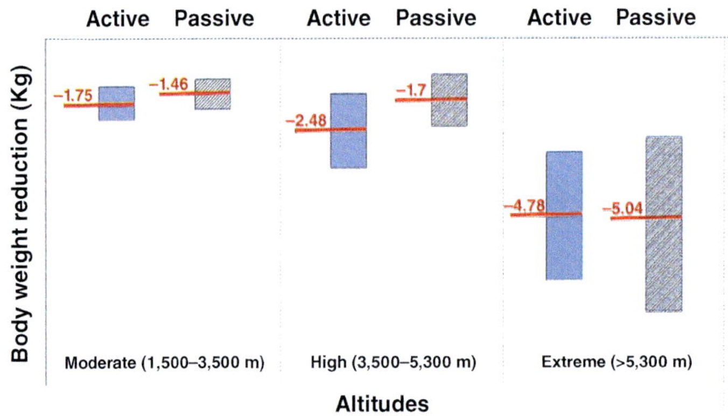

FIGURE 20.3 Reduction of pooled body weight with exposition at various mountain altitudes for periods of up to 42 days, according to a meta-analysis by Adapted from [18].

approximately 2,000 m AMSL[19] (and therefore, probably, also for physical activity carried out in the mountains), compared to similar activities performed on the plains.

Positive Effects of Exposure to Intermittent Hypobaric Hypoxia

It appears that some positive effects on various metabolic parameters in sedentary subjects can be obtained even with simple intermittent exposure to hypoxia, at simulated altitudes of 2,700–4,000 m AMSL 2–3 times a week; this is at least what is reported in a recent review of the literature.[20]

Performing moderate physical activity in a hypoxic environment can, on the one hand, favour vasodilation at the muscular level (through the release of nitric oxide, adenosine and prostaglandins by endothelial cells) and, on the other hand, it can favour the increase in circulating progenitor cells and angiogenic factors, which could induce the formation of collateral circulation at the muscular and perhaps even cardiac level. The hypothesis of hypoxia-induced increase of collateral circulation in the coronary arteries has been advanced as an explanation for the reduced cardiovascular mortality found among white citizens of 99 large American cities, which showed an inverse relationship with the altitude of residence.[21]

In hypertensive patients, performing physical activity in hypoxic conditions (at a simulated altitude of approximately 2,000 m AMSL) can induce a reduction in blood pressure greater than that obtainable with similar physical exercise performed in normoxic conditions; furthermore, it can induce the beneficial effect of reducing the overall cardiovascular risk.[21]

Abdominal obesity (visceral obesity) is characterised not only by the deposition of fat around the viscera but also, above all, by the presence of inflammatory factors, insulin resistance (and possible diabetes), endothelial dysfunction and predisposition to atherosclerosis. In obese subjects, carrying out physical activity in hypoxic conditions (even just walking at a relatively slow pace) could be more effective than brisk walking in normoxia in improving overall health;[22] furthermore, slow walking would reduce mechanical stress on the joints, and hypoxia could help reduce the sensation of hunger in obese individuals.

Reduced Prevalence of Diabetes Mellitus at High Altitudes

In Europe, the available statistics indicate that approximately 10% of the population is affected by a form of diabetes, with 65.6 million people affected in 2024, and more than one-third of the cases (33.6%) being undiagnosed.[23]

In the year 2021, it was estimated that almost 12% of the total US population and 14.7% of all adults (18 years or older) had diabetes; furthermore, 38.0% of all US adults had pre-diabetes, based on their fasting glucose or HbA1c level.[24] As we have already seen in Chapter 17, in 2022 approximately 830 million people worldwide were living with diabetes;[25] the prevalence of the disease has increased over the last 30 years, especially in low- and middle-income countries.

The above reported data refer to the general population of the various regions of the world. But what could be the prevalence of diabetes in populations living at high altitude?

It is a difficult task to ascertain: a confounding factor is that diabetes prevalence increases with age, and the average age of the population is older in high-income countries while is younger in most low-middle-income countries as well as in countries located at high average altitudes.[26]

Anyway, looking at the data collected in the International Diabetes Federation (IDF) Atlas 2025, it seems that the prevalence of diabetes in countries such as Bolivia, Ethiopia and Nepal is in the lower range of prevalence, with values of roughly 2–3, 3–4 and 7%, respectively.[27] How much this low prevalence may be related to living at moderate-high mountain altitudes or, conversely, how much it is linked to underdiagnosis or underreporting is a matter of doubt; IDF estimates that persons living with undiagnosed diabetes are 30% in the countries in South and Central America, 29% for North America and the Caribbean, 34% for Europe, 43% for countries in Southeast Asia and 37% for the Middle East and North Africa.[27]

Other data confirm that, in Peru, native male residents at altitudes of 3,250 m AMSL actually have a lower blood glucose profile than sea-level residents throughout a 12 hours of continuous monitoring,[28] probably due to faster glucose uptake and increased insulin sensitivity, as observed in experimental animals.[29] A quite large study conducted again in Peru (PERUDIAB)[30] between 2010 and 2012 confirmed the high relevance of diabetes in that country, with an estimated national prevalence of 7.0%; it was highlighted that 40% of the affected individuals were undiagnosed. The important finding of the study was that the prevalence of diabetes and pre-diabetes was higher in coastal regions than in mountainous regions (8.2 vs. 4.5% and 26.4 vs. 17.4%, respectively), explained by a probably increased insulin sensitivity due to hypoxia in high-altitude areas. Similar data have been found in other epidemiological studies, with evidence that fasting plasma glucose concentrations were inversely correlated with the altitude of residence.[31] A worrying fact is that the prevalence of diabetes was beginning to increase even in the highlands, probably due to new lifestyles progressively adopted by high-mountain populations.

In indigenous Argentinean children living at 3,750 m, insulin resistance was somewhat lower than in children living at 1,400 m, suggesting a probably lower risk of developing type 2 diabetes mellitus.[32]

Even more impressive are the findings among the Tibetan population in China. A cross-sectional study performed in 2017 made evident that altitude was negatively associated with the risk of diabetes mellitus: compared to individuals living at <3,500 m, the risk of diabetes mellitus decreased by 65% for those living at 3,500–3,999 m and by 89% for those living at ≥ 4,000 m.[33]

A genetic adaptation to decreased oxygen availability in high-altitude Tibetan populations might alter their metabolism, causing a shift in fuel preference to glucose oxidation and glycolysis, thus offering protection from diabetes at high altitude; at lower elevations and/or with the adoption of non-traditional diets, the risk of diabetes could increase.[34] In fact, in the Tibetan population, economic development and higher annual family income are associated with higher prevalence of diabetes.

Among adult Tibetans who migrated from 3,000 m (Lhasa, Tibet-China) to 1,500 m of altitude (Srinagar, India), some observations suggest that high-altitude mountain natives appear to lose their advantage when moving to lower altitudes.[35]

Also in Peruvian Amerindian women, migration from the highlands of Cuzco (3,400 m) to the lowlands of Lima (approximately 100–860 m) was associated with increased levels of glucose, insulin, and leptin as well as parameters of insulin resistance and higher diastolic blood pressure, probably due to a reduction of their physical activity.[36]

But not all people living at high altitudes have the lower plasma glucose levels described: high-altitude dwellers with chronic mountain sickness and excessive erythrocytosis (Hb ≥210 g/dL in men, Hb ≥190 g/dL in women) present elevated fasting serum glucose and insulin resistance, as shown by studies performed in the Andes, China and India.[37, 38]

In the United States, a large-scale study reported in 2014 that the odds ratio for diabetes was lower for males living at altitudes between 1,500 and 3,500 m (OR 0.88) in comparison to males living at 0–499 m AMSL, after adjustment for multiple risk factors and potential confounders; this inverse association between altitude and diabetes was not found among females.[39] The reduced prevalence of diabetes in high-altitude residents was not explained by a reduced prevalence of obesity in this population. Even ethnicity does not appear to explain the different prevalence of diabetes: in an analysis conducted in 2001 on data from the San Antonio Heart Study and the Mexico City Diabetes Study, it resulted that low-income Mexicans living at high altitude in Mexico City (2,240 m) had a lower incidence of diabetes than low-income Mexicans of similar age living at sea level (198 m of San Antonio, Texas),[40] probably due to higher insulin sensitivity[41] and despite a higher carbohydrate intake in the diet.[42]

Also in other parts of the world, the prevalence of diabetes is lower in inhabitants of moderate- or high-altitude regions.

In the European Alpine area, some data indicate that type 2 diabetes mellitus has a significantly lower incidence in mountainous areas such as Tyrol (Austria) in comparison with lowlands.[43]

In Saudi Arabia, fasting glucose levels of pregnant women were found to be lower in inhabitants of a high-altitude area (Abha, 3,000 m) than in those of a low-altitude area (Mahayil Aseer, 400 m).[44]

Reduced Mortality from Coronary Heart Disease at Moderate Altitudes

There is also an epidemiological observation conducted in New Mexico,[45] according to which mortality from coronary heart disease shows a progressive reduction among men (but not among women!) in an inverse correlation with the altitude of residence above 1,220 m AMSL (up to over 2,135 m); in that study, for every 305 m increase in living altitude CAD mortality was 98, 90, 86 and 72% compared to the group living below 1,220 m of altitude. A possible explanation of such a trend is that daily activities carried out at altitude represent greater exercise than when undertaken at lower altitudes. Similar conclusions have also been drawn by an epidemiological study conducted in Greece between 1981 and 1996,[46] which found that living in mountainous areas (even at the low altitude of about 950 m AMSL) had a 'protective effect' from total and coronary mortality; this positive effect was attributed to the increased physical activity associated with walking on rugged terrains under conditions of moderate hypoxia.

Also in the United States, living at altitude >1,000 m AMSL has been found to have a beneficial association with ischaemic heart disease mortality, which was 4–14 per 10,000 people lower than in people living within 100 m of sea level;[47] however, altitude resulted to have detrimental effects in persons with chronic obstructive pulmonary disease, with a dose-response relationship, so that living at altitude seems to have – at least in the study cited – insignificant net effects on the life expectancy of the entire population (but probably not of individual patients!).

Among other studies, in a Swiss census-based record linkage study, it has been found that mortality from both coronary heart disease and stroke was significantly lower at altitude, in an inverse relationship with residence altitude: −22% per 1,000 m for CAD, −12% per 1,000 m for stroke.[48] The effect was stronger in men than in women. The positive effect of living at altitude was explained by the authors as linked to a complex of environmental factors (reduced pollution, ultraviolet radiation, dietary composition), and not only with reduction of the prevalence of the classic cardiovascular risk factors, an effect that was instead highlighted by other investigators.[49]

However, it must be said that, while it is clear that exposure to hypoxia and physical exercise can have positive synergistic effects in patients with arterial hypertension and obesity and in sedentary subjects, it is not yet sufficiently clear what the optimal combination of physical activity (i.e. exercise intensity, type of activity) and hypoxia (altitude level, optimal hypoxic dose, normobaric or hypobaric hypoxia) could be.[50]

Could Heart Patients Also Benefit from Physical Activity at Altitude?

We must first recall here a study already cited in previous chapters, that of Schmid et al.,[51] who submitted 29 patients with moderate-severe heart failure (left ventricular ejection

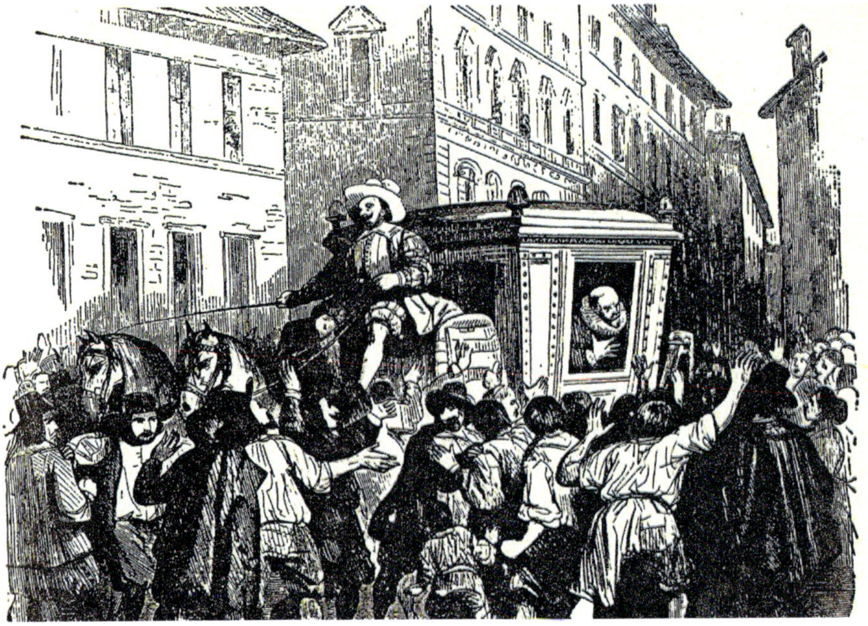

FIGURE 20.4 'Go ahead, Pedro, if you can. Go ahead, ... with judgment'. Francesco Gonin / https://commons.wikimedia.org/wiki/File:I_promessi_sposi_186.jpg / Public domain / last accessed Dec. 27, 2025.

fraction on average 28.8 ± 5.4%) to an exercise test in the high mountains (3,454 m AMSL): they observed that such an altitude is reasonably well tolerated in these patients even during physical effort.

However, while these patients do not appear to be at particularly high risk when performing controlled physical effort during a short stay at high altitude (except for a possible increase in the frequency of arrhythmias), it is nevertheless unclear whether beneficial effects could be induced in similar groups of patients when living and training at moderate or high mountain altitudes. Already in 2013, Burtscher warned that *'whereas living at higher elevations may protect from development of cardiovascular diseases, it could adversely affect mortality when heart diseases progress'* as well as in aged patients.[52]

For these patients with heart failure and other forms of heart disease, it is worth acting following the indications of the Grand Chancellor Antonio Ferrer, in 'I Promessi Sposi' ('The Betrothed') by Alessandro Manzoni, when he found himself with his carriage in the middle of a tumult: *Adelante, Pedro, si puedes. Adelante, ... con juicio*[i] (Figure 20.4).

In other words, it is essential to maintain a proper balance between types and intensity of physical exercise, on the one hand, and the mountain altitude i.e. the related hypobaric hypoxia, on the other.

[i]'Go ahead, Pedro, if you can. Go ahead,... with judgment'. Alessandro Manzoni, I Promessi Sposi [The Betrothed], 1827, Chapter 13. English translation available at: https://wellcomecollection.org/works/ve2597zr/items.

References

1 Marco Polo. The most noble and famous travels of Marco Polo, together with the travels of Nicoláo de' Conti. English translation by Frampton J. Adam and Charles Black, London, 1937. https://archive.org/details/mostnoblefamoust00polo/mode/2up.

2 Gasser BA, Hoppeler HH, Waibel M. Bergtouren als Präventivmittel von kardiovaskulären Erkrankungen? [Mountaineering for the prevention of cardiovascular diseases?]. Sportverletz Sportschaden 2016; 30(2):85–89. German. https://doi.org/10.1055/s-0035-1567024.

3 Guide Dolomiti. Rock climbing grades - different rock climbing grades across the five most popular systems. https://www.guidedolomiti.com/en/rock-climbing-grades./

4 Shephard RJ, Balady GJ. Exercise as cardiovascular therapy. Circulation 1999; 99(7):963–972. https://doi.org/10.1161/01.cir.99.7.963.

5 Hakim AA, Petrovitch H, Burchfiel CM, Ross GW, Rodriguez BL, White LR, Yano K, Curb JD, Abbott RD. Effects of walking on mortality among nonsmoking retired men. N Engl J Med 1998; 338(2):94–99. https://doi.org/10.1056/NEJM199801083380204.

6 Paffenbarger RS Jr, Hyde RT, Wing AL, Hsieh CC. Physical activity, all-cause mortality, and longevity of college alumni. N Engl J Med 1986; 314(10):605–613. https://doi.org/10.1056/NEJM198603063141003.

7 Myers J, Prakash M, Froelicher V, Do D, Partington S, Atwood JE. Exercise capacity and mortality among men referred for exercise testing. N Engl J Med 2002; 346(11):793–801. https://doi.org/10.1056/NEJMoa011858.

8 Chomistek AK, Chiuve SE, Eliassen AH, Mukamal KJ, Willett WC, Rimm EB. Healthy lifestyle in the primordial prevention of cardiovascular disease among young women. J Am Coll Cardiol 2015; 65(1):43–51. https://doi.org/10.1016/j.jacc.2014.10.024. https://www.ncbi.nlm.nih.gov/pmc/articles/PMC4291551/pdf/nihms639645.pdf.

9 Lee DC, Pate RR, Lavie CJ, Sui X, Church TS, Blair SN. Leisure-time running reduces all-cause and cardiovascular mortality risk. J Am Coll Cardiol 2014; 64(5):472–481. https://doi.org/10.1016/j.jacc.2014.04.058. Erratum in: J Am Coll Cardiol 2014; 64(14):1537. https://www.jacc.org/doi/10.1016/j.jacc.2014.08.004.

10 Rees-Punia E, Deubler E, Campbell P, Gapstur SM, Patel A. Light-intensity physical activity in a large prospective cohort of older US adults: a 21-year follow-up of mortality. Gerontology 2020; 66(3):259–265. https://doi.org/10.1159/000502860.

11 Lee DC, Lee IM. Optimum dose of resistance exercise for cardiovascular health and longevity: is more better? Curr Cardiol Rep 2023. https://doi.org/10.1007/s11886-023-01976-6.

12 Mair J, Hammerer-Lercher A, Mittermayr M, Klingler A, Humpeler E, Pachinger O, Schobersberger W. 3-week hiking holidays at moderate altitude do not impair cardiac function in individuals with metabolic syndrome. Int J Cardiol 2008; 123(2):186–188. https://doi.org/10.1016/j.ijcard.2006.11.127.

13 Gutwenger I, Hofer G, Gutwenger AK, Sandri M, Wiedermann CJ. Pilot study on the effects of a 2-week hiking vacation at moderate versus low altitude on plasma parameters of carbohydrate and lipid metabolism in patients with metabolic syndrome. BMC Res Notes 2015; 8:103. https://doi.org/10.1186/s13104-015-1066-3.

14 Lopez-Pascual A, Bes-Rastrollo M, Sayón-Orea C, Perez-Cornago A, Díaz-Gutiérrez J, Pons JJ, Martínez-González MA, González-Muniesa P, Martínez JA. Living at a geographically higher elevation is associated with lower risk of metabolic syndrome: prospective analysis of the SUN cohort. Front Physiol 2017; 7:658. https://doi.org/10.3389/fphys.2016.00658.

15 Lopez-Pascual A, Arévalo J, Martínez JA, González-Muniesa P. Inverse association between metabolic syndrome and altitude: a cross-sectional study in an adult population of Ecuador. Front Endocrinol (Lausanne) 2018; 9:658. https://doi.org/10.3389/fendo.2018.00658.

16 Pajuelo-Ramírez J, Torres-Aparcana H, Agüero-Zamora R, Quispe AM. Altitude and its inverse association with abdominal obesity in an Andean country: a cross-sectional study. F1000Res 2019; 8:1738. https://doi.org/10.12688/f1000research.20707.2. https://pmc.ncbi.nlm.nih.gov/articles/PMC6896245/pdf/f1000research-8-24140.pdf.

17 Neumayr G, Fries D, Mittermayer M, Humpeler E, Klingler A, Schobersberger W, Spiesberger R, Pokan R, Schmid P, Berent R. Effects of hiking at moderate and low altitude on cardiovascular parameters in male patients with metabolic syndrome: Austrian Moderate Altitude Study. Wilderness Environ Med 2014; 25(3):329–334. https://doi.org/10.1016/j.wem.2014.01.003. https://www.wemjournal.org/action/showPdf?pii=S1080-6032%2814%2900006-4.

18 Dünnwald T, Gatterer H, Faulhaber M, Arvandi M, Schobersberger W. Body composition and body weight changes at different altitude levels: a systematic review and meta-analysis. Front Physiol 2019; 10:430. https://doi.org/10.3389/fphys.2019.00430.

19 Nishiwaki M, Kawakami R, Saito K, Tamaki H, Takekura H, Ogita F. Vascular adaptations to hypobaric hypoxic training in postmenopausal women. J Physiol Sci 2011; 61(2):83–91. https://doi.org/10.1007/s12576-010-0126-7.

20 Lizamore CA, Hamlin MJ. The use of simulated altitude techniques for beneficial cardiovascular health outcomes in nonathletic, sedentary, and clinical populations: a literature review. High Alt Med Biol 2017; 18(4):305–321. https://doi.org/10.1089/ham.2017.0050.

21 Voors AW, Johnson WD. Altitude and arteriosclerotic heart disease mortality in white residents of 99 of the 100 largest cities in the United States. J Chronic Dis 1979; 32 (1–2):157–162. https://doi.org/10.1016/0021-9681(79)90044-4.

22 Girard O, Malatesta D, Millet GP. Walking in hypoxia: an efficient treatment to lessen mechanical constraints and improve health in obese individuals? Front Physiol 2017; 8:73. https://doi.org/10.3389/fphys.2017.00073. https://www.ncbi.nlm.nih.gov/pmc/articles/PMC5298970/pdf/fphys-08-00073.pdf

23 International Diabetes Federation. Europe - Diabetes regional report 2000 – 2050. https://diabetesatlas.org/data-by-location/region/europe.

24 CDC. National diabetes statistics report. May 15, 2024. https://www.cdc.gov/diabetes/php/data-research/index.html.

25 International Diabetes Federation. Diabetes global report 2000 – 2050. https://diabetesatlas.org/data-by-location/global.

26 NCD Risk Factor Collaboration (NCD-RisC). Worldwide trends in diabetes prevalence and treatment from 1990 to 2022: a pooled analysis of 1108 population-representative studies with 141 million participants. Lancet 2024; 404(10467):2077–2093. https://doi.org/10.1016/S0140-6736(24)02317-1. Erratum in: Lancet 2025; 405(10485):1146. https://doi.org/10.1016/S0140-6736(25)00620-8.

27 International Diabetes Federation. IDF Diabetes Atlas 11th Edition 2025. Global Factsheet. https://diabetesatlas.org/media/uploads/sites/3/2025/04/IDF_Atlas_11th_Edition_2025_Global-Factsheet.pdf and https://diabetesatlas.org/media/uploads/sites/3/2025/04/IDF_Atlas_11th_Edition_2025.pdf.

28 Castillo O, Woolcott OO, Gonzales E, Tello V, Tello L, Villarreal C, Méndez N, Damas L, Florentini E. Residents at high altitude show a lower glucose profile than sea-level residents throughout 12-hour blood continuous monitoring. High Alt Med Biol 2007; 8(4):307–311. https://doi.org/10.1089/ham.2007.8407.

29 Gamboa JL, Garcia-Cazarin ML, Andrade FH. Chronic hypoxia increases insulin-stimulated glucose uptake in mouse soleus muscle. Am J Physiol Regul Integr Comp Physiol 2011; 300(1): R85–R91. https://doi.org/10.1152/ajpregu.00078.2010.https://pmc.ncbi.nlm.nih.gov/articles/PMC3023279.

30 Seclen SN, Rosas ME, Arias AJ, Huayta E, Medina CA. Prevalence of diabetes and impaired fasting glucose in Peru: report from PERUDIAB, a national urban population-based longitudinal study. BMJ Open Diabetes Res Care 2015; 3(1):e000110. https://doi.org/10.1136/bmjdrc-2015-000110.

31 Zila-Velasque JP, Grados-Espinoza P, Challapa-Mamani MR, Sánchez-Alcántara F, Cedillo-Balcázar J, Cs AD, Hernandez-Bustamante EA, Tejada-Flores J, Piano Suárez A, Pacheco-Mendoza J, Benites-Zapata VA. Prevalence of metabolic syndrome and its components according to altitude levels: a systematic review and meta-analysis. Sci Rep 2024; 14(1):27581. https://doi.org/10.1038/s41598-024-77928-z. https://pmc.ncbi.nlm.nih.gov/articles/PMC11555074.

32 Burtscher M, Gatterer H, Burtscher J. Does growing up at high altitude pose a risk factor for type 2 diabetes? AIMS Public Health 2019; 6(1):96–98. https://doi.org/10.3934/publichealth.2019.1.96.

33 Xu S, Wang Q, Liu J, Bian B, Yu X, Yu X, Ning X, Wang J. The prevalence of and risk factors for diabetes mellitus and impaired glucose tolerance among Tibetans in China: a cross-sectional study. Oncotarget 2017; 8(68):112467–112476. https://doi.org/10.18632/oncotarget.21301. https://pmc.ncbi.nlm.nih.gov/articles/PMC5762525.

34 Ge RL, Simonson TS, Gordeuk V, Prchal JT, McClain DA. Metabolic aspects of high-altitude adaptation in Tibetans. Exp Physiol 2015; 100(11):1247–1255. https://doi.org/10.1113/EP085292. https://pmc.ncbi.nlm.nih.gov/articles/PMC10905973/pdf/nihms-1853551.pdf.

35 Riyaz MSU, Rather MK, Koul PA. Diabetes in Immigrant Tibetan Muslims in Kashmir, North India. J Immigr Minor Health 2018; 20(2):410–415. https://doi.org/10.1007/s10903-017-0558-8.

36 Lindgärde F, Ercilla MB, Correa LR, Ahrén B. Body adiposity, insulin, and leptin in subgroups of Peruvian Amerindians. High Alt Med Biol 2004; 5(1):27–31. https://doi.org/10.1089/152702904322963663.

37 Corante N, Anza-Ramírez C, Figueroa-Mujíca R, Macarlupú JL, Vizcardo-Galindo G, Bilo G, Parati G, Gamboa JL, León-Velarde F, Villafuerte FC. Excessive erythrocytosis and cardiovascular risk in Andean highlanders. High Alt Med Biol 2018; 19(3):221–231. https://doi.org/10.1089/ham.2017.0123.

38 Okumiya K, Sakamoto R, Ishimoto Y, Kimura Y, Fukutomi E, Ishikawa M, Suwa K, Imai H, Chen W, Kato E, Nakatsuka M, Kasahara Y, Fujisawa M, Wada T, Wang H, Dai Q, Xu H, Qiao H, Ge RL, Norboo T, Tsering N, Kosaka Y, Nose M, Yamaguchi T, Tsukihara T, Ando K, Inamura T, Takeda S, Ishine M, Otsuka K, Matsubayashi K. Glucose intolerance associated with hypoxia in people living at high altitudes in the Tibetan highland. BMJ Open 2016; 6(2):e009728. https://doi.org/10.1136/bmjopen-2015-009728.

39 Woolcott OO, Castillo OA, Gutierrez C, Elashoff RM, Stefanovski D, Bergman RN. Inverse association between diabetes and altitude: a cross-sectional study in the adult population of the United States. Obesity (Silver Spring) 2014; 22(9):2080–2090. https://doi.org/10.1002/oby.20800. https://pmc.ncbi.nlm.nih.gov/articles/PMC4149588/pdf/nihms-596413.pdf.

40 Burke JP, Williams K, Haffner SM, Villalpando CG, Stern MP. Elevated incidence of type 2 diabetes in San Antonio, Texas, compared with that of Mexico City, Mexico. Diabetes Care 2001; 24(9): 1573–1578. https://doi.org/10.2337/diacare.24.9.1573.

41 Belfiore F, Iannello S. Reduced insulin sensitivity in Mexican-Americans from San Antonio with elevated incidence of type 2 diabetes compared with Mexicans from Mexico City. Diabetes Care 2002; 25(5):937–938; author reply 938-9. https://doi.org/10.2337/diacare.25.5.937-a.

42 Gonzélez C, Stern MP, Mitchell BD, Valdez RA, Haffner SM, Pérez BA. Clinical characteristics of type II diabetic subjects consuming high versus low carbohydrate diets in Mexico City and San Antonio, Texas. Diabetes Care 1994; 17(5):397–404. https://doi.org/10.2337/diacare.17.5.397.

43 Eller K, Tancevski I, Eller P. Letter by Eller et al regarding article, 'Lower mortality from coronary heart disease and stroke at higher altitudes in Switzerland'. Circulation 2010; 121(14):e377. https://doi.org/10.1161/CIR.0b013e3181daaced.

44 Hassan B. Interpretation of maternal blood glucose during pregnancy at high altitude area, Abha-Saudi Arabia. J Family Med Prim Care 2020; 9(9):4633–4636. https://doi.org/10.4103/jfmpc.jfmpc_747_20. https://pmc.ncbi.nlm.nih.gov/articles/PMC7652192/pdf/JFMPC-9-4633.pdf.

45 Mortimer EA Jr, Monson RR, MacMahon B. Reduction in mortality from coronary heart disease in men residing at high altitude. N Engl J Med 1977; 296(11):581–585. https://doi.org/10.1056/NEJM197703172961101.

46 Baibas N, Trichopoulou A, Voridis E, Trichopoulos D. Residence in mountainous compared with lowland areas in relation to total and coronary mortality. A study in rural Greece. J Epidemiol Community Health 2005; 59(4):274–278. https://doi.org/10.1136/jech.2004.025510. https://www.ncbi.nlm.nih.gov/pmc/articles/PMC1733062/pdf/v059p00274.pdf.

47 Ezzati M, Murray Horwitz ME, Thomas DS, Friedman AB, Roach R, Clark T, Murray CJ, Honigman B. Altitude, life expectancy and mortality from ischaemic heart disease, stroke, COPD and cancers: national population-based analysis of US counties. J Epidemiol Community Health 2012; 66(7):e17. https://doi.org/10.1136/jech.2010.112938. Erratum in: J Epidemiol Community Health 2023; 77(11):752.

48 Faeh D, Gutzwiller F, Bopp M; Swiss National Cohort Study Group. Lower mortality from coronary heart disease and stroke at higher altitudes in Switzerland. Circulation 2009; 120(6):495–501. https://doi.org/10.1161/CIRCULATIONAHA.108.819250.

49 Burtscher M, Millet GP, Klimont J, Burtscher J. Differences in the prevalence of physical activity and cardiovascular risk factors between people living at low (<1,001 m) compared to moderate (1,001–2,000 m) altitude. AIMS Public Health 2021; 8(4):624–635. https://doi.org/10.3934/publichealth.2021050. https://pmc.ncbi.nlm.nih.gov/articles/PMC8568593.

50 Millet GP, Debevec T, Brocherie F, Malatesta D, Girard O. Therapeutic use of exercising in hypoxia: promises and limitations. Front Physiol 2016; 7:224. https://doi.org/10.3389/fphys.2016.00224.

51 Schmid JP, Nobel D, Brugger N, Novak J, Palau P, Trepp A, Wilhelm M, Saner H. Short-term high altitude exposure at 3454 m is well tolerated in patients with stable heart failure. Eur J Heart Fail 2015; 17(2):182–186. https://doi.org/10.1002/ejhf.227.

52 Burtscher M. Effects of living at higher altitudes on mortality: a narrative review. Aging Dis 2013; 5(4):274–280. https://doi.org/10.14336/AD.2014.0500274.

CHAPTER 21

Use of Drugs Acting on the Cardiovascular System at Altitude

Here, we will review the use of some of the main cardiovascular drugs at high altitude, along with their benefits and potential negative effects (see Table 21.1).

We will also provide some advice on the implications of taking drugs or substances that may affect the cardiovascular system and their legality in competitive mountain sports.

First of all, it is important to remember that many drugs may not be available in large parts of mountain areas or may be available only with considerable difficulty. A high-altitude worker, or a hiker who goes for more or less prolonged periods to mountainous areas, especially exotic ones, must remember to bring with them all the medicines they regularly use as well as those ones they may need, in amounts sufficient to ensure coverage for the entire period of the trip and for any unforeseen events. Companies that perform work at high altitudes and tourist agencies that organise high-altitude excursions in remote areas should plan to have a mobile hyperbaric chamber (portable compression chamber or CPAP helmets) available, especially in the case of ascents above 6,000 m, as well as oxygen and appropriate medications. Unfortunately, in some cases, those who organise activities of this type aim to save money and do not always have adequate tools and medicines at their disposal.[1]

It is true that in some places, such as Nepal, there is an emergency assistance system in place, such as the two first-aid points run by the Himalayan Rescue Association (HRA) in Pheriche (along the Everest valley at 4,300 m AMSL) and in Manang (3,519 m AMSL, along the Annapurna trek).[2] They are, anyway, assistance points with limited capacity and modest availability of medicines. Mountain rescue instructors from the Alpenverein Südtirol, doctors from the Institute for Mountain Emergency Medicine of EURAC (Bozen, Italy) and the International Commission for Mountain Rescue (ICAR MEDCOM) have provided and continue to provide assistance for the training of mountain guides and doctors in the Himalayas; these personnel can receive support through a telemedicine service, via satellite telephone

TABLE 21.1 Cardiovascular drugs at high altitude; a summary.

Drug	Comments	R/E
Acetazolamide	Important for the prevention of mountain sickness and high-altitude cerebral oedema (HACE) in adults	1A
	Might be helpful at high altitude in healthy subjects to reduce the risk of subendocardial ischaemia	2aC
	Can be used for prevention of acute mountain sickness (AMS) in children, but its use is discouraged due to side effects	
	Should not be used in treatment of high-altitude pulmonary oedema (HAPE)	1C
	Not recommended for prophylaxis of AMS and HACE in type 1 diabetes mellitus (increased risk of ketoacidosis)	2C
	Should be avoided in those already receiving other diuretics (UIAA)	
Alcoholic drinks	Use of alcohol should be discouraged in the high mountains, at least during medium- or high-intensity physical activity	
Angiotensin Receptor Blockers	Telmisartan is effective in lowering high blood pressure up to 3,400 m	1B
	Combination of Nifedipine–Telmisartan is effective in lowering high blood pressure up to 3,300 m	1B
Anti-arrhythmic drugs	Should be continued at usual doses	
Anti-coagulants	Should be continued; dose adaptation is recommended, to be checked carefully (UIAA)	
Aspirin	Effectively used for the prevention of headache during rapid climbing to high mountains	
	It may be used in a suspected case of acute myocardial infarction while waiting for advanced emergency services; check if patients are using anti-coagulants.	1A
Aspirin and anti-platelet drugs	In ischaemic patients ascending to high altitudes, pre-existing medications should be continued	1C
Beta-blockers	If a beta-blocker is needed, consider to switch to a selective instead of non-selective beta-blockers	2aB
	Nebivolol effectively controls high altitude-induced increase of blood pressure and preserves nocturnal blood pressure dipping	1C
Diuretics	Risk of dehydration at high altitude	
	No indication for prevention of HAPE	1C
Ivabradine	No data available for humans at high altitude	

TABLE 21.1 (continued)

Drug	Comments	R/E
Nifedipine	Drug of first choice in the treatment of HAPE when descent is impossible or delayed and reliable access to supplemental oxygen or portable hyperbaric therapy is unavailable	1C
	Useful in the prevention of HAPE	1B
	No effect in prevention of other forms of AMS	
Oxygen supplementation	In HAPE and HACE: when available, supplemental oxygen to raise SpO_2 to >90% or to relieve symptoms can be used while waiting to initiate descent or when descent is not practical	1A
	In case of rescues at altitudes >6,500 m: oxygen recommended (UIAA)	
	For climbs above 7,500 m AMSL: oxygen recommended (UIAA)	
	Patients with pulmonary hypertension in functional class III and IV should use oxygen supplementation if exposed to altitudes around 1,500–2,000 m	1C
Sildenafil, Tadalafil	Can be used for HAPE treatment when descent is impossible or delayed, access to supplemental oxygen or portable hyperbaric therapy is impossible and nifedipine is unavailable	2C
	Can be used for HAPE prevention in known susceptible individuals who are not candidates for nifedipine	1C
Statins	No specific recommendation has been issued, but it is generally recommended that patients with ischaemic heart disease should continue pre-existing medications at high altitude	1C

connections, which, however, are permitted in Nepal and Bhutan while they appear to be absolutely prohibited in India and Tibet.[3] Local emergency personnel can, therefore, be supported in recognizing and treating pathologies or risky situations, but their operational capacity is still curtailed by the limited availability of drugs and equipments.

Moving on to consider the use of drugs and recreational substances in the mountains, we recall the publication *'Drug Use and Misuse in the Mountains: A UIAA MedCom Consensus Guide for Medical Professionals'* of 2016, which constitutes the basis for the analysis of the phenomenon Drugs/Mountain.[4]

Some general considerations must be made on the pharmacokinetics of drugs at high altitude:

1. Intense physical exercise (especially if prolonged) produces changes in cardiovascular, renal and hepatic function: the reduction of blood flow in the splanchnic region reduces drug absorption through the gastrointestinal tract and drug elimination through the liver and kidneys. Particularly affected are those drugs with a narrow therapeutic range, such as digoxin, theophylline and warfarin.[5]

2. The relative dehydration that occurs at high altitude can alter plasma protein concentrations and the volume of distribution of drugs, thereby possibly affecting their absorption, distribution and elimination.
3. Reduced oxygen availability at high altitude, together with reduced plasma volume, may lead to reduced hepatic clearance by cytochrome P450 enzymes.[6, 7]
4. Reduction in body temperature also leads to a decrease in the clearance of drugs metabolised by cytochrome P450; in patients undergoing therapeutic hypothermia (no data for people with mild accidental hypothermia), it has been observed that for a reduction of 1 °C below 37 °C of body temperature, the systemic clearance of cytochrome P450 metabolised drugs decreases by 7 to 22%.[8]

Another general consideration is that, although cardiovascular diseases are present also among individuals living in high-altitude areas, there are very limited data on possible modifications of the pharmacokinetic properties of cardiovascular drugs in these populations.[9]

In our excursus, we cannot avoid starting from what, at least for a large part of Alpine populations (e.g. Venetian and Trentino people, but also Austrians and Swiss), is a kind of 'consolidated tradition': the use of **alcoholic drinks** in the mountains. Here, we will present alcohol as a 'cardiovascular drug', because some of its properties also have effects on the cardiovascular system.

It is popularly believed that the use of moderate quantities of alcohol can help provide the energy necessary to face climbs and demanding efforts at altitude, as well as allow the maintenance of an adequate body temperature despite low ambient temperatures. While it is true that alcohol causes rapid skin vasodilation (by modulation of central vasomotor control mechanisms and by direct actions on vascular smooth muscle cells) and, therefore, induces a temporary sensation of heat in the skin, this phenomenon, however, does not last long and favours the dispersion of heat. The peripheral vasodilation and consequent heat loss, together with some metabolic depression, lead to a reduction of body temperature that is a harmful effect for persons that are in a cold environment, with risk of frostbite (favoured by the concomitant reduction in the sense of attention and alertness).[10]

However, it is reported that a glass of red wine before tackling an effort in the high mountains could promote vasodilation also of the pulmonary arteries (a useful effect in this case) by inhibiting the release of the vasoconstrictor Endothelin-1 (a product released during hypoxia) and by increasing production of the vasodilator Nitric Oxide.[11]

In general, we can remember that the effects of alcohol are dose-dependent: that is, the greater the quantity consumed, the greater the effects produced (especially for blood alcohol levels >20 mmol/L, which correspond to approximately 0.9 g/L; person 'moderately intoxicated').[i] The use of alcohol:

- reduces aerobic capacity and reduces VO_2 max (the maximum oxygen consumption capacity and, therefore, the maximum sustainable work capacity),
- increases heart rate (also due to the aforementioned vasodilation); its use has also been associated with appearance of conduction abnormalities and heart rhythm disorders,[13]

[i] As a term of reference, please remember that in order to drive a car, the maximum allowed blood alcohol level in most European Countries is set at 0.5 g/L or lower, which, however, should never be reached if a person intends to drive, as the braking time doubles and the field of vision is reduced, especially the lateral one. See: Ref. [12].

- reduces the speed and force of contraction of cardiomyocytes and skeletal muscle fibres (the apparent increase in the ability to sustain physical effort after alcohol intake is linked to the person's reduced critical capacity) and
- reduces glycogen resynthesis after prolonged effort and, therefore, compromises recovery after physical effort.

As can easily be understood, these are all harmful phenomena for those who are carrying out physical activity at altitude. In addition to these cardiac and muscular effects, alcohol:

- causes a deterioration of psycho-motor skills, with marked effects on judgment and decision-making capacity; these are particularly dangerous phenomena for people who are facing challenging and potentially risky paths,
- alters reflex times and
- interferes with the control of balance and coordination. It has been seen that even one drink a week increases the risk of accidents in those who frequent the mountains, with an incidence of accidents that is approximately double compared to non-drinkers.[14]

The negative phenomena induced by alcohol are exacerbated in the mountains by the concomitant presence of other factors, such as dehydration (which alcohol can aggravate due to its diuretic effect), sleep disorders, fatigue and cold.

During mountain sports competitions, alcohol does not appear to be prohibited by the WADA (World Anti-Doping Association) in the 2023 list;[15] only in competitions that include aeronautical or archery performances, the specific Sports Associations could have maintained the prohibition.

In conclusion, the Medical Commission of the UIAA (Union Internationale des Associations d'Alpinisme) states that the use of alcohol should be discouraged in the high mountains, at least during medium-or high-intensity physical activity, because it can aggravate the debilitating effects of dehydration and hypothermia, can reduce performance during exercise, provoke a slower recovery after effort and increase the risk of traumatic injuries.[4]

We have already seen on various occasions how the partial pressure of O_2 progressively reduces with the increase in mountain altitude and how important the administration of **Oxygen** is for the treatment of high-altitude pulmonary oedema (HAPE) and other diseases linked to high altitude. In these situations, O_2 must be considered as a life-saving drug.

At extreme altitudes, hypobaric hypoxia would cause loss of consciousness within 3 minutes in people not adequately acclimatised; for this reason, oxygen supplementation has been used for high-altitude ascents since the 1922 Everest expeditions by Finch and Bruce.

However, oxygen is often prescribed and used without adequate indications and dosages, that is, without taking into account the possible negative effects caused by its administration in excessive or inadequate doses.[16] Studies on the use of oxygen compared to its non-use are very scarce, on a few heterogeneous cases, and are, therefore, difficult to evaluate.

There are many indications for O_2 supplementation:

- to reduce the risk of death from hypoxia at high altitude.[17] Experiences on Everest have highlighted a reduction in this risk from 8.3 to 3.0% with the use of O_2; on K2, reduction in risk of death from hypoxia from 18.8 to 0%.[18]
- to reduce the risk of death from various causes at extreme altitudes, especially during descent, when climbers are already exhausted and more vulnerable to accidents, with

impaired decision-making capacity; in the descent phase, fatal falls are 3 times more frequent than during the ascent.[19, 20] While 70% of the risk of death at high altitudes is due to traumatic causes, the remaining 30% (non-traumatic causes, such as HAPE and high-altitude cerebral oedema [HACE], neurological damage, but also hypoxic damage in other organs)[21] can be reduced with the administration of O_2.

- to improve effort tolerance, climbing speed and overall performance; this means that climbers may spend less time at high altitude, and, therefore, their risks of physical and mental deterioration are reduced. However, these advantages could also induce experienced climbers to overestimate their abilities and push themselves beyond their limits. (Can this phenomenon be identified as doping? Can it be considered ethical?)
- to improve SpO_2 both at rest (especially at night) and during exercise
- to reduce cognitive disorders at altitude (disorientation, poor judgment, exhaustion, poor concentration, reduced short-term memory, ability to solve problems and recognise errors)
- to reduce long-term neurological risks, which can sometimes persist even after returning to sea level with possible permanent structural damage (frontal subcortical lesions, cortical atrophy), especially in the case of repeated and prolonged exposure to extreme altitudes. This fact has been known for a long time,[22] although perhaps it is not so significant for short-term exposures and in adequately acclimatised climbers.[23, 24]

The administration of O_2 at 2 L/min at an altitude of 8,000 m is not able to optimally restore SaO_2 even at rest, and higher flows are necessary; and in climbers with muscle exhaustion, not even 4 L/min are able to normalise SaO_2, as demonstrated during the British 40th Anniversary Everest Expedition in 1993.[17]

A limitation to the administration of O_2 at high altitude is due to the possible freezing of the cylinder valves, or of the tubes or of the mask; recently, however, these components have been technically improved and are more reliable.

It is also possible to increase the O_2 concentration in tents during night rest at high altitude, bringing it to around 24 or 28%; the results are better sleep quality and greater physical performance during the day, with a lower incidence of altitude sickness.[25–27] Furthermore, it improves SpO_2 and reduces heart rate and diastolic blood pressure.[28]

In high-altitude residents with severe symptoms of Chronic Mountain Sickness (CMS), a randomised study reported that administration of O_2 via nasal catheter during lunch breaks at a flow rate of 2 L/min 7 times a week had beneficial effects after 15 and 30 days of treatment, reducing symptoms (dyspnoea, palpitations, cyanosis, headache), improving blood oxygen saturation and reducing Hb levels; the effects continued for at least 30 days after cessation of treatment. No significant effects were found in low-risk CMS populations, in which O_2 treatment does not appear to be recommended.[29]

WADA has not issued any recommendations or bans regarding the use of O_2 during climbing. The UIAA Medical Commission recommends the use of O_2 supplements for climbs above 7,500 m AMSL, and the possibility of administering O_2 should be available for treatment of HAPE and HACE and in case of rescues at altitudes >6,500 m.

A particular and somewhat curious aspect is that of the so-called 'Oxygen Bars'. In the late 1990s, 'Oxygen Bars' have been introduced in the United States, where oxygen is offered to customers who can 'sniff' it for recreational purposes, during sessions lasting from a few minutes to about 20 minutes, at an approximate cost of one dollar per minute. These Oxygen Bars may be found also in some mountain tourist resorts; in some ski resorts, 'Oxygen Lounges' offer not only the possibility of inhaling oxygen but also of having coffee, tea and soft drinks. Aside from the fact that administering oxygen without a medical prescription probably contrasts FDA regulations, inhaling oxygen for a few minutes at Oxygen Bars is unlikely to have any real beneficial physiological effects.[30, 31]

Beta-blockers are drugs widely used in adults for treatment of arterial hypertension, cardiac arrhythmias and for cardioprotection in post-myocardial infarction patients. These drugs, by partially or selectively blocking the beta receptors of catecholamines, reduce myocardial oxygen consumption by slowing heart rate, reducing blood pressure (reducing cardiac 'afterload') and slightly reducing cardiac inotropism (i.e. the contractile force of the heart). The most common beta-blockers currently in use are (among various others) **Atenolol**, **Bisoprolol**, **Carvedilol**, **Metoprolol**, **Nebivolol** and **Propranolol**. As already mentioned above, the indications for their use are essentially to obtain a reduction in heart rate, reduction in O_2 consumption (an important factor in patients with ischaemic heart disease), improvement in myocardial perfusion (coronary flow occurs during diastole; therefore – with its lengthening due to bradycardia – the coronary flow increases), control of ventricular and supraventricular arrhythmias, control of blood pressure (reduction of sympathetic effects, a phenomenon that is maintained even at high altitude) and reduction of physical symptoms related to stress and anxiety.

The main side effects of this category of drugs (especially for non-selective beta-blockers) are asthma and bronchospasm (from β_2 receptor blockade), peripheral vasoconstriction with Raynaud's phenomena or cold hands and feet (from β_2 receptor blockade and – in part – from reduction in cardiac output), possible appearance of intermittent claudication (due to skeletal muscle vasoconstriction), tiredness, fatigue, hypotension, bradycardia and reduction in the maximum heart rate achievable during effort and reduction in maximum sustainable work. It should also be remembered (especially in relation to the possible abuse of these drugs in sports competitions) that the abrupt suspension of beta-blockers can create a rebound phenomenon, i.e. a sudden increase in heart rate and blood pressure, with possible serious deleterious effects.

What happens if these drugs are used (either for therapeutic purposes or for voluntary intake or doping) by those who go to high altitudes?

Since these drugs are widely used in the clinical practice,[ii] it is very likely that many people who use them will travel to moderate or high altitudes. To date, however, the percentage of people who climb to altitude and use beta-blockers is not known. Additionally, some 'athletes' resort to the use of beta-blockers to reduce their basic heart rate, thus trying to increase their cardiac reserve.

Beta-blockers, precisely because of their effects, limit the cardiac response to hypoxia; the heart rate, therefore, does not increase adequately in the early stages of exposure to hypoxia, while the ventilatory response remains unchanged. By not allowing the heart rate to increase beyond certain levels, it is possible that the cardiac output at maximum effort is modestly reduced; this, therefore, leads to a reduction in maximal effort capacity (Figure 21.1) and the possible appearance of O_2 desaturation during maximal effort, especially in older people who perform physical activity at moderate altitudes.[33]

The performance of submaximal physical exercise (such as during activities in the mountains) has variable effects on the plasma concentrations of oral bisoprolol[34, 35] and propranolol[36, 37] and no substantial effect on concentrations of atenolol,[38] carvedilol[39] and nebivolol.[35]

[ii]For instance, in Italy, the prevalence of beta-blocker use in the general population was 61 per 1,000 inhabitants in 2013 and rose to more than 90 per 1,000 inhabitants in 2019; from: Ref. [32].

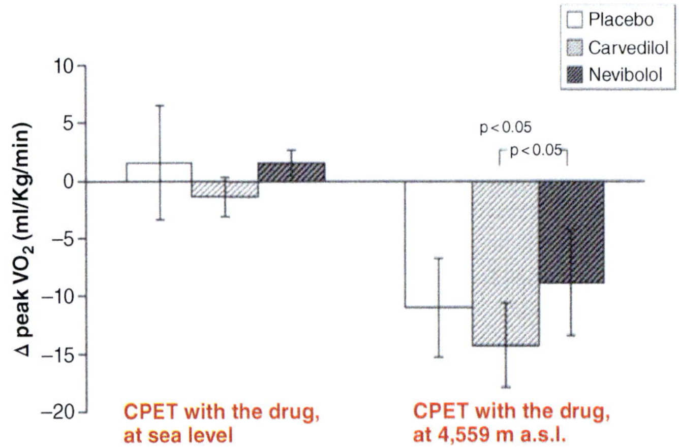

FIGURE 21.1 Reduction of peak O_2 consumption during cardiopulmonary exercise testing performed at high altitude compared to that performed at sea level; differences between beta-blockers and placebo. [41] / John Wiley & Sons / CC BY 3.0

In sensitive subjects, a certain degree of bronchospasm may be produced, which at high altitudes may be accentuated by the concomitant inhalation of cold air and by exertion.

The use of beta-blockers does not modify the risk of developing mountain sickness phenomena.

The subjects in whom the use of beta-blockers (especially non-selective ones) at high altitude is mainly contraindicated are those who suffer from Raynaud's disease; in these cases, the peripheral vasoconstriction that is usually induced by exposure to cold can become so accentuated and prolonged as to cause possible frostbite of the extremities. These drugs may reduce the ability to self-regulate body temperature during exposure to cold.[40]

If it is necessary to continue using beta-blockers, it would be preferable to use Nebivolol, which – in addition to being a selective beta-blocker, which, therefore, interferes little with bronchial regulation – has peripheral vasodilatory effects through the stimulation of endothelial production of Nitric Oxide; at peak effort, it also allows better conservation of O_2 consumption and adequate increase in ventilation (Evidence: 2aB).[41]

In winter sports, WADA prohibits the use of beta-blockers during sports competitions in the following cases: skiing and snowboarding in the case of ski jumping, 'freestyle', 'halfpipe' and 'big air' jumps. It also appears that the use of beta-blockers is prohibited during competitions and even outside of competitions in sports that include shooting, such as winter biathlon. The use of beta-blockers is accepted during climbs even if competitive.

The use of beta-blockers is recommended in patients already being treated with this category of drugs, who should not interrupt treatment.

Some people may be on chronic treatment with **Ivabradine**, a relatively recently introduced drug, which is intended to control inappropriately high heart (sinus) rate. During physical effort, ivabradine reduces the Double Product (i.e. the product between Heart Rate and Systolic Pressure), which leads to a reduction in myocardial O_2 consumption and improves effort capacity, even in patients with chronic obstructive pulmonary disease.[42, 43]

To date, no studies appear to have been conducted on individuals taking Ivabradine and climbing to high altitudes. In experimental animals with laboratory-induced pulmonary hypertension, one study suggests that ivabradine may exert beneficial effects, improving right ventricular systolic and diastolic function;[44] at present, there are no data in humans with primary or secondary (and high-altitude-induced) pulmonary hypertension.

The drug is not included in the WADA guide of prohibited substances in competitions.

ACE inhibitors (ACE-Is) (ramipril and similar drugs) and **angiotensin-II receptor blockers (ARBs)** (sartans) are drugs widely used in the treatment of hypertension; they also play an important role in the treatment of heart failure and have significant nephroprotective effects in hypertensive patients and in patients with diabetic nephropathy.

Regarding the use of these drugs at high altitude, the data available at rather scarce. While at sea level, they have undisputed positive effects; at high altitude, they can reduce the kidneys' ability to produce erythropoietin and, therefore, reduce the compensatory increase in haematocrit (and consequently O_2 transport) in response to hypoxia.

In normotensive individuals, treatment with **Telmisartan** has been demonstrated to be effective to control high-altitude-induced hypertension even at high altitude: it can control the increase of blood pressure induced by hypobaric hypoxia up to 3,400 m; its effect is present both during day-time and night-time (Evidence: 1B). At higher altitudes, Telmisartan seems to be ineffective, because of the concomitant suppression of the renin–angiotensin system and the increased plasma noradrenaline at those altitudes.[45] In case of increase of blood pressure values during exposure to high altitude, hypertensive patients already under treatment with Telmisartan may add long-acting Nifedipine to achieve better pressure control (Evidence: 1B).[46]

ACE-Is and ARBs are the most commonly used antihypertensive medications, even among high-altitude residents, as observed among a Pamirs population (average altitude level of 4,500 m).[47]

ACE-Is and ARBs are not included in the WADA list of prohibited substances.

Many patients with various types of heart disease and some patients with arterial hypertension must chronically take **diuretics**, both loop or drastic diuretics (**furosemide, torasemide and ethacrynic acid**) and thiazide or thiazide-like diuretics (**hydrochlorothiazide, chlorthalidone and indapamide**).

These drugs can aggravate the dehydration that already occurs when climbing to altitude, due to physical effort, low air humidity and possible episodes of vomiting and diarrhoea. In addition to the appearance of hypotension (with the possibility of related dizziness), this also leads to the possible onset of hypokalaemia, which predisposes individuals to the possibility of serious and potentially fatal cardiac consequences (arrhythmias).

Patients who need to travel to altitude must be instructed to bring with them adequate quantities of liquids and oral rehydration solutions or salts (or fruit such as apricots and bananas).

Exposure to an altitude of 3,600 m (both acute exposure for 15 hours and prolonged exposure for 6 months) increases plasma concentrations of Furosemide,[48] a fact that could have clinical implications.

WADA has included diuretics (all types) in the list of prohibited substances at all times (both in and out of competition), because these drugs are considered 'masking agents'. In fact, since diuretics increase the quantity of urine produced, they create a dilution of any doping agents, making their identification in the urine more difficult. They also modify urinary pH, and this can also modify the elimination of substances used for doping purposes.[49]

A particular issue is represented by **Acetazolamide**, which is not generally used in the treatment of heart disease but is extremely important for the prevention of mountain sickness and HACE (Evidence 1A).[50] In persons with CMS, it has been found that acetazolamide (250 mg/day) decreases haematocrit, serum EPO and serum transferrin, while it increases serum ferritin; it increases ventilation, PaO_2 and SpO_2. In particular, acetazolamide increases nocturnal SpO_2 and reduces the number of apnoea–hypopnoea episodes and the pulmonary vascular resistance.[51] Acetazolamide has also been found to contribute to the control of blood pressure at high altitude, as well as to reduce the risk of subendocardial ischaemia at high altitude (Evidence: 2aC).[52]

In a group of subjects usually living at low altitudes, a significant reduction of plasma concentrations of free Acetazolamide was observed during acute (24 hours) and long-term (10 months) exposure to an altitude of 4,360 m; hence, the hypothesis has been raised that dosage adjustments may be necessary in some subjects.[53]

The drug itself does not substantially change the ability of athletes to sustain physical effort, or perhaps reduces it moderately, even if many subjects who take it feel better, without headaches or other symptoms of altitude sickness. However, WADA still considers acetazolamide a masking substance (i.e. capable of hiding the effects of other prohibited substances) and prohibits its use by athletes both in competition and outside of competition. Athletes who need to take for therapeutic purposes one of the drugs listed and banned by WADA should submit an application for 'Therapeutic Use Exemption – TUE' to their sports federation or to WADA.[54]

Canrenone, a drug prescribed to patients with heart failure and also to hypertensive patients, is also included in the WADA list among diuretics that are always prohibited, both during competitions and outside of them.

Aspirin (ASA, acetylsalicylic acid) is a drug very commonly used in the population, due to its analgesic, antipyretic and anti-inflammatory effects; for preventive and therapeutic purposes, it is administered daily at a low dose (from 75 to 160 mg/day) to patients with ischaemic heart disease, diabetes, carotid stenosis and atherosclerotic peripheral vascular disease.

Altitude-related hypoxia induces the production of prostaglandins, which cause headaches in 20–90% of hikers who are not acclimatised to altitudes between 2,500 and 5,000 m AMSL; ASA, by irreversibly blocking the Cyclooxygenases COX-1 and COX-2 (which are found in many tissues, essentially in endothelial cells), leads to a block in the production of Prostaglandins, and – consequently – it is able to prevent hypoxia headache; for this reason, ASA is effectively used for the prevention of headache during rapid climbing to high mountains at a dose of 320 mg for a total of 3 doses administered every 4 hours.[55]

Furthermore, blocking the production of Prostaglandins leads to blocking the production of Thromboxane A_2; this, therefore, produces an anti-platelet effect. However, the anti-platelet effect produced by ASA has almost no effect on the risk of deep vein thrombosis, which – as we have seen – exists during activities at altitude for various reasons (traumas, tight clothing). It is not effective in subjects suffering from atrial fibrillation, who instead require oral anti-coagulant therapy.

The major negative effect of taking ASA is that it is potentially gastro-erosive, i.e. it can lead to the appearance of gastritis or gastric and duodenal ulcers, even with acute bleeding, especially in cases where ASA is taken together with dexamethasone (as in the case of preventive treatment of altitude sickness).

While taking acetazolamide for the prevention of acute mountain sickness (AMS), aspirin should be used with caution, due to an increased risk of metabolic acidosis and aspirin toxicity.

Ibuprofen also has similar effects to those of ASA; at a dose of 400–600 mg in a single dose, it is effective in preventing altitude sickness, reducing the inflammatory response to hypoxia.

Neither drug (ASA and ibuprofen) is included in the list of prohibited drugs by WADA.

Another drug frequently used in cardiology is **Nifedipine**, together with other di-hydro-pyridine Ca-antagonist drugs (**Amlodipine**, **Lercanidipine** and **Barnidipine**, etc.). The main indications for its use include, among others:

- inhibition of coronary spasm, for which it is used in cases of vasospastic angina;
- dilation of the systemic arteries, which leads to a reduction in blood pressure (sometimes abruptly and symptomatically with Nifedipine), useful in case of hypertensive crisis associated with symptoms of heart failure or neurological symptoms;
- reduction of cardiac work, linked to the effect of reducing peripheral vascular resistances, useful in case of exertional angina;
- reduction of pulmonary hypertension, in those cases in which it is sensitive to Ca-antagonists.

Its use is often burdened by side effects, which can sometimes be significant:

- reflex increase in heart rate, linked to the reduction in blood pressure induced by the drug;
- headache (especially with nifedipine administered sublingually, 10–23%);
- appearance of peripheral oedema (lower limb oedema, 7–30% of subjects under treatment; less frequent with newer Ca-antagonists with a less abrupt and more prolonged effect). During exposure to cold, the presence of oedema can favour the appearance of skin lesions;
- dizziness (10–27%), faintness and weakness;
- facial flushing (10–25%);
- nausea;
- episodes of chest pain with atypical characteristics; they can often make the clinical picture difficult to interpret, especially in coronary or suspected coronary heart disease patients (10%);
- marked and symptomatic hypotension (abrupt reduction in blood pressure, especially following sublingual administration of nifedipine), accompanied by a sense of fainting and difficulty speaking.

The use of Nifedipine in the high mountains is mainly linked to its effects on the pulmonary arteriolar vasculature; as indicated above, it allows to reduce hypoxic pulmonary vasoconstriction. Therefore, it is very useful in the treatment of HAPE, in which it is able to rapidly reduce the pressure in the pulmonary artery and improve alveolar gas exchange. Nifedipine is, therefore, the drug of first choice in the treatment of HAPE (Evidence: 1C), at a dose of 20 mg in the form of slow-release tablets, administered every 6–8 hours; it allows to gain the time that is necessary to organise the transport of the patient to a lower altitude (which constitutes the main intervention). It is also useful in the prevention of HAPE, when administered – alone or associated with Acetazolamide – at a dose of 20 mg (always in the form of slow-release tablets) every 8 hours, starting 24 hours before climbing to altitude and continuing until descent to medium-low mountain altitudes.

However, it is essential to remember that nifedipine does NOT prevent other forms of altitude sickness.[56]

Attention is also drawn to the fact that, before administering nifedipine, it is necessary to verify that the subject is not already being treated with other di-hydro-pyridine Ca-antagonists: in this case, the concomitant administration of nifedipine could lead to severe hypotension. A similar risk of severe hypotension exists in a dehydrated person (as often happens at high altitudes), or if the patient is taking **Sildenafil/Tadalafil** to prevent mountain sickness, as well as in those who are simultaneously taking β-blockers (see above) or α-blockers (e.g. Doxazosin for the treatment of arterial hypertension, or Tamsulosin for the treatment of benign prostatic hypertrophy). Alcohol also accentuates the hypotensive effects of nifedipine.

It is worth noting that there appears to exist an interethnic variably in the metabolism of Nifedipine: after oral administration, Mexican and Japanese populations show higher peak levels of the drug in comparison to European and North American subjects.[57]

At least in experimental animals exposed to acute and chronic hypobaric hypoxia (equivalent to an altitude of 4,300 m), the pharmacokinetic parameters of nifedipine (as well as of bosentan and sildenafil) resulted to be significantly affected.[9] No clear data are yet available on possible pharmacokinetic modifications of these drugs in mountaineers and in high-altitude populations, although one study has recently reported modifications of the clearance of the drug in hypertensive patients living at moderate-high altitudes.[58]

Nifedipine is not included in the WADA list of substances prohibited for athletes.

The Calcium-channel blocker **Verapamil** is often used for prevention of recurrent supraventricular arrhythmias and for slowing of ventricular response in atrial fibrillation patients; due to its effects of dilation of systemic and coronary vessels, reduction of heart rate and modest reduction of myocardial contractility, it is used also in the management of chronic stable angina, in vasospastic angina and as add on therapy in systemic hypertension. Very few data exist about its use in high-altitude situations; an old experimental study suggests that verapamil has no effect on high-altitude-induced right ventricle hypertrophy.[59] Physical effort does not modify the plasma concentrations of Verapamil;[6] some data suggest that exposure to hypoxia (oxygen level reduced to 12% in a hypobaric chamber, equivalent to 4,500 m above sea level) does not change significantly the clearance of the drug,[6] but the issue still needs further investigations. Verapamil is not included in the WADA list of drugs prohibited to athletes.[15]

The pharmacokinetics of the widely used Statins also appear to be influenced by high altitude: in one study, the steady-state peak plasma concentrations of **Atorvastatin** were found to be higher in subjects living at moderate-high altitudes than in those living at low altitudes;[60] similar data have also been reported for Simvastatin in experimental animals.[9]

Patients who are being treated with **anti-arrhythmics** should take special precautions when travelling to high altitudes and engaging in physical activity, due to the risk that hypobaric hypoxia may increase the risk of onset or exacerbation of arrhythmias. Anti-arrhythmic drugs should be continued at the usual doses, without self-made changes; increasing dosages of the drugs can induce potential pro-arrhythmic effects by altering the duration of the action potential of myocardial cells.

Patients being treated with **oral anti-coagulants** for the prevention or treatment of systemic embolisms (e.g. patients suffering from atrial fibrillation) or pulmonary embolic relapses (e.g. patients with previous deep vein thrombosis) should be advised to pay attention to the risk of trauma or injuries when they find themselves carrying out physical activity in the mountains, especially if in isolated areas or at high altitude.

It is necessary to evaluate whether there may be interference on the level of anticoagulation from other drugs they may take during the climb; furthermore, before undertaking a stay in the high mountains, it is necessary to ascertain the feasibility of carrying out checks on the level of anticoagulation (when these are necessary: e.g. in the case of treatment with Warfarin or Acenocoumarol; not so with the New Oral Anti-coagulants).[61]

Physical activity, such as that performed by high-altitude residents or during prolonged stays at altitude, has been reported to be associated with the need for an increase in warfarin doses of approximately 5–7% (perhaps due to increased hepatic perfusion or improved metabolism).[62, 63]

It is known that there is a risk of developing deep vein thrombosis among individuals who undertake travels or activities at high altitude, due to the procoagulant effect given by the combination of inflammation, hypobaric hypoxia, endothelial dysfunction and reduced fibrinolysis;[64] in this case, anti-coagulant prophylaxis could reduce the risk of dangerous complications, but the precise indications and the most appropriate treatment schemes are not yet clear.[65]

For further details and for other drugs not directly of cardiac interest, please refer to the aforementioned publications *'Drug Use and Misuse in the Mountains: A UIAA MedCom Consensus Guide for Medical Professionals'* of 2016[4] and the WADA manual (World Anti-Doping Association) of 2023.[15]

References

1 Pattenden HA, Shah NM, Hillebrandt D, Rodger M, Windsor JS. Do British commercial mountaineering expeditions carry drugs to treat high altitude illnesses? J Travel Med 2012; 19(4):250–252. https://doi.org/10.1111/j.1708-8305.2012.00610.x.

2 Himalayan Rescue association Nepal: https://www.himalayanrescue.org. And: Nepal e medicina in montagna, una lunga storia nel campo della ricerca in quota [Nepal and mountain medicine, a long history in the field of research at altitude]: https://www.montagna.tv/136271/nepal-e-medicina-in-montagna-una-lunga-storia-nel-campo-della-ricerca-in-quota/ [article in Italian].

3 Dätwyler T. Quand le médecin d'expédition reste à la maison. Télémédecine en montagne. Club Alèine Suisse. At: https://www.sac-cas.ch/fr/les-alpes/quand-le-medecin-dexpedition-reste-a-la-maison-23567/ [article in French, German and Italian].

4 Donegani E, Paal P, Küpper T, Hefti U, Basnyat B, Carceller A, Bouzat P, van der Spek R, Hillebrandt D. Drug use and misuse in the mountains: a UIAA MedCom consensus guide for medical professionals. High Alt Med Biol 2016; 17(3):157–184. https://doi.org/10.1089/ham.2016.0080.

5 Lenz TL. The effects of high physical activity on pharmacokinetic drug interactions. Expert Opin Drug Metab Toxicol 2011; 7(3):257–266. https://doi.org/10.1517/17425255.2011.553190.

6 Streit M, Göggelmann C, Dehnert C, Burhenne J, Riedel KD, Menold E, Mikus G, Bärtsch P, Haefeli WE. Cytochrome P450 enzyme-mediated drug metabolism at exposure to acute hypoxia (corresponding to an altitude of 4,500 m). Eur J Clin Pharmacol 2005; 61(1):39–46. https://doi.org/10.1007/s00228-004-0886-1.

7 Zhou X, Nian Y, Qiao Y, Yang M, Xin Y, Li X. Hypoxia plays a key role in the pharmacokinetic changes of drugs at high altitude. Curr Drug Metab 2018; 19(11):960–969. https://doi.org/10.2174/1389200219666180529112913.

8 Tortorici MA, Kochanek PM, Poloyac SM. Effects of hypothermia on drug disposition, metabolism, and response: a focus of hypothermia-mediated alterations on the cytochrome P450 enzyme system. Crit Care Med 2007; 35(9):2196–2204. https://doi.org/10.1097/01.ccm.0000281517.97507.6e.

9 Zhu J, Duan Y, Duo D, Yang J, Bai X, Liu G, Wang Q, Wang X, Qu N, Zhou Y, Li X. High-altitude hypoxia influences the activities of the drug-metabolizing enzyme CYP3A1 and the pharmacokinetics of four cardiovascular system Drugs. Pharmaceuticals (Basel) 2022; 15(10):1303. https://doi.org/10.3390/ph15101303.

10 Istituto Superiore di Sanità. Bere alcol aiuta a scaldarsi?. 28 marzo 2019 [Italian Higher Institute of Health. Does drinking alcohol help you keep warm?. March 28, 2019]. https://www.issalute.it/index.php/falsi-miti-e-bufale/fumo-alcol-droghe-dipendenze/bere-alcol-aiuta-a-scaldarsi?highlight=WyJiZXJlIiwiYWxjb2wiLCJiZXJlIGFsY29sIl0=. [article in Italian].

11 Wallerath T, Li H, Gödtel-Ambrust U, Schwarz PM, Förstermann U. A blend of polyphenolic compounds explains the stimulatory effect of red wine on human endothelial NO synthase. Nitric Oxide 2005; 12(2):97–104. https://doi.org/10.1016/j.niox.2004.12.004.

12 European Transport Safety Council. Blood Alcohol Content (BAC) Drink Driving Limits across Europe. At: https://etsc.eu/issues/drink-driving/blood-alcohol-content-bac-drink-driving-limits-across-europe/

13 Wong CX, Tu SJ, Marcus GM. Alcohol and Arrhythmias. JACC Clin Electrophysiol 2023; 9(2): 266–279. https://doi.org/10.1016/j.jacep.2022.10.023.

14 Roeggla G, Roeggla H, Roeggla M, Binder M, Laggner AN. Effect of alcohol on acute ventilatory adaptation to mild hypoxia at moderate altitude. Ann Intern Med 1995; 122(12):925–927. https://doi.org/10.7326/0003-4819-122-12-199506150-00006.

15 World Anti-Doping Association. International Standard Prohibited List 2023. https://www.wada-ama.org/en/prohibited-list.

16 Bateman NT, Leach RM. ABC of oxygen. Acute oxygen therapy. BMJ 1998; 317(7161):798–801. https://doi.org/10.1136/bmj.317.7161.798.

17 Garrido E, Soria JM, Salisbury R. Breathless and dying on Mount Everest. Lancet Respir Med 2019; 7(11):938–939. https://doi.org/10.1016/S2213-2600(19)30281-4. Erratum in: Lancet Respir Med 2019; 7(11):e36. https://www.thelancet.com/journals/lanres/article/PIIS2213-2600(19)30283-8/fulltext.

18 Huey RB, Eguskitza X. Supplemental oxygen and mountaineer death rates on Everest and K2. JAMA 2000; 284(2):181. https://doi.org/10.1001/jama.284.2.181-a. Erratum in: JAMA 2000; 284(23):2999.

19 Huey RB, Eguskitza X, Dillon M. Mountaineering in thin air. Patterns of death and of weather at high altitude. Adv Exp Med Biol 2001; 502:225–236.

20 Salisbury R, Hawley E. The Himalaya by the Numbers: A Statistical Analysis of Mountaineering in the Nepal Himalaya. Kathmandu, Nepal: Vajara Publications; 2011. http://www.himalayandatabase.com/downloads/hbnsampl.pdf.

21 Basnyat B, Cumbo TA, Edelman R. Acute medical problems in the Himalayas outside the setting of altitude sickness. High Alt Med Biol 2000; 1(3):167–174. https://doi.org/10.1089/15270290050144163.

22 Regard M, Oelz O, Brugger P, Landis T. Persistent cognitive impairment in climbers after repeated exposure to extreme altitude. Neurology 1989; 39(2 Pt 1):210–213. https://doi.org/10.1212/wnl.39.2.210.

23 Taylor L, Watkins SL, Marshall H, Dascombe BJ, Foster J. The impact of different environmental conditions on cognitive function: a focused review. Front Physiol 2016; 6:372. https://doi.org/10.3389/fphys.2015.00372.

24 Li L, Zhou Y, Zou S, Wang Y. The Effects of high-altitude mountaineering on cognitive function in mountaineers: a meta-analysis. Int J Environ Res Public Health 2023; 20(6):5101. https://doi.org/10.3390/ijerph20065101.

25 Luks AM, van Melick H, Batarse RR, Powell FL, Grant I, West JB. Room oxygen enrichment improves sleep and subsequent day-time performance at high altitude. Respir Physiol 1998; 113(3):247–258. https://doi.org/10.1016/s0034-5687(98)00068-1.

26 McElroy MK, Gerard A, Powell FL, Prisk GK, Sentse N, Holverda S, West JB. Nocturnal O_2 enrichment of room air at high altitude increases daytime O_2 saturation without changing control of ventilation. High Alt Med Biol 2000; 1(3):197–206. https://doi.org/10.1089/15270290050144190.

27 West JB. Commuting to high altitude: value of oxygen enrichment of room air. High Alt Med Biol 2002; 3(2):223–235. https://doi.org/10.1089/15270290260131948.

28 Moraga FA, López I, Morales A, Soza D, Noack J. The effect of oxygen enrichment on cardiorespiratory and neuropsychological responses in workers with chronic intermittent exposure to high altitude (ALMA, 5,050 m). Front Physiol 2018; 9:187. https://doi.org/10.3389/fphys.2018.00187.

29 Feng B, Xu WH, Gao YQ, Liu FY, Li P, Zheng SJ, Gai LY, Zhang G. Intermittent oxygen inhalation with proper frequency improves overall health conditions and alleviates symptoms in a population at high risk of chronic mountain sickness with severe symptoms. Chin Med J (Engl) 2016; 129(11):1322–1329. https://doi.org/10.4103/0366-6999.182831.

30 Bren L. Oxygen bars: is a breath of fresh air worth it? FDA Consum 2002; 36(6):9–11. https://permanent.access.gpo.gov/lps1609/www.fda.gov/fdac/features/2002/602_air.html.

31 Walsh C, Thimmesch AR, D'Achiardi A, Pierce JD. Oxygen bar effectiveness: a randomised quantitative study. J Complement Integr Med 2011; 8. https://doi.org/10.2202/1553-3840.1424.

32 Calabria S, Piccinni C, Ronconi G, Dondi L, Cinconze E, Esposito I, Addesi A, Pedrini A, Maggioni AP, Martini N. Uso cronico dell'associazione estemporanea ACE-inibitori e beta-bloccanti in Italia dal 2013 al 2019 attraverso i dati amministrativi sanitari [Chronic use of the extemporaneous association ACE-inhibitors and beta-blockers in Italy from 2013 to 2019 through health administrative data]. Recenti Prog Med 2021; 112(10):678–686. https://doi.org/10.1701/3679.36659.

33 Faulhaber M, Flatz M, Burtscher M. Beta-blockers may provoke oxygen desaturation during submaximal exercise at moderate altitudes in elderly persons. High Alt Med Biol 2003; 4(4): 475–478. https://doi.org/10.1089/152702903322616227.

34 Le Coz F, Sauleman P, Poirier JM, Cuche JL, Midavaine M, Rames A, Lecocq B, Jaillon P. Oral pharmacokinetics of bisoprolol in resting and exercising healthy volunteers. J Cardiovasc Pharmacol 1991; 18(1):28–34. https://doi.org/10.1097/00005344-199107000-00005.

35 Stoschitzky K, Stoschitzky G, Klein W, Müller F, Bühring K, Lamprecht G, Lindner W. Different effects of exercise on plasma concentrations of nebivolol, bisoprolol and carvedilol. Cardiovasc Drugs Ther 2004; 18(2):135–138. https://doi.org/10.1023/B:CARD.0000029031.87129.05.

36 Arends BG, Böhm RO, van Kemenade JE, Rahn KH, van Baak MA. Influence of physical exercise on the pharmacokinetics of propranolol. Eur J Clin Pharmacol 1986; 31(3):375–377. https://doi.org/10.1007/BF00981142.

37 Hurwitz GA, Webb JG, Walle T, Bai SA, Daniell HB, Gourley L, Boyd Loadholt C, Gaffney TE. Exercise-induced increments in plasma levels of propranolol and noradrenaline. Br J Clin Pharmacol 1983; 16(6):599–608. https://doi.org/10.1111/j.1365-2125.1983.tb02228.x.

38 van Baak MA, Mooij JM, Schiffers PM. Exercise and the pharmacokinetics of propranolol, verapamil and atenolol. Eur J Clin Pharmacol 1992; 43(5):547–50. https://doi.org/10.1007/BF02285100.

39 Stoschitzky K, Zweiker R, Klein W, Zitta S, Gruber L, Lamprecht G, Lindner W. Unpredicted lack of effect of exercise on plasma concentrations of carvedilol. J Cardiovasc Pharmacol 2002; 39(1):58–60. https://doi.org/10.1097/00005344-200201000-00007.

40 Mieske K, Flaherty G, O'Brien T. Journeys to high altitude--risks and recommendations for travelers with preexisting medical conditions. J Travel Med 2010; 17(1):48–62. https://doi.org/10.1111/j.1708-8305.2009.00369.x.

41 Valentini M, Revera M, Bilo G, Caldara G, Savia G, Styczkiewicz K, Parati S, Gregorini F, Faini A, Branzi G, Malfatto G, Magrì D, Agostoni P, Parati G. Effects of beta-blockade on exercise performance at high altitude: a randomized, placebo-controlled trial comparing the efficacy of nebivolol versus carvedilol in healthy subjects. Cardiovasc Ther 2012; 30(4):240–248. https://doi.org/10.1111/j.1755-5922.2011.00261.x.

42 Alshammari TM. Ivabradine: do the benefits outweigh the risks? J Cardiovasc Pharmacol Ther 2017; 22(3):210–218. https://doi.org/10.1177/1074248416672008.

43 Kaleem M, Kaushley A, Agrawal V, Singh TB. Effect of ivabradine on heart rate, functional capacity and pulmonary artery pressure in patients of COPD with cor pulmonale. Indian Heart J 2021; 73(3):369–371. https://doi.org/10.1016/j.ihj.2021.03.009.

44 Ishii R, Okumura K, Akazawa Y, Malhi M, Ebata R, Sun M, Fujioka T, Kato H, Honjo O, Kabir G, Kuebler WM, Connelly K, Maynes JT, Friedberg MK. Heart rate reduction improves right ventricular function and fibrosis in pulmonary hypertension. Am J Respir Cell Mol Biol 2020; 63(6):843–855. https://doi.org/10.1165/rcmb.2019-0317OC.

45 Parati G, Bilo G, Faini A, Bilo B, Revera M, Giuliano A, Lombardi C, Caldara G, Gregorini F, Styczkiewicz K, Zambon A, Piperno A, Modesti PA, Agostoni P, Mancia G. Changes in 24 h ambulatory blood pressure and effects of angiotensin II receptor blockade during acute and prolonged high-altitude exposure: a randomized clinical trial. Eur Heart J 2014; 35(44):3113–3122. https://doi.org/10.1093/eurheartj/ehu275.

46 Bilo G, Villafuerte FC, Faini A, Anza-Ramírez C, Revera M, Giuliano A, Caravita S, Gregorini F, Lombardi C, Salvioni E, Macarlupu JL, Ossoli D, Landaveri L, Lang M, Agostoni P, Sosa JM, Mancia G, Parati G. Ambulatory blood pressure in untreated and treated hypertensive patients at high altitude: the High Altitude Cardiovascular Research-Andes study. Hypertension 2015; 65(6): 1266–1272. https://www.ahajournals.org/doi/epub/10.1161/HYPERTENSIONAHA.114.05003.

47 Wang L, Li N, Heizhati M, Abulikemu S, Zhang D, Luo Q, Zhou L, Hong J, Hu J, Cai L, Zhao X, Sun L, Shao L. Prevalence, awareness, treatment, control, and related factors of hypertension among Tajik nomads living in Pamirs at high altitude. Int J Hypertens 2020; 2020:5406485. https://doi.org/10.1155/2020/5406485.

48 Arancibia A, Nella Gai M, Paulos C, Chávez J, Pinilla E, Angel N, Ritschel WA. Effects of high altitude exposure on the pharmacokinetics of furosemide in healthy volunteers. Int J Clin Pharmacol Ther 2004; 42(6):314–320. https://doi.org/10.5414/cpp42314. Erratum in: Int J Clin Pharmacol Ther 2004; 42(9):526.

49 Cadwallader AB, de la Torre X, Tieri A, Botrè F. The abuse of diuretics as performance-enhancing drugs and masking agents in sport doping: pharmacology, toxicology and analysis. Br J Pharmacol 2010; 161(1):1–16. https://doi.org/10.1111/j.1476-5381.2010.00789.x.

50 Nieto Estrada VH, Molano Franco D, Medina RD, Gonzalez Garay AG, Martí-Carvajal AJ, Arevalo-Rodriguez I. Interventions for preventing high altitude illness: Part 1. Commonly-used classes of drugs. Cochrane Database Syst Rev 2017; 6(6):CD009761. https://doi.org/10.1002/14651858.CD009761.pub2.

51 Villafuerte FC, Corante N. Chronic Mountain Sickness: Clinical Aspects, Etiology, Management, and Treatment. High Alt Med Biol 2016; 17(2):61–69. https://doi.org/10.1089/ham.2016.0031.

52 Parati G, Agostoni P, Basnyat B, Bilo G, Brugger H, Coca A, Festi L, Giardini G, Lironcurti A, Luks AM, Maggiorini M, Modesti PA, Swenson ER, Williams B, Bärtsch P, Torlasco C. Clinical recommendations for high altitude exposure of individuals with pre-existing cardiovascular conditions: A joint statement by the European Society of Cardiology, the Council on Hypertension of the European Society of Cardiology, the European Society of Hypertension, the International Society of Mountain Medicine, the Italian Society of Hypertension and the Italian Society of Mountain Medicine. Eur Heart J. 2018; 39(17):1546–1554. https://doi.org/10.1093/eurheartj/ehx720.

53 Ritschel WA, Paulos C, Arancibia A, Agrawal MA, Wetzelsberger KM, Lücker PW. Pharmacokinetics of acetazolamide in healthy volunteers after short- and long-term exposure to high altitude. J Clin Pharmacol 1998; 38(6):533–539. https://doi.org/10.1002/j.1552-4604.1998.tb05791.x.

54 WADA, Therapeutic Use Exemptions (TUEs): https://www.wada-ama.org/en/athletes-support-personnel/therapeutic-use-exemptions-tues. As an example: in Italy: Organizzazione Nazionale Antidoping (NADO): https://www.nadoitalia.it/images/documenti/2022/Therapeutic_Use_Exemption_Application_Procedure.pdf. In Germany: https://www.nada.de/en/medicine/in-case-of-disease-therapeutic-use-exemption-tue. In England: https://www.ukad.org.uk/tue-application.

55 Burtscher M, Likar R, Nachbauer W, Philadelphy M. Aspirin for prophylaxis against headache at high altitudes: randomised, double blind, placebo controlled trial. BMJ 1998; 316(7137):1057–1058. https://doi.org/10.1136/bmj.316.7137.1057.

56 Hohenhaus E, Niroomand F, Goerre S, Vock P, Oelz O, Bärtsch P. Nifedipine does not prevent acute mountain sickness. Am J Respir Crit Care Med 1994; 150(3):857–860. https://doi.org/10.1164/ajrccm.150.3.8087361.

57 Castañeda-Hernández G, Hoyo-Vadillo C, Palma-Aguirre JA, Flores-Murrieta FJ. Pharmacokinetics of oral nifedipine in different populations. J Clin Pharmacol 1993; 33(2):140–145. https://doi.org/10.1002/j.1552-4604.1993.tb03934.x.

58 Li Y, Mu S, Huang Q, Jin J, Tong Y, Wang R, Li W. Population pharmacokinetics of nifedipine in high-altitude and plain patients with hypertension. J Clin Pharmacol 2025; 65(12):1757–1766. https://doi.org/10.1002/jcph.70087.

59 Vaughan Williams EM. Ventricular hypertrophy--physiological mechanisms. J Cardiovasc Pharmacol 1986; 8(Suppl 3):S12–S16. https://doi.org/10.1097/00005344-198608003-00004.

60 Li Y, Huang Q, Zeng X, Wang R, Li W. Population pharmacokinetics of atorvastatin in high-altitude and plain patients with hyperlipidemic. J Clin Pharmacol 2024; 64(3):345–352. https://doi.org/10.1002/jcph.2376.

61 DeLoughery TG. Anticoagulation Considerations for Travel to High Altitude. High Alt Med Biol 2015; 16(3):181–185. https://doi.org/10.1089/ham.2015.0058.

62 Shendre A, Beasley TM, Brown TM, Hill CE, Arnett DK, Limdi NA. Influence of regular physical activity on warfarin dose and risk of hemorrhagic complications. Pharmacotherapy 2014; 34(6):545–554. https://doi.org/10.1002/phar.1401.

63 Rouleau-Mailloux É, Shahabi P, Dumas S, Feroz Zada Y, Provost S, Hu J, Nguyen J, Bouchama N, Mongrain I, Talajic M, Tardif JC, Perreault S, Dubé MP. Impact of regular physical activity on weekly warfarin dose requirement. J Thromb Thrombolysis 2016; 41(2):328–335. https://doi.org/10.1007/s11239-015-1248-9.

64 Nair V, Singh S, Ashraf MZ, Yanamandra U, Sharma V, Prabhakar A, Ahmad R, Chatterjee T, Behera V, Guleria V, Patrikar S, Gupta S, Vishnoi MG, Rigvardhan, Kalshetty K, Sharma P, Bajaj N, Khaling TD, Wankhede TS, Bhattachar S, Datta R, Ganguli LP. Epidemiology and pathophysiology of vascular thrombosis in acclimatized lowlanders at high altitude: a prospective longitudinal study. Lancet Reg Health Southeast Asia 2022; 3:100016. https://doi.org/10.1016/j.lansea.2022.05.005.

65 Chaudhry WAR, Ahmad BA, Waqas MS, Khan JR, Khan MHUH, Khiyam U, Malik J. Altitude-related venous thrombosis with heart disease: an updated review. Curr Probl Cardiol 2023; 49(1 Pt A):102018. https://doi.org/10.1016/j.cpcardiol.2023.102018.

CHAPTER 22

Special Aspects of Basic Life Support at Altitude

This chapter presents only some peculiar aspects of cardiopulmonary resuscitation performed at high altitude or, in any case, in a harsh environment. For the general notions and necessary in-depth information, we invite you to **refer to the documents produced by the Scientific Societies**,[1–4] in particular with regard to interventions on avalanche victims.

Short Time Means Saving Brain and Life

A first aspect to consider is the **time factor**. We all remember how, in the event of a cardiac arrest, the chances of survival rapidly decrease as the minutes pass between the arrest itself and the start of appropriate resuscitation activities (Figure 22.1). It has long been known that the chance of survival decreases by approximately 6–10% with every passing minute, until it almost disappears when resuscitation measures are started 10 minutes after the onset of the event.[5, 6] In the absence of cerebral perfusion, irreversible brain damage appears already after 4–6 minutes of circulation arrest. It is therefore essential that bystanders are able to initiate basic life support (BLS) manoeuvres as soon as possible;[7] and – obviously – this is extremely important also for events that occur in mountainous or isolated areas. However, there are studies that highlight how a significant percentage (from 11 to 23%) of people, even those trained to perform basic resuscitation, do not feel capable of starting the necessary manoeuvres, due to their emotional state, their feeling of poor preparation or inability to carry out the required role, or concern of causing damage[8, 9] or fear of contracting diseases.[10] In Europe, the bystander CPR rate is 58 % with significant regional variations (from 13 to 82 %).[3]

An often discussed issue in the case of witnessed circulatory arrest is whether these 'lay people' (i.e. non-healthcare workers) are legally authorised to initiate basic cardiopulmonary resuscitation manoeuvres. This is particularly true for cases occurring in the mountains, where it is therefore difficult to have adequately and specifically trained healthcare personnel available. Obviously, witnesses of a cardiac arrest must contact the Health Rescue Center

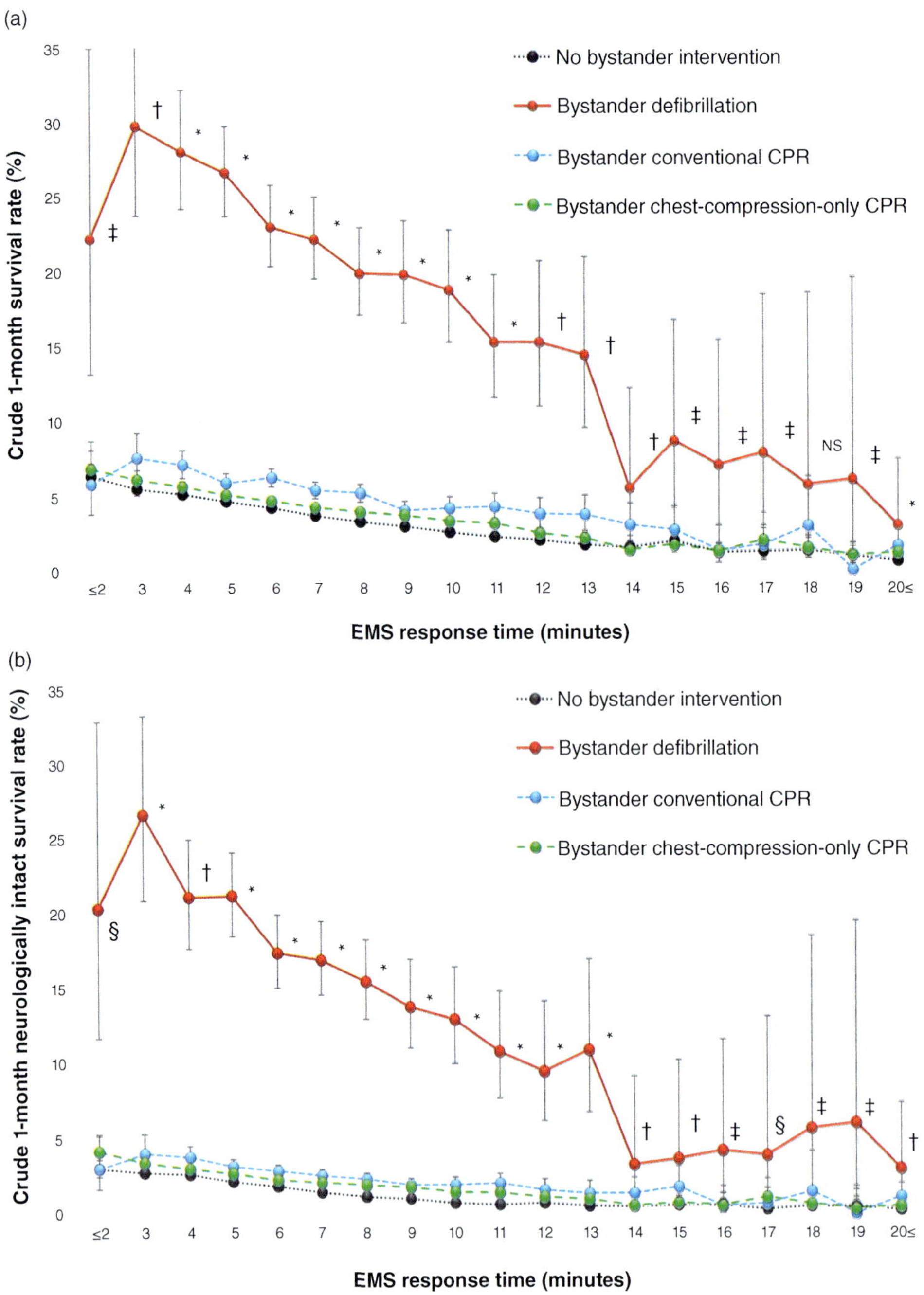

FIGURE 22.1 Reduction in the possibility of survival (a) and neurologically intact survival (b) as time passes from the event and the start of resuscitation manoeuvres (CPR). [7] / American Heart Association / CC BY 4.0

(in the European Union and other countries, calling the standard emergency phone number 112; in the USA, the number 911) to ask for help and start the rescue chain. This centre will provide adequate guidance on the actions that bystanders will be able to gradually implement, while awaiting the arrival of advanced medical assistance. Some centres have set up a telemedicine system, through which information and clinical data can be exchanged between remote mountain refuges and the central rescue service.[11]

At high altitude, however, it happens that a cardiac arrest may occur in a very cold environment, or may be secondary to burial by a snow avalanche or drowning in very cold water. In these cases, **cooling** of the victim's body allows for a marked reduction in the brain's oxygen demands and can make survival possible without significant neurological damage, even if very prolonged resuscitation manoeuvres are required.[12, 13] Although the literature on this topic is quite scarce, it seems that the chances of survival of a victim of cardiac arrest in hypothermia are approximately double (50 vs. 27%) than those of a patient in normothermia.[14, 15]

To our knowledge, the longest duration of resuscitation followed by complete neurological recovery (after progressive rewarming of the patient) is reported to be 390 minutes.[14] In a recent literature review, Zafren and Mechem[13] indicate: *"Cardiopulmonary resuscitation (CPR), including chest compressions, should be initiated in patients with accidental hypothermia who sustain a cardiac arrest. Contraindications to chest compressions include verified do not resuscitate (DNR) status, obviously lethal injuries, a frozen chest wall that is not compressible, and the presence of any signs of life. Always assume that some perfusion is occurring when any sign of life is present. Fixed and dilated pupils are not a contraindication to starting CPR. Apparent rigor mortis is not a reliable sign of death. Mandibular rigidity can simulate rigor mortis."*

We highly recommend referring to the paper by Lott C et al. 2021,[1] that includes precious flow charts reporting to the resuscitation behaviours to be applied in patients with hypothermia and cardiac arrest.

Remember that in the case of a victim with severe hypothermia, it can be very difficult to identify any vital signs, as breathing and peripheral pulses can be very weak, irregular and slow. While in the normothermic victim the search for vital signs should not exceed 10 seconds, in the hypothermic victim it is recommended to search for vital signs for up to 1 minute.[3, 16]

First Evaluation: Safety for Rescuers

Once the victim of cardiac arrest is reached, it is essential to assess the **safety** for the rescuers (as well as for the patient); if needed, it is important to quickly move the patient to a more suitable place to allow operators to begin resuscitation manoeuvres safely. The terrain in which the accident occurs is often rough, wet or snowy and slippery, or at risk of a further falling of snow or stones: these are all situations that can make it difficult to start adequate cardiopulmonary resuscitation manoeuvres on site, or can even put the rescuers at risk. For example, if it is necessary to use a defibrillator, the presence of water on the ground is a danger factor.

Check Airways Patency

An essential factor to check at the beginning of cardiopulmonary resuscitation manoeuvres is – as always – the **patency of the airways**. In cases of cardiac arrest at high altitude, in subjects who have been buried by an avalanche, it is common for the upper airways to be clogged by snow.

In these situations, what is generally recommended (i.e. extending the patient's head backwards and lifting the jaw; be careful with trauma victims, who may have cervical spine injuries) may often not be sufficient, and it is therefore necessary to ensure that the airways are clear of obstructing materials.

If they were available (in the first aid kits usually present in alpine refuges or on ski slopes), the use of supraglottic tubes could then prove useful to facilitate subsequent ventilation and reduce the risk of the victim inhaling foreign bodies; but even these relatively simple devices require a certain degree of training.

Adequate Ventilation: Mouth-to-mouth?

Ventilation performed by first responders has been shown to significantly improve survival of victims of cardiac arrest in general, as well as of cardiac arrest linked to hypoxia, such as in avalanche victims.[17–19]

However, some studies have highlighted that first responders are often hesitant to perform mouth-to-mouth ventilation, even on a family member or a friend (74% declared they would be available to a family member, but only 15% would be available to a stranger), mostly due to fear of the possible transmission of diseases.[20] As a valid alternative to mouth-to-mouth ventilation, mouth-to-mask ventilation could be effective if available in first aid kits in mountain facilities (shelters, ski slopes). Using a mask and Ambu bag would obviously provide better ventilation.

Adequate ventilation is important to stabilise the myocardium (and reduce the risk of ventricular fibrillation if the patient still has a spontaneous rhythm). If available, O_2 administration should be implemented, with the use of a mask or intranasal cannula, in order to achieve an SpO_2 of 92–98%.

Adequate Chest Compressions Essential, Although Difficult in Mountain Areas

An aspect that is always highlighted in cardiopulmonary resuscitation manoeuvres is the need to maintain **adequate chest compressions** in terms of depth and rate.[i] This aspect in the mountains is particularly crucial for a number of reasons:

- Resuscitation manoeuvres are sometimes initiated by non-medical professionals or by people with little experience.

[i]Compress to a depth of at least 5 cm, but not more than 6 cm (in adults); compress the chest at a rate of 100–120 per minute with as few interruptions as possible.[3] These recommendations are valid also for obese patients, without deviations from standard BLS and ALS; in patients with pectus excavatum, consider reduced chest compression depth of 3–4 cm.

- Rescuers are faced with a difficult logistical situation, with the victim often lying on a non-horizontal or uneven surface. For example, during the extrication of a patient buried in an avalanche, the start of resuscitation manoeuvres may be delayed for up to 10 minutes before the patient can be positioned supine; in these conditions, CPR has proven to be effective, even if the rescuer performs the manoeuvres from atypical positions (such as astride the patient's pelvis or above his head).[21]
- Environment may often be cold, a fact which contributes to easier fatigue for rescuers, who are also working with tight and bulky clothing.
- Hypobaric hypoxia, which becomes relevant for rescuers ascending rapidly to high altitudes: at altitudes above 3,000 m AMSL, the depth of chest compressions decreases rapidly within a few minutes. Such physical effort can prove hard and sometimes endanger even the experienced rescuer.[22–24]
- Need to transport the patient on a stretcher, sometimes even for long distances on foot until reaching the emergency vehicle (ambulance, helicopter), moments in which manual chest compressions often have to be interrupted for short periods (thus losing effectiveness, unless the patient is in profound hypothermia).
- Prolonged times for an equipped medical emergency team to transfer the patient to a hospital for advanced treatment.

A help in providing chest compressions adequate in terms of frequency, depth and duration can come from the use of **external chest compressors** (Figure 22.2). While these compressors have not proven to be significantly useful for resuscitation procedures carried out in an urban environment (the results in terms of survival without brain damage are comparable to those obtained by resuscitation with manual chest compressions only),[25–27] they appear to be particularly effective when the manoeuvres take place

- in a mountain[3, 28] or otherwise hostile environment,
- on victims of arrest due to accidental hypothermia,
- on victims of arrest which occurred without witnesses, and
- with the need for prolonged transport on a stretcher and
- long travel times to reach an equipped health centre.[29]

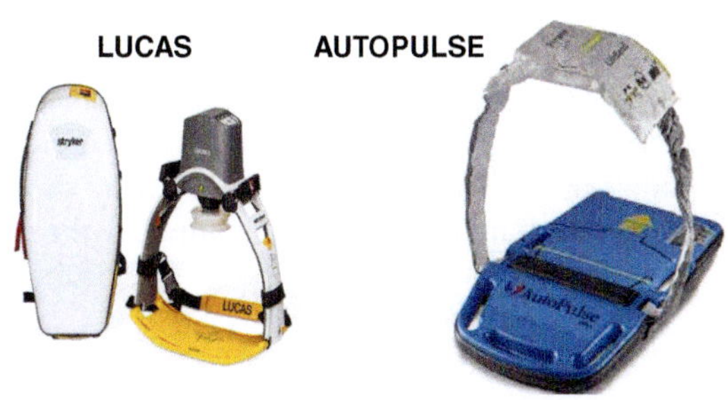

FIGURE. 22.2 Two models of automated external chest compressors.

The use of mechanical chest compressors allowed for prolonged resuscitation manoeuvres of up to 8 hours and 42 minutes[30] (which would have been almost impossible with exclusively manual manoeuvres!), in a case of hypothermic cardiac arrest that occurred on the Marmolada (Italian Alps) in the summer of 2018.

Mechanical chest compressors also appear to be particularly useful even in cases where helicopter transport of the victim is necessary,[31, 32] allowing the resumption of spontaneous heart rhythm in about one-third of cases, instead of about a quarter of the patients submitted to manual cardiac massage.[33]

Regarding the frequency of chest trauma caused by manual or mechanical compressions during resuscitation manoeuvres,[34] there are no data relating to resuscitations performed in the mountains; during stretcher transport, manual compressions can easily cause thoracic parietal trauma (rib fractures, pneumothorax), which could perhaps be less frequent if the compressions were performed by a mechanical compressor.

We have already seen in Chapter 9 how approximately 25% of deaths among those who carry out physical activity in the mountains (hikers, skiers) occur due to ventricular fibrillation; the percentage could be even higher, reaching 30% of deaths among hikers and 52% of deaths among skiers, according to a study by Windsor et al.[35]

Life-saving early defibrillation

It is therefore extremely important that **automated external defibrillators (AEDs)** be installed in 'sensitive' areas, such as on ski slopes, in major mountain refuges, and in restaurants, so that AEDs are readily available in case of an emergency and the delay of intervention on the victim of cardiac arrest can therefore be minimised. To reach this goal, every sports facility must be equipped with a semi-automatic or more advanced technology defibrillator (and during competitions there must be a person trained in the use of the AED), as – for instance – is mandatory in Italy following the legislative decree of 26 June 2017.[36]

This need for rapid intervention may somehow clash with local legislation on the use of AEDs, which is still heterogeneous between the European countries. According to the ENSURE study published in 2021,[37] in 15 European countries every citizen is allowed to use an AED, whereas a training certificate is required in three countries (Italy, as seen above, Spain, Greece). In the Russian Federation, only EMS personnel are authorised to use an AED. An AED mapping system and first responders equipped with an AED are available in only 11 countries.

However, this situation is evolving, and the legal requirements for the use of an AED are often superseded by the 'Good Samaritan law'. In Italy, for instance, in the absence of trained healthcare or non-healthcare personnel, in cases of suspected cardiac arrest the use of a semi-automated or automated defibrillator is permitted even by those without specific training;[38] in fact, article 54 of the Italian Penal Code, relating to the 'state of necessity', applies.[39] This is similar, for instance, to the Necessity Defense in Criminal Law Cases of the US legislation,[40] as well as in legislations of other countries.

Current AEDs can be used easily, with only a minimum of training, and in any case even untrained people are able to carry out the operations that are signalled by the automatic voice of the AED.

The chance of survival of a victim of cardiac arrest increases significantly if, in addition to basic resuscitation manoeuvres, defibrillation is performed quickly. A Danish study[41] (note: carried out in a mixed urban–rural area; clearly not mountainous!) demonstrated that defibrillation performed by a bystander resulted in survival free from major neurological damage in 81% of cases, compared to 65% of patients defibrillated only upon the arrival of a trained rescuer. There are very few reports on the results of resuscitation and defibrillation manoeuvres in mountain areas: in an Austrian national registry, only 8 victims out of 136 rescued cases had survived primary cardiac arrest, but all 8 had received immediate resuscitation manoeuvres and defibrillation from bystanders.[42] Similar results were also found for cases of cardiac arrest that occurred in the Tatra mountains in Poland.[43]

Recently, in Sweden and Germany, and most recently also in Italy, the possibility of delivering AEDs via drones has been evaluated.[44] With this system, a defibrillator would have been made available in about 3 minutes less (in another simulated rescue study: even 16 minutes earlier)[45] compared to its arrival by ambulance. The arrival of the drone also made it possible to maintain telephone communication with the emergency rescue operations centre even in areas not covered by the normal network; this intervention has increased the confidence of the rescuers on the ground. The limitations of the method, however, include potential flight bans issued by air traffic control authorities, unreachable areas, and hours of darkness.

When a defibrillator needs to be used, it seems safe to operate on a patient lying on snow or ice; however, the presence of water on the ground can be a complicating factor, although not a prohibiting factor. If possible, the patient should be moved safely and quickly to a dry surface, spending no more than a few (<10) seconds. In additions to checking the correct application of the self-adhesive pads, rescuers should ensure that the surface of the patient's chest is dry with no water between the pads.[46]

As regards electrical defibrillation in hypothermic patients, it is likely not to be effective if the victim's body temperature is below 30 °C.[12] If the defibrillation attempt is not effective (the guidelines suggest up to 3 defibrillation attempts in patients with body temperature <30 °C, to avoid excessive risk of myocardial damage),[3] resuscitation manoeuvres must still be continued, even for hours, until the victim is adequately warmed up.

The American Heart Association guidelines recommend that resuscitation of a witnessed cardiac arrest be continued by bystanders (healthcare or otherwise) until.

Continuation vs. Interruption of Reanimation Manoeuvres in the Mountains

1. restoration of effective spontaneous circulation
2. the intervention of a rescue team with advanced life support
3. the rescuer is no longer able to continue, due to muscle exhaustion, or due to presence of dangerous environmental conditions, or when the continuation of resuscitation manoeuvres may place other people at risk
4. valid and clear criteria for irreversible death are present, or signs of certain death are identified, or criteria for suspension of resuscitation manoeuvres are met.

Any of the following conditions are considered valid for **not undertaking or terminating resuscitative measures** in a victim without evidence of vital signs:[4]

1. unacceptable risk to the rescuer, or physical exhaustion of the rescuer
2. decapitation of the victim or loss of brain tissue, or truncation of the chest, or incineration, or decomposition of the entire body, or penetrating wound to the heart
3. the whole body is frozen rigid
4. avalanche victim in cardiac arrest due to asystole, with obstructed airways (e.g. by compact snow) and a burial time >60 minutes.

All the following criteria, however, must be met in order to **terminate resuscitation manoeuvres** in a victim of unwitnessed cardiac arrest:

- no recovery of spontaneous circulation during 20 minutes of resuscitation manoeuvres,
- + no indication given by the automatic defibrillator at any time to give shock, or observation of only asystole on the ECG,
- + no hypothermia (i.e. no clinical evidence of accidental hypothermia with internal temperature <35 °C) or other conditions that indicate prolonging resuscitation manoeuvres, e.g. victim of lightning or poisoning or overdose (in the latter two cases, contact the Poison Control Center before suspending the manoeuvres).

If a defibrillator is not available, resuscitation manoeuvres can be interrupted after 20 minutes of ineffective manoeuvres.[4]

References

1 Lott C, Truhlář A, Alfonzo A, Barelli A, González-Salvado V, Hinkelbein J, Nolan JP, Paal P, Perkins GD, Thies KC, Yeung J, Zideman DA, Soar J; ERC Special Circumstances Writing Group Collaborators. European Resuscitation Council Guidelines 2021: Cardiac arrest in special circumstances. Resuscitation 2021; 161:152–219. https://doi.org/10.1016/j.resuscitation.2021.02.011. Erratum in: Resuscitation 2021; 167:91–92. https://doi.org/10.1016/j.resuscitation.2021.08.012.

2 Wyckoff MH, Greif R, Morley PT, Ng KC, Olasveengen TM, Singletary EM, Soar J, Cheng A, Drennan IR, Liley HG, Scholefield BR, Smyth MA, Welsford M, Zideman DA, Acworth J, Aickin R, Andersen LW, Atkins D, Berry DC, Bhanji F, Bierens J, Borra V, Böttiger BW, Bradley RN, Bray JE, Breckwoldt J, Callaway CW, Carlson JN, Cassan P, Castrén M, Chang WT, Charlton NP, Phil Chung S, Considine J, Costa-Nobre DT, Couper K, Couto TB, Dainty KN, Davis PG, de Almeida MF, de Caen AR, Deakin CD, Djärv T, Donnino MW, Douma MJ, Duff JP, Dunne CL, Eastwood K, El-Naggar W, Fabres JG, Fawke J, Finn J, Foglia WE, Folke F, Gilford E, Goolsby CA, Granfeldt A, Guerguerian AM, Guinsburg R, Hirsch KG, Holmberg MJ, Hosono S, Hsieh MJ, Hsu CH, Ikeyama T, Isayama T, Johnson NJ, Kapadia VS, Kawakami MD, Kim HS, Kleinman M, Kloeck DA, Kudenchuk PJ, Lagina AT, Lauridsen KG, Lavonas EJ, Lee HC, Lin YJ, Lockey AS, Maconochie IK, Madar RJ, Malta Hansen C, Masterson S, Matsuyama T, McKinlay CJD, Meyran D, Morgan P,

Morrison LJ, Nadkarni V, Nakwa FL, Nation KJ, Nehme Z, Nemeth M, Neumar RW, Nicholson T, Nikolaou N, Nishiyama C, Norii T, Nuthall GA, O'Neill BJ, Gene Ong YK, Orkin AM, Paiva EF, Parr MJ, Patocka C, Pellegrino JL, Perkins GD, Perlman JM, Rabi Y, Reis AG, Reynolds JC, Ristagno G, Rodriguez-Nunez A, Roehr CC, Rüdiger M, Sakamoto T, Sandroni C, Sawyer TL, Schexnayder SM, Schmölzer GM, Schnaubelt S, Semeraro F, Skrifvars MB, Smith CM, Sugiura T, Tijssen JA, Trevisanuto D, Van de Voorde P, Wang TL, Weiner GM, Wyllie JP, Yang CW, Yeung J, Nolan JP, Berg KM; Collaborators. 2022 International consensus on cardiopulmonary resuscitation and emergency cardiovascular care science with treatment recommendations: summary from the basic life support; advanced life support; pediatric life support; neonatal life support; education, implementation, and teams; and first aid task forces. Resuscitation 2022; 181:208–288. https://doi.org/10.1016/j.resuscitation.2022.10.005.

3 Greif R, Lauridsen KG, Djärv T, Ek JE, Monnelly V, Monsieurs KG, Nikolaou N, Olasveengen TM, Semeraro F, Spartinou A, Yeung J, Baldi E, Biarent D, Djakow J, van Gils M, van Goor S, Gräsner JT, Hogeveen M, Karageorgos V, Lott C, Madar J, Nabecker S, de Raad T, Raffay V, Rogers J, Sandroni C, Schnaubelt S, Smyth MA, Soar J, Wittig J, Perkins GD, Nolan JP; European Resuscitation Council Guidelines 2025 Collaborator Group. European Resuscitation Council Guidelines 2025 Executive Summary. Resuscitation 2025; 215(Suppl 1):110770. https://doi.org/10.1016/j.resuscitation.2025.110770.

4 Lugnet V, McDonough M, Gordon L, Galindez M, Mena Reyes N, Sheets A, Zafren K, Paal P. Termination of cardiopulmonary resuscitation in mountain rescue: a scoping review and ICAR MedCom 2023 recommendations. High Alt Med Biol 2023; 24(4):274–286. https://doi.org/10.1089/ham.2023.0068.

5 Cummins RO, Eisenberg MS, Hallstrom AP, Litwin PE. Survival of out-of-hospital cardiac arrest with early initiation of cardiopulmonary resuscitation. Am J Emerg Med 1985; 3(2):114–119. https://doi.org/10.1016/0735-6757(85)90032-4.

6 Cummins RO. Emergency medical services and sudden cardiac arrest: the 'chain of survival' concept. Annu Rev Public Health 1993; 14:313–333. https://doi.org/10.1146/annurev.pu.14.050193.001525.

7 Goto Y, Funada A, Goto Y. Relationship Between emergency medical services response time and bystander intervention in patients with out-of-hospital cardiac arrest. J Am Heart Assoc 2018; 7(9):e007568. https://doi.org/10.1161/JAHA.117.007568.

8 Riccò M, Berrone M, Vezzosi L, Gualerzi G, Canal C, De Paolis G, Schallenberg G. Factors influencing the willingness to perform bystander cardiopulmonary resuscitation on the workplace: a study from North-Eastern Italy. Acta Biomed 2020; 91(4):e2020180. https://doi.org/10.23750/abm.v91i4.8593.

9 Farquharson B, Dixon D, Williams B, Torrens C, Philpott M, Laidlaw H, McDermott S. The psychological and behavioural factors associated with laypeople initiating CPR for out-of-hospital cardiac arrest: a systematic review. BMC Cardiovasc Disord 2023; 23(1):19. https://doi.org/10.1186/s12872-022-02904-2.

10 Scquizzato T, Olasveengen TM, Ristagno G, Semeraro F. The other side of novel coronavirus outbreak: Fear of performing cardiopulmonary resuscitation. Resuscitation 2020; 150:92–93. https://doi.org/10.1016/j.resuscitation.2020.03.019.

11 Martinelli M, Moroni D, Bastiani L, Mrakic-Sposta S, Giardini G, Pratali L. High-altitude mountain telemedicine. J Telemed Telecare 2022; 28(2):135–145. https://doi.org/10.1177/1357633X20921020.

12 Paal P, Gordon L, Strapazzon G, Brodmann Maeder M, Putzer G, Walpoth B, Wanscher M, Brown D, Holzer M, Broessner G, Brugger H. Accidental hypothermia-an update: the content of this review is endorsed by the International Commission for Mountain Emergency Medicine (ICAR MEDCOM). Scand J Trauma Resusc Emerg Med 2016; 24(1):111. https://doi.org/10.1186/s13049-016-0303-7.

13 Zafren K, Mechem CC. Accidental hypothermia in adults. UpToDate April 13, 2023. https://www.uptodate.com/contents/accidental-hypothermia-in-adults#disclaimerContent.

14 Brown DJ, Brugger H, Boyd J, Paal P. Accidental hypothermia. N Engl J Med 2012; 367(20): 1930–1938. https://doi.org/10.1056/NEJMra1114208. Erratum in: N Engl J Med 2013; 368(4):394.

15 Parati G, Pellegrini D. Cardiovascular emergencies at Altitude. In: Brugger H, Zafren K, Festi L, Paal P, Strapazzon G (Eds). Mountain Emergency Medicine. Chapter 31. Milan: Edra; 2021. pp. 399–418.

16 Rauch S, Paal P. Cardiac arrest in Mountain Areas. In: Brugger H, Zafren K, Festi L, Paal P, Strapazzon G (Eds). Mountain Emergency Medicine. Chapter 37. Milan: Edra; 2021. pp. 493–504

17 Paal P, Beikircher W, Brugger H. Der Lawinennotfall. Eine aktuelle Ubersicht [Avalanche emergencies. Review of the current situation]. Anaesthesist 2006; 55(3):314–324. https://doi.org/10.1007/s00101-006-0997-4.

18 Brugger H, Paal P, Boyd J. Prehospital resuscitation of the buried avalanche victim. High Alt Med Biol 2011; 12(3):199–205. https://doi.org/10.1089/ham.2011.1025.

19 Rauch S, Strapazzon G, Brugger H. On-site medical management of avalanche victims-a narrative review. Int J Environ Res Public Health 2021; 18(19):10234. https://doi.org/10.3390/ijerph181910234.

20 Locke CJ, Berg RA, Sanders AB, Davis MF, Milander MM, Kern KB, Ewy GA. Bystander cardiopulmonary resuscitation. Concerns about mouth-to-mouth contact. Arch Intern Med 1995; 155(9):938–943. https://doi.org/10.1001/archinte.155.9.938.

21 Wallner B, Moroder L, Salchner H, Mair P, Wallner S, Putzer G, Strapazzon G, Falk M, Brugger H. CPR with restricted patient access using alternative rescuer positions: a randomised cross-over manikin study simulating the CPR scenario after avalanche burial. Scand J Trauma Resusc Emerg Med 2021; 29(1):129. https://doi.org/10.1186/s13049-021-00944-9. Erratum in: Scand J Trauma Resusc Emerg Med 2021; 29(1):143.

22 Wang JC, Tsai SH, Chen YL, Hsu CW, Lai KC, Liao WI, Li LY, Kao WF, Fan JS, Chen YH. The physiological effects and quality of chest compressions during CPR at sea level and high altitude. Am J Emerg Med 2014; 32(10):1183–1188. https://doi.org/10.1016/j.ajem.2014.07.007.

23 Carballo-Fazanes A, Barcala-Furelos R, Eiroa-Bermúdez J, Fernández-Méndez M, Abelairas-Gómez C, Martínez-Isasi S, Murciano M, Fernández-Méndez F, Rodríguez-Núñez A. Physiological demands of quality cardiopulmonary resuscitation performed at simulated 3250 meters high. Am J Emerg Med 2020; 38(12):2580–2585. https://doi.org/10.1016/j.ajem.2019.12.048.

24 van Veelen MJ, Brugger H, Falla M, Strapazzon G. Chest compressions at altitude are of decreased quality, require more effort and cannot reliably be self-evaluated. Scand J Trauma Resusc Emerg Med 2023; 31(1):92. https://doi.org/10.1186/s13049-023-01149-y.

25 Gates S, Quinn T, Deakin CD, Blair L, Couper K, Perkins GD. Mechanical chest compression for out of hospital cardiac arrest: systematic review and meta-analysis. Resuscitation 2015; 94:91–97. https://doi.org/10.1016/j.resuscitation.2015.07.002.

26 Gates S, Lall R, Quinn T, Deakin CD, Cooke MW, Horton J, Lamb SE, Slowther AM, Woollard M, Carson A, Smyth M, Wilson K, Parcell G, Rosser A, Whitfield R, Williams A, Jones R, Pocock H, Brock N, Black JJ, Wright J, Han K, Shaw G, Blair L, Marti J, Hulme C, McCabe C, Nikolova S, Ferreira Z, Perkins GD. Prehospital randomised assessment of a mechanical compression device in out-of-hospital cardiac arrest (PARAMEDIC): a pragmatic, cluster randomised trial and economic evaluation. Health Technol Assess 2017; 21(11):1–176. https://doi.org/10.3310/hta21110.

27 Zhu N, Chen Q, Jiang Z, Liao F, Kou B, Tang H, Zhou M. A meta-analysis of the resuscitative effects of mechanical and manual chest compression in out-of-hospital cardiac arrest patients. Crit Care 2019; 23(1):100. https://doi.org/10.1186/s13054-019-2389-6.

28 Rupp SL, Overberger RC. Manual vs mechanical cardiopulmonary resuscitation for out-of-hospital cardiac arrest on a ski slope: a pilot study. Wilderness Environ Med 2023; 34(3):289–294. https://doi.org/10.1016/j.wem.2023.03.006.

29 Sheraton M, Columbus J, Surani S, Chopra R, Kashyap R. Effectiveness of mechanical chest compression devices over manual cardiopulmonary resuscitation: a systematic review with meta-analysis and trial sequential analysis. West J Emerg Med 2021; 22(4):810–819. https://doi.org/10.5811/westjem.2021.3.50932.

30 Forti A, Brugnaro P, Rauch S, Crucitti M, Brugger H, Cipollotti G, Strapazzon G. Hypothermic cardiac arrest with full neurologic recovery after approximately nine hours of cardiopulmonary resuscitation: management and possible complications. Ann Emerg Med 2019; 73(1):52–57. https://doi.org/10.1016/j.annemergmed.2018.09.018.

31 Putzer G, Braun P, Zimmermann A, Pedross F, Strapazzon G, Brugger H, Paal P. LUCAS compared to manual cardiopulmonary resuscitation is more effective during helicopter rescue-a prospective, randomized, cross-over manikin study. Am J Emerg Med 2013; 31(2):384–389. https://doi.org/10.1016/j.ajem.2012.07.018.

32 Pietsch U, Reiser D, Wenzel V, Knapp J, Tissi M, Theiler L, Rauch S, Meuli L, Albrecht R. Mechanical chest compression devices in the helicopter emergency medical service in Switzerland. Scand J Trauma Resusc Emerg Med 2020; 28(1):71. https://doi.org/10.1186/s13049-020-00758-1.

33 Hu J, Xu X, Hu C, Xia S, Xu L. [Effects of mechanical cardiopulmonary resuscitation during vertical spatial pre-hospital transport in patients with cardiac arrest: a historical cohort study]. Zhonghua Wei Zhong Bing Ji Jiu Yi Xue 2023; 35(4):362–366. Chinese. https://doi.org/10.3760/cma.j.cn121430-20230221-00160.

34 Preda T, Nafi M, Villa M, Cassina T. Traumatic injuries after manual and automatic mechanical compression during cardiopulmonary resuscitation, a retrospective cohort study. Resusc Plus 2023; 16:100465. https://doi.org/10.1016/j.resplu.2023.100465.

35 Windsor JS, Van Der Kaaij J, Rodway GW, Mukherjee R, Montgomery HE. Sudden cardiac death in the mountain environment. Medicina Sportiva 2009; 13(4):197–202. https://www.researchgate.net/publication/244936900_Sudden_Cardiac_Death_in_the_Mountain_Environment.

36 Ministero della Salute. Decreto 26 giugno 2017. Linee guida sulla dotazione e l'utilizzo di defibrillatori semiautomatici e di eventuali altri dispositivi salvavita da parte delle associazioni e delle società sportive dilettantistiche (17A04597) [Italian Ministry of Health. Decree of 26 June 2017. Guidelines on the provision and use of semi-automatic defibrillators and any other life-saving devices by amateur sports associations and clubs]: https://www.trovanorme.salute.gov.it/norme/dettaglioAtto?id=59789.

37 Baldi E, Grieco NB, Ristagno G, Alihodžić H, Canon V, Birkun A, Cresta R, Cimpoesu D, Clarens C, Ganter J, Markota A, Mols P, Nikolaidou O, Quinn M, Raffay V, Ortiz FR, Salo A, Stieglis R, Strömsöe A, Tjelmeland I, Trenkler S, Wnent J, Grasner JT, Böttiger BW, Savastano S. The automated external defibrillator: heterogeneity of legislation, mapping and use across Europe. New insights from the ENSURE study. J Clin Med 2021; 10(21):5018. https://doi.org/10.3390/jcm10215018.
38 Ministero della Salute. 118 e Pronto Soccorso. Defibrillatori automatici esterni. Chi può usare il DAE [Italian Ministry of Health. Emergency Medical Services. Automatic external defibrillators. Who can use the AED]. https://www.salute.gov.it/new/it/tema/112-118-e-pronto-soccorso/defibrillatori-automatici-esterni-dae/.
39 Italian Penal Code. Article 54 (State of necessity). - *Anyone who has committed the act because he was forced to do so by the need to save himself or others from the current danger of serious harm to the person, a danger not caused by him voluntarily, nor otherwise avoidable, is not punishable, provided that the act is proportionate to the danger.* It is indisputable that the use of an AED by a non-healthcare person is absolutely proportionate to the existing danger, also due to the fact that current AEDs provide clear indications on the procedures to follow.
40 The Necessity Defense in Criminal Law Cases: https://www.justia.com/criminal/defenses/necessity/.
41 Sarkisian L, Isse YA, Gerke O, Obling LER, Paulin Beske R, Grand J, Schmidt H, Højgaard HF, Meyer MAS, Borregaard B, Hassager C, Kjaergaard J, Møller JE. Survival and neurological outcome after bystander versus lay responder defibrillation in out-of-hospital cardiac arrest: A sub-study of the BOX trial. Resuscitation 2023; 110059. https://doi.org/10.1016/j.resuscitation.2023.110059.
42 Ströhle M, Vögele A, Neuhauser P, Rauch S, Brugger H, Paal P. Sudden cardiac arrest and cardiopulmonary resuscitation with automated external defibrillator in the Austrian mountains: a retrospective study. High Alt Med Biol 2019; 20(4):392–398. https://doi.org/10.1089/ham.2018.0134.
43 Mikiewicz M, Polok K, Szczeklik PW, Górka A, Kosiński S. Sudden cardiac arrests in the Polish Tatra mountains: a retrospective study. Wilderness Environ Med 2023; 34(2):128–134. https://doi.org/10.1016/j.wem.2022.11.005.
44 Schierbeck S, Nord A, Svensson L, Ringh M, Nordberg P, Hollenberg J, Lundgren P, Folke F, Jonsson M, Forsberg S, Claesson A. Drone delivery of automated external defibrillators compared with ambulance arrival in real-life suspected out-of-hospital cardiac arrests: a prospective observational study in Sweden. Lancet Digit Health 2023; 5(12):e862–e871. https://doi.org/10.1016/S2589-7500(23)00161-9.
45 Claesson A, Bäckman A, Ringh M, Svensson L, Nordberg P, Djärv T, Hollenberg J. Time to delivery of an automated external defibrillator using a drone for simulated out-of-hospital cardiac arrests vs emergency medical services. JAMA 2017; 317(22):2332–2334. https://doi.org/10.1001/jama.2017.3957.
46 Baldi E, Contri E. Using an AED in particular environments: is it safe or not? Suggestions for lay people and their instructors. Resuscitation. 2016 Sep; 106:e25. https:doi.org/10.1016/j.resuscitation.2016.06.037.

Appendix 1

Classes of Recommendations and Levels of Evidence

Providing evidence-based recommendations is always of great importance; anyway, the paucity of existing studies, often conducted on small numbers of cases, and the limited evidence available on individuals exposed to high altitudes make it difficult to present robust recommendations. In the book, the level of evidence is reported only when the Authors of the original papers or reviews have clearly stated it; in the other cases, the recommendations are based on consensus or on personal experience of experts and are not accompanied in the book by statements on the strength of evidence. However, the recommendations given are usually considered reasonable to ensure patient safety.

Classes of Recommendations	Definition
Class 1	Benefit >>> Risk. Evidence and/or general agreement that a given treatment or procedure is beneficial, useful and effective. It is recommended/indicated. Strong recommendation.
Class 2	Conflicting evidence and/or a divergence of opinion about the usefulness/efficacy of the given treatment or procedure.
Class 2a	Benefit >> Risk. Weight of evidence/opinion is in favour of usefulness/efficacy. It should be considered. Reasonable to do. Moderate recommendation.
Class 2b	Benefit ≥ Risk. Usefulness/efficacy is less well established by evidence/opinion. It may be considered. Weak recommendation.
Class 3	Benefit = Risk, or Risk > Benefit. No benefit or harmful. Evidence or general agreement that the given treatment or procedure is not useful/effective and, in some cases, may be harmful. It is not recommended.

(continued)

(continued)

Levels of Evidence		
A		High-quality evidence. Data derived from: - multiple randomised clinical trials, or - meta-analysis of high-quality randomised clinical trials, or - randomised clinical trials confirmed by high-quality registry studies.
B		Moderate-quality evidence.
	B-R	Data derived from: - a single randomized clinical trial or moderate quality randomised clinical trials. - meta-analysis of moderate-quality randomised clinical trials.
	B-NR	Data derived from: - one or more large non-randomized studies. - one or more well-designed and well-performed observational or registry studies. - meta-analysis of such studies.
C		Limited data or expert opinion.
	C-LD	Limited data derived from: - randomised or non-randomised observational or retrospective or registry studies with limitations of design or execution. - meta-analysis of such studies. - physiological or mechanistic studies in human subjects.
	C-EO	Expert opinion: Consensus of expert opinion based upon clinical experience.

Index

Note: Page numbers in *italics* and **bold** refers to figures and tables respectively.

C

D

M

N

O

P

Printed and bound by CPI Group (UK) Ltd, Croydon, CR0 4YY

10/08/2026

14939131-0001